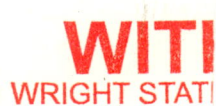

DATE DUE			
~~JUN 6 1994~~			
~~JUN 1 3 1994~~			
~~DEC 1 4 1995~~			
10/25/96			

HIGHSMITH 45-220

SUICIDE IN ALCOHOLISM

SUICIDE IN ALCOHOLISM

George E. Murphy

New York   Oxford
OXFORD UNIVERSITY PRESS
1992

Oxford University Press

Oxford New York Toronto
Delhi Bombay Calcutta Madras Karachi
Kuala Lumpur Singapore Hong Kong Tokyo
Nairobi Dar es Salaam Cape Town
Melbourne Auckland

and associated companies in
Berlin Ibadan

Copyright © 1992 by Oxford University Press, Inc.

Published by Oxford University Press, Inc.,
200 Madison Avenue, New York, New York 10016

Oxford is a registered trademark of Oxford University Press

All rights reserved. No part of this publication may be reproduced,
stored in a retrieval system, or transmitted, in any form or by any means,
electronic, mechanical, photocopying, recording, or otherwise,
without the prior permission of Oxford University Press.

Library of Congress Cataloging-in-Publication Data
Murphy, George E. (George Earl), 1922–
Suicide in alcoholism / George E. Murphy. .
p. cm.
Includes bibliographical references and index.
ISBN 0-19-507153-0
1. Alcoholics—Suicidal behavior—Case studies. 2. Alcoholism—
Case studies. 3. Suicide—Case studies. I. Title.
[DNLM: 1. Alcoholism—case studies. 2. Suicide—case studies.
WM 274 M978s]
RC565.M9 1992
362.2'8—dc20
DNLM/DLC
for Library of Congress   91-32161
ISBN 0-19-507153-0

2 4 6 8 9 7 5 3 1

Printed in the United States of America
on acid-free paper

To Eli Robins, M.D.—Mentor,
Friend, and Personal Hero

Preface

Case histories have always fascinated me. They supply the human quality that cold statistics lack. The 50 case histories at the core of this book have been nudging me to write them up for a good many years—not just because I like case histories. Dr. Eli Robins, my mentor, taught me to present *all* of the data so that readers could draw their own conclusions. It always seemed the best way to go. But the circumstances of publishing in the periodical literature require a narrow focus. That means leaving things out. A book is the solution, and here it is, at last.

But case histories are not enough. Some very interesting and potentially helpful ideas have emerged from the detailed examination of the mass of data. With input from my colleagues, particularly Dr. Lee Robins, I have been able to compare my observations with a data base of living alcoholics. The result is exciting news with the potential for reducing suicides of alcoholics.

In a book of this scope there are, inevitably, issues of a more technical nature that may be of interest to the specialist but not to the general reader. I have chosen to put at least some of these comments and discussions into reference notes to be found at the end of the book. A reference note is designated in the text by a superscript numeral at the appropriate place.

Further in the interest of the general reader, I have prepared a brief glossary of medical and psychiatric terms that are not found in a standard college dictionary. It is my intention that readers without professional training will find the contents of this book accessible, while professionals will find the information useful both clinically and for research purposes.

Statistical analyses are an inevitable and necessary part of demonstrating the extent to which findings are removed from the ordinary. Except as specifically noted, all comparisons are tested by the χ^2 statistic with Yates's correction for small numbers. A probability $P < 0.05$ is taken as statistically meaningful, or "significant." That figure corresponds to a likelihood of the finding having occurred by chance only 5% of the time, or 1 time in 20 samples. A P value of 0.01 equates to 1 chance in 100 of the finding reflecting other than a true difference.

St. Louis G.E.M.
July 1991

Acknowledgments

No work of consequence can be claimed as the sole product of one person's effort. There are always essential antecedents and indispensable helpers. I want, first and foremost, to recognize and thank Dr. Eli Robins, who introduced me to the fascinating problem of suicide, fostered and encouraged my academic interests, taught me the methodology of clinical investigation and clarity in data presentation. He has always exemplified uncompromising intellectual and personal integrity. He has given me continued access both to his suicide data and his personal library, as well as to his wise counsel.

Richard Wetzel, Ph.D., has been my statistical consultant and frequent collaborator, in matters concerning suicide and in other research areas as well, for many years. Wherever there are statistical calculations in this book, he has both advised me and carried them out. Throughout the study and after, I received the generous support and cooperation of the late Dr. George Gantner, then St. Louis County Coroner, later Chief Medical Examiner for St. Louis County and for the City of St. Louis until 1988. His official support was crucial to carrying out the study. Dr. Lucas Van Orden, while in residency training at Washington University, rough drafted many of the case histories, thus giving me a strong boost at the start of this undertaking.

I thank Lee N. Robins, Ph.D., for her valuable comments and for making available to me pertinent data from the St. Louis portion of the Epidemiological Catchment Area Study. Larry McEvoy, M.A., taught the computer to find the appropriate data. I thank Kathleen Bucholz, Ph.D., and John Helzer, M.D., for giving me access to data from the moderate drinking study (Helzer et al., 1985). Without those data for comparison, my findings would be much less persuasive.

We must all be grateful for the generosity of bereaved relatives and others for taking the time and bearing the strain of answering our many questions. John Armstrong, M.D., William Clendenin, M.D., John Fischer, M.D., and Steven Hermele, M.D., did the bulk of the interviewing.

In carrying out my search of the international literature, I have received invaluable help with translations. Miklos Biro, Ph.D., of Novi Sad, Jugoslavia, clarified details of interest to me in a paper on which he was a coauthor. Ole Bratfos, M.D., of the Sentralsykehuset, Akershus, Norway, supplied me with an English abstract of his book in Norwegian. Sven Eliasson, M.D., of Washington University translated a paper from

Danish. I am indebted to Vera Hauptfeld, Ph.D., of Washington University for translations from Czechoslovakian; Professor Michael Linden, M.D., of the Free University of Berlin, for putting a paper in Viennese German into idiomatic English; Edelpraud Romvari, R.N., of Barnes Hospital for translations from German and Slavica Selaković-Buršić, M.D., of Novi Sad, Jugoslavia, for translation of a long paper from Serbo-Croatian. Michele Van Eerdeweg, M.D., Washington University Department of Psychiatry, translated some passages from French for me. Ralph Johnson, M.D., provided unpublished information concerning treatment of patients in the Lambie, Whiteside, Bell, and Johnson (1983) study (personal communication, March 4, 1991). Professor Dr. Med. Nils Retterstøl, Director of Gaustad Hospital, Oslo, supplied me with useful references as well as advance information on the findings of the Nordic Planning Group for Research into Suicide in Scandinavia; Charles Rich, M.D., performed a similar service regarding his published work; I am also grateful to the many researchers whose work is cited in this volume. Without them, many of my observations would be mere speculation.

I am indebted to C. Robert Cloninger, M.D., Professor and Head of the Department of Psychiatry, for allowing me the continued use of my office and the services of my secretary since my retirement from academia in 1990. Finally, I want to thank Sandy Kroenig, my valued secretary, for her prompt, perceptive, and patient typing and retyping of myriad tables and versions of this manuscript.

Some of my data were developed under NIMH Research Grants MH05938, 07126, and 09247.

Contents

I BACKGROUND

1 Introduction   3
   Background of the Study   3
   A Predictor Beyond Clinical Diagnosis   5
   Decision to Replicate   6

2 Some Fundamental Considerations in the Study of Suicide Data   8
   The Role of Alcoholism in Suicide   8
   What Is a Suicide?   10
   The Reliability of Suicide Rates   11
   Cross-Cultural Differences in Suicide Rates   12
   Do Missed Cases Invalidate the Research Findings?   14
   Is Alcoholism a Disease?   15

II THE STUDY

3 Description and Limitations of the Study   21
   Rationale for the Study   21
   The Procedure   21
   The Interview   23
   Diagnostic Criteria   23
   Loss Events   24
   Limitations of the Investigation   25
   Potential Sources of Bias   27
   Outcome of the Investigation   30

III ALCOHOLICS WHO KILL THEMSELVES: CASE HISTORIES

4   Men with Onset of Alcoholism Before Age 25   33
    Case Histories   34
    Discussion   93

5   Men with Onset of Alcoholism from Age 25 to 44   100
    Case Histories   100
    Discussion   148

6   Men with Onset of Alcoholism at Age 45 Years or Later   150
    Case Histories   150
    Discussion   161

7   Alcoholic Women   163
    Case Histories   163
    Discussion   186

IV FINDINGS AND IMPLICATION

8   Why They Do It   189
    Interpersonal Loss   189
    Drinking   192
    Psychiatric Comorbidity   192
    Lack of Social Support   194
    Unemployment/Underemployment   196
    Health Problems   197
    Legal Troubles   198
    Psychoactive Substance Abuse   199
    Communication of Suicidal Thoughts   199
    Family History   200
    Discussion of the Findings   201

9   Seven Risk Factors for Suicide in Alcoholics   212
    General Considerations   212
    Reverse Replication of the Findings   213
    Are the Findings Predictive or Merely Descriptive of
        Alcoholic Suicides?   215
    A Replication Sample   220
    Conclusions   225

10 What Can Be Done About Suicide in Alcoholics?   226
    Spontaneous Remission   226
    The Remainder   226
    Treatment Considerations   229
    Suicide Prevention Efforts   233
    Risk Prediction Is Not Suicide Prediction   233

CONTENTS

11 What Is the Lifetime Risk of Suicide in Alcoholism? 236
  Existing Estimates of Lifetime Risk of Suicide 236
  Follow-Up Studies as a Data Base 239
  Suicide Risk from Follow-Up Studies 240
  Problems with Recent Prevalence Estimates 246
  Alcoholics at Risk of Suicide 246
  Comorbidity as a Risk Factor 247
  The Meaning of Lifetime Risk of Suicide in Alcoholism 248
  Alcoholics at Greatest Risk 249

12 Some Final Thoughts on the Final Act 250
  Risk Factors for Suicide 250
  Is Suicide an Impulsive Act? 251
  Is Suicide an Ambivalent Act? 252
  Personality Disorder and Suicide 253
  Psychoactive Substance Abuse and Suicide 254
  The Future 255

Appendix A: DSM-III-R Diagnostic Criteria 257
Appendix B: Suicide Interview 259
Glossary 283
Notes 285
References 297
Index 311

I

BACKGROUND

1

Introduction

BACKGROUND OF THE STUDY

"Sure, I'd left him before—but this time I meant it!" She was a rather plain-looking woman in her mid-40s, slender and neatly groomed. I interviewed her in the living room of her one-bedroom flat above a row of shops in a low-income part of town. In response to my questioning, she told me about her husband's chronic alcoholism, the days and nights he didn't come home, the paychecks that didn't come home, the bills that didn't get paid, the frequent verbal abuse, the infrequent but increasing physical abuse that had driven her to leave him. She'd leave him and he'd find her. Somehow, he was always able to persuade her that he was truly sorry for what he had done and that he had changed. Against her better judgment, helplessly, she would take him back. The last time but one, she had made the mistake of giving her sister-in-law her telephone number. He found her again and the story was repeated. This time, she told no one. She changed jobs. She got another unlisted telephone number, which she kept entirely to herself. She kept contact with friends and relatives by telephoning out. She picked up her mail at the post office. When her husband died, the police were able to locate her only through the telephone company.

Unusual? Only in the details. I conducted this interview as a part of a systematic study of suicides, designed and led by Dr. Eli Robins. He was then an associate professor, later head of the Department of Psychiatry at the Washington University School of Medicine. I was a psychiatric resident at the time. The study plan was simple. The St. Louis City and St. Louis County coroners' offices were contacted weekly for any new suicides. We were allowed to take the record to a table and copy the information from the coroner's report. A police investigation report might also be present.

Then we telephoned the closest family member identified in the report, explained why we wanted to talk with them and tried to set up an appointment. Not everyone was eager to talk with us. Some flatly refused. A few made repeated promises of an interview "later," but later never arrived. Some made appointments and didn't keep them. The great majority did make appointments and kept them. Occasionally the outcome was strange.

One hot summer evening I climbed the wooden back steps to a second-floor apartment in a thoroughly seedy neighborhood to keep an appointment with a recent widow.

I was met by the widow and her boyfriend—and two uniformed policemen with their hands on their unlimbered service revolvers. After overcoming my astonishment, I satisfied the police as to the legitimacy of my mission and they left. The boyfriend wouldn't go. Then I elicited a fantastic tale of an angel with everything to live for. She'd tell a lie and he'd swear to it. Then he'd tell one and she would endorse it. It was clear that I wasn't getting the truth.

The police investigation was more informative. The victim was well known to the city psychiatric hospital as an alcoholic and ne'er-do-well. He had an arrest record for petty offenses. He had recently gotten another woman pregnant and had apparently contracted a sexually transmitted disease in the process, as we learned from the City Health Department. He wasn't one of our better class of customers. Whether his wife had thrown him out was, of course, not forthcoming.

It wasn't any fun. After initial refusal and several canceled appointments in another case, I was able to gain agreement from a widower that he would talk with me about his wife, who had taken her life several months earlier. I went to his house at the appointed time to find a short, apologetic note tacked to the door. It said that he had been called away. "Called away" is putting it nicely. He had followed his wife in suicide that day.

Did the prospect of my inquiry cause that? I hope not, but I'll never know. Was the interview usually upsetting to the informants? Of course it was. Reliving the final days or hours often brought tears. Sometimes the interview brought enlightenment. Almost always it brought some degree of relief as well as the knowledge that the information supplied might help others in the future. We are most grateful for the generous cooperation afforded us by our informants.

"I'd left him before—but this time I meant it!" The words kept coming back to my mind. I had heard them again and again. And it wasn't just from that one woman. Other widows had said nearly the same thing. Could that circumstance have some special significance? I had to go back to the data. After all, I was not the only interviewer. There were five of us: Jack Kayes, Seymour Gassner, Robert Wilkinson, all medical students; myself; and Dr. Robins. In our systematic interview, we had asked 17 specific questions about the events in the year preceding the suicide. These are found on pages 265 to 266 of the interview protocol (Appendix B). They were designed to elicit history that might not otherwise be forthcoming concerning possible upsetting or precipitating events. For each of these events, we had asked informants not only about whether they had occurred, but when they had occurred in calendar time. We calculated the temporal relationship to the suicide for ourselves. In going back into the data I was interested in whether there was a preponderance of any type of potentially upsetting life event as well as the occurrence of events shortly before the suicides.

We had learned that nearly all of the suicides were psychiatrically ill when they took their lives. Two psychiatric diagnoses accounted for nearly two-thirds of all of the cases. Major depressive disorder (we called it manic-depressive disease back then) accounted for 40% of the total, and alcoholism for another 23%. The remainder was a miscellaneous group including four persons with a principal or only diagnosis of chronic brain syndrome (denoting structural brain damage), three with schizophrenia, two with drug addiction (one of those had hysteria or Briquet's syndrome as well)

INTRODUCTION

(Goodwin & Guze, 1989). In 20 cases the information conflicted or was insufficient to allow a confident diagnosis, but the psychiatric nature of the case was not in doubt. In five cases there was insufficient information for any diagnosis. Five suicides were not evidently psychiatrically ill but were suffering the terminal phase of cancer. Three were apparently well (Robins, Murphy, Wilkinson, Gassner, & Kayes, 1959).

A PREDICTOR BEYOND CLINICAL DIAGNOSIS

In order to see whether my impression regarding social disruption preceding suicide in alcoholics had any merit, we compared the experiences of the suicides with the two most common diagnoses, depressive disorder and alcoholism. We found that loss of a close interpersonal relationship had been experienced within a year of their deaths by 48% of those with alcoholism and by only 15% of those with a diagnosis of depressive disorder (Murphy & Robins, 1967) (Table 1.1). The difference was statistically significant ($P < 0.01$). (This figure means that the statistical probability [P] of such a difference occurring by chance in a sample of this size is less than 1%, i.e., it should occur less than once in 100 trials.) No one should be surprised that the alcoholics had had a lot of social disruption in their lives. That is in the nature of the disorder. What was surprising, however, was the recency of this particular type of event. Nearly one-third (32%) of the alcoholics had experienced interpersonal loss *within 6 weeks of their suicide*.

That was not true of those with affective disorder (major depressive disorder). The difference in frequency of these events in the final 6 weeks was highly significant statistically ($P < 0.001$; less than 1 chance in 1,000). Looked at in another way, there are 8⅔ six-week periods in a year, yet two-thirds of all of the interpersonal loss within the year had confronted the alcoholics in the final 6 weeks of their lives. The probability of that maldistribution occurring by chance is less than 1 in 50 ($P < 0.02$). So however one looks at it, the alcoholics but not the depressives had experienced a major disruption in their personal relationships very shortly before their self-termination. We

Table 1.1 Loss of Affectional Relationships Preceding Suicide

	Within 1 year		Within 6 Weeks	
	Affective Disorder	Alcoholism	Affective Disorder	Alcoholism
Separated	3	9	2	7
Divorced	2	1	0	0
Widowed	0	1	0	0
Bereaved	3	1	0	0
Apart (other)	1	3	0	3
Total with affective loss	9	15	2	10
Percentage of population affected	15%	48%[a]	3%	32%[b]

[a]Significantly different from affective disorder; $P < 0.01$.
[b]Significantly different from affective disorder; $P < 0.001$; significantly different from that expected; $P < 0.02$.
Note: From G. E. Murphy and E. Robins. Social Factors in Suicide. *JAMA*, 1967, *199*:303–308. Copyright 1967, American Medical Association.

reported it as a potential predictor of increased suicide risk for alcoholics (Murphy & Robins, 1967).

This finding strongly suggested a unique risk factor for suicide in alcoholics not shared by non–substance abusing depressives. The relative absence of social stressors among the depressives was in keeping with the now generally recognized endogenous (i.e., intrapersonal) nature of the suicidal urge in depression. The evidence for reactivity to social stressors on the part of the alcoholics was also consistent with clinical experience. It was not simply a matter of alcoholics bringing a lot of interpersonal problems down upon themselves by their behavior; there was a sufficient amount of that. Nearly half of them were so affected in the final year of their lives. What was striking was the frequent close temporal contiguity of the suicide to the loss event.

DECISION TO REPLICATE

We were well aware that what we reported was a chance finding, not one that had been predicted. Robust as the probability was, it was still only a correlation. No other predictors of suicide having this degree of statistical significance had been found (or have been reported up to this time). It was important to know whether it was a reliable finding.

For maximum credibility, a replication study in the clinical domain should have a statistically adequate number of probands (subjects) as like those initially studied as possible, and investigated in the same way as before. A consecutive series of candidates of the appropriate sort is generally considered acceptable. Our task then was to study all suicides by alcoholics occurring in our area (St. Louis City and County) until a reasonable number—say 50—had been accumulated. I sought and received grant support for the study as part of an NIMH Alcoholism Study Grant (MH 09247).

It was our impression from the original study that we could readily identify the alcoholics from the reports of the coroners' investigations. Salient parts of the drinking history came readily to the fore from a range of informants. The death investigators for the St. Louis County Coroner and the St. Louis City Coroner asked the right kinds of questions. We occasionally found grounds to reject a suspected diagnosis of alcoholism when a more detailed history was obtained. When interview confirmed the diagnosis, it had always been clearly foreshadowed by the postmortem blood alcohol level (when available) and/or an informant's comment about "heavy drinking" or the like. Alcoholics tended to have quite high postmortem blood levels of alcohol in contrast to other suicides. We had turned up no alcoholics by our interviewing that we had not already suspected of being so on the basis of the death investigation record.

That being the case, a replication of the original finding should be possible with great economy of effort. It would not be necessary to investigate four suicides to turn up one alcoholic, roughly the ratio in the original study. As it turned out, we conducted interviews concerning only 58 putative alcoholics to find 50 that met our diagnostic criteria. The representativeness of this sample is discussed in Chapter 3.

To ensure that comparable data are collected concerning each subject, a set of questions must be preplanned and printed to guide the interviewer. In that way, each question is asked and answered in each case. Responses are recorded verbatim, either by hand, as we did, or by the more recently available tape recorder. Surviving family members, attending physicians, and others, are interviewed in this fashion. This method of studying suicide was pioneered by Eli Robins in 1956 and 1957 (Robins, Gassner, Kayes, Wilkinson, & Murphy, 1959; Robins, Murphy, et al., 1959; Robins, 1981). Death investigation of this type has come to be characterized as a "psychological autopsy" (Litman, Curphey, Shneidman, Farberow, & Tabachnik, 1963). In fact, the relevant issues are chiefly medical, sociological, and psychiatric, much more than psychological, as will be seen in this book. But the term "psychological autopsy" has come into common usage and is likely to persist, despite its descriptive shortcomings.

2

Some Fundamental Considerations in the Study of Suicide Data

THE ROLE OF ALCOHOLISM IN SUICIDE

In order to appreciate fully the importance of the subject at hand, one must be clear about the contribution alcoholism makes to suicide. There are now 11 published independent retrospective studies of unselected (usually consecutive) series of suicides from seven countries that include a diagnostic breakdown of the subjects (probands) (Table 2.1). They total 1,562 cases investigated in substantially the same way, through interviews with surviving spouses, family, and friends. These interviews, augmented by physicians' and hospital records, official records, and other data sources, yield a consensus that nearly all suicides were psychiatrically ill at the time they took their lives. A brief description of each study is found in the Notes for this chapter, preceding the appendices.

Studies of Community Samples

The various retrospective studies of community samples of suicides are methodologically similar. Except for that of Hagnell and Rorsman (1979), the sample sizes are quite substantial. Suicide studies up through 1980 all employed a system of diagnostic precedence, resulting in a single diagnosis per case. That is also true of Åsgård's 1990 study of women. They show a considerable range of findings, with alcoholism being identified in 7–31% of the suicides. The extreme values can readily be accounted for. Women have much lower rates of alcoholism than men, and somewhat lower rates of suicide among those alcoholics (Table 7.1), hence Åsgård's low figure. Beskow's (1979) investigation concerned only men, who consistently have a higher rate of alcoholism than women. Barraclough's (1974) population, with the lowest representation of alcoholics among studies including both sexes, was older and presumably more stable than the others. The other early studies show a narrower range of 19–27% of alcoholics among the suicides.

Most studies reported later than 1980 listed multiple rather than hierarchical diagnoses. This reveals the high level of comorbidity in the suicide population but obscures

Table 2.1 Proportions of Selected Diagnoses in Community Samples of Suicide

Reference	N	Affective Disorder (%)	Alcohol-ism (%)	Schizo-phrenia (%)	Substance Abuse/ Dependency (%)	No Psychiatric Illness (%)
Robins, Murphy, et al. (1959a), United States[a,1]	134	45	24 (30)[b]	2	25	6
Dorpat & Ripley (1960), United States[2]	114	30	27	12	31	0
Barraclough et al. (1974), United Kingdom[3,4]	100	70	15	3	19	7
Beskow (1979), Sweden[5]	270♂	28 (45)[b]	31	3	37	4
Hagnell & Rorsman (1979), Sweden[6]	28	50	19	7	39	7
Chynoweth et al. (1980), Australia[7]	135	33 (55)[b]	20	4	22 (34)[b]	2
Mitterauer (1981), Austria[8]	94	63[b]	30	5[e]	45[b]	0
Kapamadžija et al. (1982), Jugoslavia[9]	100	61[b]	41[b]	3[b]	44[b]	0?
Rich et al. (1986), United States[10]	283	44[b]	29[f] (54)[b]	3[b]	60[b]	5
Arató et al. (1988), Hungary[c,11]	200	51[b]	20[b]	8[b]	20	14
Åsgård (1990), Sweden[d,12]	104♀	59	7	3	12[b]	5

[a]Superscript numbers refer to notes at the end of the book.
[b]Diagnoses inclusive, not hierarchical.
[c]19% were considered to be without psychiatric illness.
[d]14% were diagnosed as suffering from an adjustment disorder without other psychiatric diagnosis.
[e]19% additional with paraphrenia and paranoid syndromes.
[f]Rich, Fowler, & Young, 1989.

the incidence of primary psychiatric diagnoses, just as the hierarchical diagnoses obscure comorbidity. Comorbidity is common in alcoholism (see Morrison, 1982) and more common among alcoholic suicides. Mitterauer (1981) found a depressive syndrome in 28 of his 30 alcoholic suicides. Rich, Fowler, Fogarty, and Young (1988) report a diagnosis of alcoholism in 54% of their probands, but alcoholism with no other diagnosis was found in only 15 cases. Alcohol abuse in conjunction with other substance abuse was most common. To a certain extent, this may be a phenomenon of a California coastal city and the methodologically inflated size of the younger group. The rate of drug abuse in the young group, usually combined with alcohol abuse, was 66%. Drug use often came first. In the older group it came later, if at all, and was found in "only" 26%. Combined substance abuse was not a frequent finding in earlier studies.

Although the diagnostic limits of alcoholism are not uniform throughout the studies reviewed, the general concept seems to prevail that those so diagnosed will have a history not only of excessive alcohol consumption but of multiple personal, social, economic, and legal troubles as a consequence. In general, alcoholism contributes between one-fifth and one-fourth of the suicides as determined in various countries at various times. It ranks second only to depressive disorder in this regard. In the United States 7,000–8,000 suicides a year are traceable to alcoholism and its consequences. We will see shortly (Chapters 4–7) how this has come about in a series of 50 cases. But first, it would be well to address a number of issues that are of recurring concern among those interested in the subject at hand. They relate to the meaning of the suicide figures. What is a suicide? How comparable are the international suicide rates? What is the impact of missed cases? Is alcoholism a disease?

WHAT IS A SUICIDE?

Three umpires were discussing a central issue of their profession, the pitched ball. "Some are balls and some are strikes and I call 'em the best I can," said the first. "I call 'em the way I see 'em," said the second. The third of this company, older and wiser, said, "They ain't either one 'til I call 'em!" For the official record, so it is with coroners and medical examiners. But others may question the calls without being thrown out of the game. As a consequence there is a vigorous, at times contentious, literature on the reliability of coroners' and medical examiners' decisions.

Suicide is the act of taking one's own life voluntarily and intentionally. Since the deceased cannot testify as to his or her intent, the conclusion must be drawn by inference. Between 11% (McCarthy & Walsh, 1966) and 40% (Rich, Young, & Fowler, 1986) of *adjudicated* suicides leave one or more notes. As final communications, the messages characteristically consist of apologies, protestations of love, or instructions for disposition of property or of the body (Robins, Gassner, et al., 1959; E. Robins, unpublished data). Intent must still be inferred, even if alternative explanations would be difficult to sustain. In the remainder of cases, the evidence to be considered is still more circumstantial. It is at this point that tradition, as well as personal and professional philosophies, enters the picture.

In England, for many centuries, suicide was a legal issue—a crime punishable by forfeiture of the decedent's property to the crown. Thus, according to legal principles, the judgment of suicide must be based upon evidence considered to be "beyond reasonable doubt." In the Scandinavian countries, in contrast, the determination of suicide has been regarded as a public health matter to be decided by physicians on the "preponderance of evidence," the customary basis of medical decisions (Brooke & Atkinson, 1974, p. 17).

The situation is less clear-cut in the United States, where the responsibility has been left to the individual states. Consequently, organizational structures, financial support, and investigational practices vary widely from state to state (Nelson, Farberow, & MacKinnon, 1978). A coroner system with at least nominal ties to the British system was the norm for a very long time. The post was commonly appointive and political, without formal qualifications. In some jurisdictions, the coroner is the local undertaker—a social role burdened with conflict of interest in the case of suicide ascertainment. The medical examiner system has gradually replaced the coroner system in the more populous areas of the country (including St. Louis and St. Louis County), but many local coroners, some with minimal qualifications, are still to be found.[13]

Official suicide figures are far from uniform but can be safely assumed to underestimate the true state of affairs. Recently, a collaborative effort by representatives of a number of agencies under the U.S. Department of Health and Human Services, together with the American Academy of Forensic Sciences, the National Association of Medical Examiners, the International Association of Coroners and Medical Examiners, the American Association of Suicidology, and others, published "Operational Criteria for the Determination of Suicide" (Rosenberg et al., 1988). This work offers clear quidelines for coroners and medical examiners on the classification of suicide. The medically conventional "reasonable probability" rule is to be the guide rather than the legalistic "beyond reasonable doubt." In time, these guidelines may bring about a more uniform decision-making process, but currently existing data will remain of uncertain accuracy.

Given that suicides are defined differently in different places, a proponent of the beyond reasonable doubt criterion might conclude that some countries overestimate their suicides. However, I have never seen or heard this view expressed by a serious student of the subject, let alone documented. Rather, there is a small but impressive body of investigative literature indicating that suicide is officially underestimated as a rule.

THE RELIABILITY OF SUICIDE RATES

Brent, Perper, and Allman (1987) reviewed coroners' records leading to verdicts of suicidal, accidental, and undetermined manner of death among children and adolescents aged 10–19 years from 1960 through 1983 in Allegheny County (Pittsburgh), Pennsylvania. Some but not all records contained pertinent information regarding circumstances of death suggesting intent to die, as well as evidence of a recent stressor, a psychiatric history, or previous suicidal behavior. Records of deaths ruled accidental and meeting these requirements were found for 95% of hangings, 76% of deaths from carbon monoxide asphyxia, 62% of falls, and 46% of deaths from firearms. The 355 vehicular deaths in this age range were not investigated from a comparable standpoint. In addition to 159 suicide verdicts in the 24-year period, 30 of 66 cause-undetermined deaths and 8 of 89 accidental deaths were reclassified as suicide. The conclusion was that suicide in children and adolescents was underreported by 23.9%. Intoxicating blood levels of alcohol were found with increasing frequency over the 24-year period of study, but there was no increase in the initially infrequent occurrence of other intoxicants.

Apart from this study regarding adolescents, few quantitative data have been developed for the United States. Jobes, Berman, & Josselson (1987) found that 100 United States medical examiners did not reach complete consensus on mode of death (mode being suicide, accident, homicide, natural, or undetermined) in a series of test cases presented to them individually. The investigators reported opinions from a variety of sources but no direct data that suicides are underdiagnosed in the United States. Warshauer and Monk (1978) reported that the introduction of a category of death by "cause undetermined" in the eighth revision of the International Classification of Diseases (ICD 8; World Health Organization, 1977) was followed by a marked transfer of deaths of black males out of the suicide category in New York. They also showed a differential effect for certain causes of death. These differences are far less striking when statistics from the entire United States are considered (O'Carroll, 1989).

CROSS-CULTURAL DIFFERENCES IN SUICIDE RATES

Davies and Kaplan-Dinur found that in Israel, "during the years 1954–58, less than two-thirds of the cases of suicide [as determined by police reports] were so recorded by the attending physician," that is, on death certificates (1962, p. 33). Physicians addressing the question intellectually (as opposed to instantially) characteristically approach it from the balance of probabilities or preponderance of evidence viewpoint. When confronted with the necessity for an unwelcome decision regarding their own patient, however, objectivity may be a casualty.

McCarthy and Walsh (1966), using the balance of probabilities criterion, examined the records of all sudden deaths in the City and County of Dublin (Ireland) over the period of 1954–1963. They found double the number of suicides officially recognized. Carrying their investigation 5 years further, 1964–1968, they were surprised to find the discrepancy to have become greater than threefold (McCarthy & Walsh, 1975). They note that "the two coroners responsible for the area under consideration during the period of the earlier study are dead, and the present series was adjudicated by their replacements" (p. 306). But even allowing fully for the suggested discrepancy, the suicide rate in Ireland was still substantially below that in England. Subsequently, and not altogether attributable to improved ascertainment practices, Ireland's suicides have climbed to 8 per 100,000 population in 1985, very near to that of England (Kelleher & Daly, 1990).

Ovenstone (1973) reviewed death records of Edinburgh residents above the age of 11 years, except for those judged to have arisen from natural causes, over an 18-month period between October 1969 and March 1971. She employed as her definition of suicide "a deliberate initiation of an act of self-poisoning or self-injury which resulted in death, irrespective of whether there was evidence of intent to die" (p. 16). Again, this is the "balance of probabilities" philosophy of ascertainment. Based on extensive record search, Ovenstone concluded that over the 18-month period the Scottish Crown Counsel underdiagnosed suicide by 37.7%. For 1970 alone, the Registrar General (the final authority) underreported suicide by 32%. "The addition of the researcher-diagnosed suicides increased the suicide rate for the city of Edinburgh by approximately 50 per cent for both sexes" (p. 17). "Cause-undetermined" deaths, and not accidents, were the source of nearly all of the misclassifications.

There is also evidence that the means of dying may affect ascertainment. Atkinson, Kessel, and Dalgaard (1975) found wide interborough differences in the proportion of poisoning deaths given a verdict of suicide in England and Wales. The range was from 10 to 100% (p. 254). Not only does the legalistic English coroner tradition set a higher threshold for ascertaining suicide (Brooke & Atkinson, 1974); it seems to lend itself to a broad range of interpretations, at least where poisoning is concerned.

These and other studies leave little doubt that, from a medical perspective, suicide rates in the various countries are underestimates. Misclassification of other modes of death (homicide, accident) as suicide is thought to be 1% or less.

Despite the widespread evidence of underestimation of suicides, as well as different conceptual approaches to ascertainment, there do seem to be transnational differences that have been stable over fairly long periods (Dreyer, 1959). Religion is a factor. The suicide rate in Muslim countries is very much lower than in the Western world. Jews in the West have lower suicide rates than Christians. Other aspects of culture may be important as well.

The suicide rate in the Scandinavian countries is generally much higher than among Anglo-Saxons. Norway is the exception. Throughout at least the first half of the 20th century the suicide rate in Norway remained very substantially below that of the others. This difference has been a source of much speculation and debate, largely centering around differences in ascertainment methods and practices (Bolander, 1972). Since Norway consistently reports a higher proportion of deaths of undetermined cause than do the other Scandinavian countries, it is here that the presumed deficit in suicides has been thought to be hidden (Retterstøl, 1972).

To investigate this question, a team of Nordic experts on suicide was assembled in 1977; it was known as the Planning Group for Research into Suicide in Scandinavia (Juel-Nielsen, Retterstøl, & Bille-Brahe, 1987). Their documented conclusion is that "the demonstrated differences between the Scandinavian countries with regard to the registered suicide rates reflect a true difference between the countries when it is a question of the frequency of suicide" (Kolmos & Bach, 1987, p. 41).

A plausible explanation for the persistently lower Norwegian suicide rates is that Norway enjoys a higher lever of social integration than the other Scandinavian countries (Bille-Brahe, 1987). Whether it is legitimate to assume that alcoholics share in the social integration of the larger society is a matter for conjecture. Yet there may be something about being Norwegian, or living as Norwegians do, that reduces the propensity to suicide.

In an earlier effort to test the hypothesis of a cultural basis for differences in a broader sampling of national rates, Sainsbury and Barraclough (1968) compared the rank order of suicide rates among immigrants to the United States from 10 countries

Table 2.2 Suicide Rates of Immigrants to the United States Related to the Rates of Their Countries of Origin

	Suicide Rates per 100,000[a]		Rank Order	
Country	(1) Foreign-Born In U.S.	(2) Country of Origin	(1)	(2)
Sweden	34.2	18.1	1	4
Austria	32.5	24.8	2	2
Czechoslovakia	31.5	24.9	3	1
Germany (Federal Republic)	25.7	18.7	4	3
Poland	25.2	8.0	5	6
Norway	23.7	7.8	6	7
England and Wales	19.2	11.5	7	5
Italy	18.2	6.2	8	9
Canada	17.5	7.4	9	8
Ireland	9.8	2.5	10	10
Mexico	7.9	2.1	11	11
United States		10.4		

[a] $r = 0.90, P < 0.01$.

Note: From P. Sainsbury. Suicide: Opinions and Facts. *Proc. R. Soc. Med.*, 1973, 66:10, Reproduced by permission of the publisher.

to the rank order of rates in their countries of origin (Table 2.2). The rationale was that any institutionalized national bias in ascertainment in the various countries would be nullified by the ascertainment practices in the United States. The rank order correlation was strikingly high ($P < 0.01$).

By reorganizing Whitlock's (1971) data, Sainsbury (1973) was later able to replicate this finding on immigrants from 14 countries to Australia *by sex*. The rank order correlation was 0.79 for men and 0.76 for women ($P < 0.01$). In a study of immigrants to Canada, Kliewer and Ward (1988) also found "a significant positive correlation between the standardized [suicide] mortality ratios in the origin countries and those of the immigrants."

It seems safe to say that there simply are differences in national suicide rates that are not artifacts of ascertainment.

DO MISSED CASES INVALIDATE THE RESEARCH FINDINGS?

The *magnitude* of lost data is not a crucial issue for an understanding of the nature and antecedents of suicide. What *is* crucial is the question of whether, and in what ways, the missed cases might differ from those identified. For if cases are missed because of some systematic aspect of their nature and not by random investigative laxity or constraint, then our picture of the natural history of suicide is flawed and incomplete. The issue has been addressed in some respects.

Self-initiated violent deaths are likely to be ruled unequivocally as suicide, whereas deaths by poisoning (excluding carbon monoxide inhalation) fall as, or more often into the equivocal or open verdict category (Ovenstone, 1973; Atkinson et al., 1975; McCarthy & Walsh, 1975; Nuttal, Evenson, & Cho, 1980). Such a circumstance, to the extent that it hides suicides, might lead to an underestimation of the number of female suicides, since women, even according to official records, are twice as likely as men to choose self-poisoning. That did not appear to have been the case, however, in either Ovenstone's or Nuttal and Evenson's study. It is unclear in Atkinson et al. and McCarthy and Walsh. In any event, narrowing the sex ratio of suicides would have no appreciable impact on the findings concerning the antecedents of suicide unless there is something besides sex-related choice of method that leads to being overlooked.

Holding and Barraclough (1978) examined 110 cases with verdicts of "undetermined" cause of death that had been rendered in a 2-year period by one coroner of West London. They matched those cases as to sex, age, and cause of death with like numbers of cases adjudicated as suicide and as accident during the same period or near it, to test the hypothesis that undetermined deaths were mostly concealed suicides. No attempt was made to reach conclusions independent from those of the coroner. Given the repeatedly demonstrated high (i.e., 90–100%) correlation of suicides with psychiatric illness (Table 2.1), it would be expected that concealed suicides would be among those *having* a history of psychiatric treatment, of psychiatric hospital admission, of a diagnosis of depression, or of any mental illness.

The proportion of undetermined cases with a history of psychiatric treatment (42%) lay midway between that of suicide (59%) and of accident (28%) cases. Results were similar with respect to history of psychiatric hospital admission (46% of suicides, 33% of the undetermined, and 20% of accidents, respectively), a diagnosis of depression (73%, 41%, 27%) and the authors' assessment of presence of mental illness (87%, 73%, 60%). The balance of the undetermined cases could not be diagnosed either sick or well. With respect to number under current psychiatric care, either inpatient or outpatient, the undetermined resembled the suicides (29 versus 30) but not accidents ($N = 8$). The hypothesis was not confirmed entirely, but it appeared likely to be true for a proportion of the cases.

Ovenstone (1973), in her 1970 sample, compared official suicides with those identified by her criteria as missed cases of suicide on a variety of demographic and social variables. She found no differences in civil state, household composition, social class, employment, overcrowding and substandard housing, debts, criminal record, general practitioner consultations, previous psychiatric treatment, suicidal behavior, physical illness, alcohol abuse, or psychiatric and personality diagnoses. Missed suicides included more women aged 55 years and older. The data base of 40 missed suicides provides no support for concern that missed cases are very different from those recognized.

Brent et al. (1987) noted that reclassified cases were similar to adjudicated suicides with respect to age, sex, circumstances and method of suicide or positive blood alcohol concentration at the time of death. Reclassified cases "were much more similar to the cases of completed suicide than they were to the remaining accidents and undetermined verdicts."[14]

These are critical dimensions with respect to the question of whether missed cases are like or unlike identified cases. If one does not take the extreme position that *all* undetermined cases are hidden suicides, the evidence seems clear that there is enough similarity of findings to give at least a balance of probabilities that the lost are not unlike the found.[15]

IS ALCOHOLISM A DISEASE?

Strongly held opinions differ as to whether alcoholism is a disease. Such a debate asks the wrong question. Diseases are not entities in the sense that plants or animals are. Instances of a disease bear a much more relativistic relationship to the disease named than does, for example, a duck to the class *Galinaceae*. Collections of symptoms and items of clinical history comprise the framework against which a given case is compared for purposes of diagnosis. Diagnoses are conceptual conveniences, ways of ordering the observations that give them heightened meaning and utility. Their purpose is twofold: to make a prognosis (a prediction of outcome) and to direct therapy. The "right" question is, therefore, Is it clinically useful to regard alcoholism as a disease?

By defining the diagnostic term "alcoholism," a group of patients can be identified who are alike in critical respects. That permits surrounding issues to be examined. The answer, then, is "Yes." Regarding alcoholism as a disease "has meant that characteristic strategies applied to the rest of medicine to understand etiology, pathogenesis, clinical course, outcome, response to treatment, and epidemiology are appropriate for alcoholism as well" (Guze, Cloninger, Martin, & Clayton, 1988, p. 83). Both the present author and those reviewed in these pages find it useful to regard alcoholism as a disease.

It was not until after the publication of "Diagnostic Criteria for Use in Psychiatric Research" (Feighner et al., 1972) that American psychiatrists other than ourselves had the means to be very specific about their populations under study. They could not agree with one another at better than a chance level regarding diagnosis (Beck, 1962; Beck, Ward, Mendelson, Mock, & Erbaugh, 1962). Scientific communication, especially on this side of the Atlantic Ocean, was not meaningful. The situation was not much better in the United Kingdom (Kreitman, 1961).

Particularly within the field of psychiatry, the borders between adjacent diseases (those similar in some respects) are rarely, if ever, clear-cut. There is a degree of arbitrariness in establishing them. Where those borders are drawn is determined largely by the purposes for which the classification is intended. The research diagnostic criteria of the Washington University Department of Psychiatry (Feighner et al., 1972) seek to achieve clinical homogeneity under the various rubrics at a cost of some cases being left uncertain or unclassified. Criteria for a diagnosis of alcoholism are given in Table 2.3.

Table 2.3 Research Criteria for the Diagnosis of Alcoholism

A "definite" diagnosis is made when symptoms occur in at least three of the four following groups. A "probable" diagnosis is made when symptoms occur in only two groups.
A. Group One:
  1. Any manifestation of alcohol withdrawal such as tremulousness, convulsions, hallucinations, or delirium.
  2. History of medical complications, e.g., cirrhosis, gastritis, pancreatitis, myopathy, polyneuropathy, or Wernicke-Korsakoff's syndrome.
  3. Alcoholic blackouts, i.e., amnesic episodes during heavy drinking not accounted for by head trauma.
  4. Alcoholic binges or benders (48 hours or more of drinking associated with default of usual obligations; must have occurred more than once to be scored as positive).
B. Group Two:
  1. Patient has not been able to stop drinking when he wanted to do so.
  2. Patient has tried to control drinking by allowing himself to drink only under certain circumstances, such as only after 5:00 p.m., only on weekends, or only with other people.
  3. Drinking before breakfast.
  4. Drinking non–beverage forms of alcohol, e.g., hair oil, mouthwash, Sterno.
C. Group Three:
  1. Arrests for drinking.
  2. Traffic difficulties associated with drinking.
  3. Trouble at work because of drinking.
  4. Fighting associated with drinking.
D. Group Four:
  1. Patient thinks he drinks too much.
  2. Family objects to his drinking.
  3. Loss of friends because of drinking.
  4. Other people object to his drinking.
  5. Feels guilty about his drinking.

Note: From J. P. Feighner, E. Robins, S. B. Guze, R. A. Woodruff, Jr., G. Winokur, and R. Munoz. Diagnostic Criteria for Use in Psychiatric Research. *Arch. Gen. Psychiatry,* 1972, 26:57–63. Copyright 1972, American Medical Association.

DSM-III and DSM-III-R (American Psychiatric Association [APA], 1980, 1987) cast a wider net to maximize the number of cases classifiable for clinical and record-keeping purposes. DSM-III (APA, 1980) cast aside all but a vestige of a syndrome (collection of characteristic and defining features of a recognized disorder) in the case of alcohol *abuse* (Appendix A). The characteristic symptoms and consequences are listed, but no minimum number or pattern was specified—only a minimum duration of 1 month. Alcohol dependence criteria were similarly nonspecific. The DSM-III-R (APA, 1987) criteria aspired to a common definition for all psychoactive substance abuse disorders. In doing so, they sacrificed clarity so far as modern concepts of alcoholism are concerned. Criteria for a substance abuse diagnosis are less detailed than in DSM-III, with either continued or recurrent use required (Appendix A). The criteria have a syndromic quality, but again lack the specificity characterizing our diagnostic categories.

Evidence for the utility of the distinction between psychoactive substance *abuse* and *dependence* is inconclusive (Schuckit, Zisook, & Mortola, 1985; Kleber, 1990). Despite my dissatisfaction with it, it is the official standard today. I do not find the distinction clinically meaningful and will not employ it here. As Vaillant and Milofsky (1982) propose, "alcoholism, like hypertension, represents a continuum."

II
THE STUDY

3

Description and Limitations of the Study

RATIONALE FOR THE STUDY

The data that form the core of this book were gathered for the single purpose of testing a finding from our earlier study of a consecutive series of suicides in St. Louis and St. Louis County (Robins, Murphy, et al., 1959). That finding was described in Chapter 1 and Table 1.1.

THE PROCEDURE

The study embraced all of the alcoholic suicides in two time periods: all of 1968 and 1969 and February through October 1971. This had exclusively to do with whether there were, at a given time, any psychiatric residents in our training program willing to devote a substantial amount of time to this inquiry. The residents who participated most intensively were Drs. John W. Armstrong, William W. Clendenin, John R. Fischer, and Steven L. Hermele. Drs. Bruce Crane, Michael Johnson, Marijan Herjanic, and I each completed one primary interview. I also had the assistance of Mrs. Bonnie Walbran during the first two years of the study for obtaining records and coding and entering data.

The process of choosing the probable alcoholics from among all of the suicides in the City of St. Louis and St. Louis County during the periods of study was as follows. A research assistant or interviewer visited each coroner's office every week or two and abstracted the contents of each coroner's report carrying a verdict of suicide. In addition to demographic data, the account of the suicidal act and the antecedent circumstances were transcribed verbatim from the coroner's death investigation report, together with any notation concerning current or past medical or psychiatric treatment. Names and addresses of identified physicians, family members, and other informants were recorded, as were pertinent physical and toxicologic findings. Suicide notes were copied verbatim.

Based on that information, I carried out the following selection process, together with one or more of the interviewers:

1. If either alcoholism or heavy drinking as a practice was mentioned, the subject was identified as putatively alcoholic and listed for inclusion in the study.
2. Subjects in whom the blood alcohol concentration was 0.10 gram % (g%) or greater and those reported to have been drinking just before the suicide were considered putative alcoholics.
3. If another diagnosis or diagnostic description (such as "schizophrenic" or "despondent over heart condition") without mention of alcohol was recorded, the subject was identified as not alcoholic and removed from consideration.

Blood alcohol concentration was reported in 55% of the adjudicated suicides. It was least likely to have been done where death was by gunshot wound or hanging, as well as where death was not immediate but followed a period of hospital treatment.

To test my belief that we could readily recognize the alcoholics among the adjudicated suicides, we sought our own evidence for or against the presence of alcoholism in every case during 1968 where the inquest information was insufficient to indicate probable alcoholism. There were 137 coroners' verdicts of suicide in the City of St. Louis and St. Louis County in that year. Based on information suggesting alcohol abuse in the coroners records, we sought and secured primary interviews in 27 cases; 24 proved to be alcoholics. In 5 cases, coroner's evidence suggested the presence of alcoholism, but the family refused to be interviewed.

In 29 cases, the inquest contained an explicit statement of a diagnosis other than alcoholism, usually "despondent" or "depression." We obtained information from medical sources (family physicians, psychiatrists, hospital records) stating another psychiatric diagnosis and no evidence of an alcohol problem in 51 cases, and from family members in 20 cases. (In one case, a landlady was the only existing source.) In the remaining cases, we sought further information from available sources by telephone concerning alcohol abuse. A denial of knowledge of an alcohol problem was accepted at face value unless some other evidence pointed toward alcoholism. Equivocal responses were treated like affirmative ones, and the case was scheduled to be studied by interviewing a family member.

To avoid biasing the outcome by sample selection, what was specifically *not* considered as evidence of alcoholism was any information concerning disruptions of relationships, actual or threatened. In all, we identified one possible alcoholic through our case by case inquiry who would have been missed from coroner's records alone. The family physician reported that his 67-year-old male patient had been an alcoholic *earlier in his life*. We failed to secure an interview through inadvertence.[1]

Having thus verified our ability to identify alcoholics from the record (24 true positives and 3 false positives by interview, 1 missed case, 5 refusals of interview, 2 probables with no informant) we were satisfied that we no longer needed to follow behind the coroners and gather our own information. The proportion of confirmed alcoholics in the suicide pool for 1968 was 19%; for probable alcoholics, 23%. This latter figure is the same as the proportion of alcoholics in our original study.

THE INTERVIEW

The method of investigation we followed was a replication of that used in our 1957 study (Robins, Gassner, et al., 1959; Robins, Murphy, et al., 1959, Robins, 1981). Potential informants were identified from the police investigation report and the record of the coroner's investigation. The informant most closely associated with the deceased was contacted by telephone when possible. The nature and purpose of the study was explained and an appointment for the interview was requested. Most interviews were conducted in the informant's home, although occasionally the informant chose to come to the medical center for it. When the primary informant refused or could not be located, another informant was sought.[2] Securing cooperation for interviewing was not always an easy task. It required both dedication and perseverance.

Our last interviewer was particularly ingenious. When refused an interview by a potentially appropriate informant, he would identify from the death certificate the site of burial of the subject, go to the cemetery, and learn from the custodian what cleric had performed the obsequies. The minister, priest, or rabbi was asked for help in securing the family's cooperation in our work. By this method, he completed a number of cases we had given up on, including one secured 126 weeks after the suicide (Case 32). I conducted one primary interview by telephone, with a psychiatrist who knew the subject quite well. The family, living at some distance from St. Louis, had declined to give information.

I went over each interview together with the interviewer, usually within 24 hours of its accomplishment, to be certain that it was as complete as possible and that I could read and understand it fully without recourse to the interviewer's memory. Occasionally, there would be contradictions or seeming contradictions in the text. The interviewer would clarify them on the spot if possible or call the respondent back. Missing information could be secured in the same way. It was important to clear up all of this before the trail grew cold. As I write this book, I am glad we made that effort, and I now wish it had been even more rigorous. Today, it is much too late.

The interview itself was semistructured. It followed a printed interview guide designed to ensure that each question would be asked in each case. Responses were recorded substantially verbatim, including whatever elaboration was obtained. The interview guide is reproduced as Appendix B. It is very similar to the one used in 1957 (Robins, 1981, pp. 26–46). The emphasis was on doing as nearly as possible what had been done before.

DIAGNOSTIC CRITERIA

At the time I undertook this study, we had been using explicit criteria for all of the major psychiatric diagnoses for a number of years at Washington University. They underwent modifications from time to time as we gained more experience with them. The criteria I used for diagnosing alcoholism (Table 3.1) were a precursor to those published in "Diagnostic Criteria for Use in Psychiatric Research" (Feighner et al., 1972).

Table 3.1 Criteria for Alcoholism Originally Used in This Study: One Symptom in at Least Three Groups or Two Symptoms in Two Groups

I. Personal concern
   1. Thought he drank too much?
   2. Felt guilty about drinking?
   3. Wanted to stop but couldn't?
II. Interpersonal problems
   4. Family objected to drinking?
   5. Informant thought he drank too much?
   6. Others thought so?
   7. Lost friends because of drinking?
   8. Marital problems?
III. Social-legal problems
   9. Trouble at work?
   10. Lose a job?
   11. Driving trouble?
   12. Arrested?
   13. Fighting?
IV. Medical problems
   14. DTs, shakes, etc.?
   15. Impotence?
   16. Hospitalized because of drinking or its complications?
V. Pattern
   17. Drink before breakfast?
   18. Benders?

I have a certain fondness for this particular schedule. It seems to me to be just a bit more rational than the criteria that were published (Table 2.3). For example, I don't think that binges or benders belong in the category of physical consequences of alcohol abuse. They represent loss of control and belong in Feighner's Group Two. I also question the utility of "drinking non-beverage forms of alcohol" as a criterion symptom. It seems to me that it occurs only in individuals who have already accumulated such a plethora of other negative consequences in several areas that it adds nothing to the sensitivity or the specificity of the criteria. The Feighner criteria have been published, so I used them as the final arbiter of strict diagnosis.

The impact of these criteria on my 50 cases is that 2 subjects are reclassified as "probable alcoholic." All 50 subjects easily meet DSM-III and DSM-III-R criteria for alcohol dependence and/or abuse. I have recorded each criterion symptom elicited for a diagnosis of alcoholism in the subject's history (Chapters 4–7).

Concerning other psychiatric diagnoses, again I followed the departmental criteria (Feighner, et al., 1972). The case histories show how each subject does or does not meet criteria for affective disorder. All of the eight subjects whom I diagnosed as "probable" affective disorder by our research criteria meet the somewhat less rigorous but appropriately syndromic DSM-III-R criteria for definite major depressive disorder.[3]

LOSS EVENTS

In asking about antecedent loss events, interviewers adhered strictly to the original policy of asking the informant to date each event in calendar time, not in temporal relation to the suicide. We determined the temporal relationship by subtracting the date of occurrence from the date of the suicidal act. Sometimes the informant's memory was inexact. If timing was uncertain, the event was assumed to have occurred more than 6 weeks before the suicide. Events that were anticipated, whether realistically or uncertainly, were carefully distinguished from those that had occurred. To avoid overdiagnosing losses, only those that had actually occurred were counted for the comparison, as in the original study (Murphy & Robins, 1967).

LIMITATIONS OF THE INVESTIGATION

The most significant limitation on any study of individual suicides is the unavailability of the victim for questioning. For self-evident reasons, that will always be the case. Prospective studies of suicide are not feasible for two compelling reasons. The first is the statistical rarity of suicide: roughly 1 in 8,000 persons per year. Even in an "enriched" population—such as alcoholics or depressives (persons at higher risk of suicide)—the rate is low, so very large populations would be required to generate a suicide sample of statistically meaningful size. The second problem pertains to our responsibility to the members of such a study. When we apprehend a patient's serious consideration of suicide, we must make every effort to dissuade the patient, to treat and to protect him or her. If that effort is successful, it cannot be proven to have been so. A prevented suicide is a nonevent, statistically (Murphy, 1984). *A successful prevention cannot be distinguished from a nonsuicidal crisis, so nothing can be said about the antecedents of such a crisis that can unequivocally be related to suicide.* Therefore, our only recourse in studying suicide is to secondary sources, retrospectively.

The interview was designed to give a broad picture of the history, experiences, and behavior of each subject. Many questions were asked concerning psychiatric symptoms and behaviors. That is the basis for making the diagnosis of alcoholism as well as other psychiatric diagnoses. This array of questions antedated the full formulation of the Washington University Department of Psychiatry diagnostic criteria for use in research, the so-called Feighner Criteria (Feighner et al., 1972). But the fact that not all of the questions that we would ask today were systematically asked is not altogether attributable to when the study was done.

In following the 1957 interview schedule, I failed to update fully the list of symptoms to be inquired about. In particular, regarding the diagnosis of alcoholism, blackouts were not systematically included, nor were efforts to *control* drinking as distinguished from abstinence. Consumption of non–beverage alcohol was also omitted, but I regard that question as redundant in any event. Two symptoms relevant to the diagnosis of major depressive disorder were not systematically investigated. The presence of agitation or retardation was not asked about. "Trouble thinking" was asked about in a general way, but impaired concentration was not. Often there was a question in my mind in this belated review as to how diligently the key symptoms had been pursued. It was a long interview, and not every response was probed fully in every case. Interviewers did sometimes record the presence of symptoms not included in the interview. To the extent that a diagnosis is made, it is a minimum estimate.

The inquiry as to symptoms required for a diagnosis of antisocial personality disorder (ASPD) was also incomplete. Drinking, drugs, arrests, and marital and job instability were adequately covered. Early symptoms such as lying, stealing, school discipline, running away from home, and vagabondage were not. Had they been included, it is unlikely that much confidence could be placed in a diagnosis of ASPD, because few informants had known the deceased in adolescence, and our criteria require onset of symptoms before age 15. It is unfortunate that this information is lacking, because of the frequently reported association of ASPD (variously defined) with alcoholism (Fremming, 1951; Helgason, 1964; Sundby, 1967; Dubourg, 1969; Woodruff, Guze, Clayton, & Carr, 1973; Berglund, 1984; Martin, Cloninger, Guze, & Clayton, 1985b; Penick, Powell, Liskow, Jackson, & Nickel, 1988).

Age of onset of alcoholism is not easy to identify historically, even under ideal circumstances.[4] I used my best judgment in assessing it, aiming to be moderately conservative. All of the pertinent data are presented for the reader's consideration.

Overall, there is the question of how complete the informant's knowledge might have been of the symptoms we were interested in (to say nothing of other aspects of the victim's life). Owing to the social isolation in which many of these subjects lived toward the end of their lives, the informant's knowledge of relevant symptoms was often deficient. Selecting the closest relative for interview—the spouse in 74% of cases—generally seemed to be satisfactory. Additional informants, except for attending physicians, were rarely interviewed.

Attending physicians are better at reporting medical complaints and treatment than psychiatric symptoms (Murphy, 1975). They often seemed unsure about the presence or degree of alcohol abuse. A spouse was more likely to know of both psychiatric symptoms and drinking pattern. On the other hand, physicians and hospitals keep records. Hospital records (obtained in 34% of the cases) fixed dates of admissions and included historical detail obtained from the eventual victim. They sometimes documented symptoms not known to or recalled by our primary informant. Often, however, they were dismayingly sparse. That is not surprising, as the study far antedates wide acceptance and teaching of criterion-based psychiatric diagnosis in the United States. Without necessarily believing that alcoholics are fully reliable informants, I chose to rely on first-person contemporaneous accounts of problematic behavior and symptoms preserved in the hospital record over informants' accounts when they conflicted. In the infrequent instance of an informant's report of hospitalization (DTs, for example) not documented by otherwise seemingly complete records, the discrepancy is noted in the case vignette.

In interviews with spouses there was at times a flavor of self-exculpation or denial. It was most clear in comparing the report of the coroner's investigation closely following the death to our later interview with the same informant. In case of conflict in chronology or other details, I chose to rely on the earlier report unless more than one source contradicted it. My experience is that informants are more forthcoming in the immediate wake of the tragedy than they are after they have had time to reflect.

In general, the kinds of details we asked about were well enough known to our informants: spouses (74%), siblings (10%), friends (6%), parents (4%), other family, including in-laws (4%), one paramour (2%), and one psychiatrist/acquaintance (2%). None of the eight cases studied that were not diagnosed as alcoholism or probable alcoholism was on the borderline of inclusion. They are not included in any aspect of the study except by being mentioned in this chapter.

DESCRIPTION AND LIMITATIONS OF THE STUDY

An area of neglect that will prove to be of considerable importance is that of social ties. Given the large amount of information we set out to obtain, and the two or more hours required to obtain it, a careful history of social integration might not have been feasible in any event. We had put relatively little emphasis on that area in the original investigation and I did not enlarge it in the replication.[5] That the histories are incomplete is inevitable. That they may be biased in some respects is likely. However, I have taken pains to record as completely as possible the information obtained in each case, relying entirely on the record. My inferences are clearly identified in the case histories.

POTENTIAL SOURCES OF BIAS

Missed Cases

Over the course of the study, 81 individuals whose deaths were ruled suicide by the coroners of St. Louis or of St. Louis County were considered to be putative alcoholics and slated for study. Of these cases, 22 were not investigated further: 13 because of refusal by the only prospective informant identified in the investigation reports, 5 because the only known informant had moved out of town (3 cases) or there was no informant at all (2 cases). Four were missed through inadvertence. Were the missed cases different from those studied?

First, the sex ratio is different. Males outnumber females by a margin of only 2:1 among missed cases, but by 6:1 in those studied (Table 3.2). The latter ratio is consistent with the sex ratio of alcoholics identified in the Epidemiologic Catchment Area (ECA) study of psychiatric disorders in the community (Robins, Helzer, Przybeck, & Regier, 1988, Table 3, p. 19). A higher proportion of widowers than widows refused to be interviewed (4 of 5 versus 5 of 9). On the other hand, we have no evidence that women are more or less likely than men to show the type of reactivity we were investigating.

The mean age of the missed cases is slightly higher (51.7 years versus 47.9 years), again without obvious significance. More missed cases were divorced. The absence of a spouse as informant accounts for some of them being missed. However, living alone was not more likely to lead to being missed. About the same proportion in each group was living alone, 32% and 30%, respectively, substantially fewer than the 52% living alone in the original study. Of 9 subjects whom interview showed not to be alcoholic, 2 (22%) lived alone.

Among the 7 women missed, 5 were married and 4 husbands refused interview. The other married woman was described at inquest as "despondent." Her reported blood alcohol concentration (BAC) of 0.15 g% was the only reason to consider her a possible alcoholic. (A BAC $\geq$ 0.10 g% represents *legal* evidence of intoxication in Missouri.) One woman was divorced and neither her former husband nor her sister would agree to being interviewed. There may have been good reason. She had shot her husband in the leg 8 years earlier and had made an attempt on her own life at that time. They had been divorced for 2 years but continued to live in the same house. Earlier on the day of her death, *she and her ex-husband had been arguing about whether he would remarry her. He refused and she threatened to leave him*. In fact,

Table 3.2 Descriptive Characteristics of Missed Cases vs. Those Studied

	Missed Cases		Alcoholic by Study		Not Alcoholic by Study	
	N = 22	%	N = 50	%	N = 9	%
Sex						
Male	15	68	43	86	9	100
Female	7	32	7	14		
Age (mean)		51.7		47.9		41.0
25–34	3	14	3	6	3	33
35–44	4	18	13	26	5	56
45–54	4	18	22	44		
55–64	7	32	10	20		
65+	4	18	2	4	1	11
Civil state						
Married	14	64	42	84	6	67
Separated	2	9	8	16		
Widowed	0	0	1	2		
Divorced	7	32	4	8	1	11
Single	1	4	3	6	2	22
Living alone	7	32	15	30	2	22
Method						
Gunshot	11	50	25	50	6	67
CO	2	9	8	16	0	
Ingest	5	23	7	14	0	
Hang	4	18	3	6	2	22
Cut/stab	0		4	8	0	
Leap/collide	0		2	4	1	11
More than 1 method	0		1	2	0	

she did so, by ingesting a fatal overdose of a barbiturate prescribed to him. Her physician told me she had a quick temper, boyfriends, and a problem with alcohol.

Among the 15 males missed, 9 were married. The wife refused to be interviewed in 5 instances and 2 had moved away. One wife was never located despite repeated efforts. She, too, may have moved away. *One married man had been separated for about 2 months because of his drinking.* My notes do not explain our failure to obtain an interview. The remaining 6 men were divorced. In 2 cases, the family refused to give an interview. In another case, *divorce had preceded the suicide by less than 6 weeks*. The victim, a 70-year old retired machinist, was reported to have been despondent over the divorce. The widow remarried and moved out of state within 3 weeks after his death. A BAC of 0.12 g% was the only reason for his planned inclusion. The ex-wife having moved away, there was no one to interview.

A BAC of 0.11 g% was the only evidence suggesting alcoholism in another case where there was no family member to interview. That man was described by a neighbor at inquest as despondent over divorce from his second wife 9 months earlier. The other two divorced men were inadvertently not followed up. One was described as a heavy drinker, drinking heavily the night of his death. The other was described as *despondent and drinking heavily since the death of his ex-wife 1 month prior to his suicide.*[6] (She had married again.)

Some of the refusals to be interviewed were justified by prospective informants on grounds of their being upset. In others, no explanation was given. In at least two instances, refusal was only implicit by repeated postponement of a commitment to meet. I had the distinct impression in several cases that conflict between the informant and the deceased was the reason for the refusal to discuss, but that, of course, is only speculation. Based on what we did learn, this group was not without interpersonal troubles. I conclude it is unlikely, had they all been interviewed, that they would have diluted away our positive finding.

Era of the Study

It is doubtful whether the important characteristics of suicide have changed much over the years, but in thinking about the findings, and particularly the case histories, it is well to keep in mind certain sociological changes. This study was conducted 20 years ago, and the mean age of the subjects at death was about 48 years. One consequence is a lower mean level of academic attainment than would be true today. There is no basis for thinking that limited education contributes to suicide, although early onset of abusive drinking might adversely affect educational attainment in a few cases.

Because of when the study was done, military service was much more widespread than it is today. A great many of the subjects were of draft age during World War II, a few during the Korean conflict; hence a certain emphasis on military service or its absence. Of the 43 men in the study, 28 (65%) did have military service. Few used Veterans Administration facilities for their psychiatric hospitalizations, and only 4 were on any disability status. It is also likely that psychiatric attention was both less available and less acceptable at that time. Certainly, treatment for alcoholism and substance abuse problems was less widely available than it is today.

Interval Between Suicide and Interview

As a matter of respect for the grieving, we approached no one until 4 weeks had elapsed from the date of death. Primary interviews were secured in a range of intervals from 4 to 126 weeks, with a mean of 28 weeks and a median of 16 weeks. To what extent did the time gap between the event and the interview affect reliability and accuracy of the information? There can be no sure answer to that question. There was, in every case, a record of an interview by trained investigators from the coroner's office, conducted in most cases within hours of discovery of the death. In a few, death followed the terminal act by days or even weeks, so the coroner's investigation, too, was delayed. As a result of delay in interviewing, some information was probably lost or diminished in specificity, yet there is a richness of detail in nearly every case that expands greatly on what is available from official records alone.

The informant's perception of the reason(s) for the suicide was often less specific than mine (see case histories, Chapters 4–7). Threatened separations were almost certainly underreported, and actual separation, if participated in by the informant, was recognized as relevant to the suicidal outcome only once. There is a certain amount of understandable self-exculpation or self-protection in this.

OUTCOME OF THE INVESTIGATION

The principal findings of this replication were that again, half of the alcoholic suicides had experienced loss of a close interpersonal relationship in the last year of their lives (Murphy, Armstrong, Hermele, Fischer, & Clendenin, 1979, Table 3.3). Again, the observed number affected within 6 weeks of suicide (13 of 50) significantly exceeds the number expected by chance ($P < 0.01$) in the final one-ninth of the year. The total of 13 of 50 (26%) is not significantly different from 11 of 32 (32%; Table 1.1) (χ^2 with Yates's correction, 1 df = 0.433). This investigation was a maximally stringent test of the original observation. The methods were the same, and so was the outcome, as required by the hypothesis being tested. Much more was learned, as will be discussed in Chapter 8.

Table 3.3 Loss of Affectional Relationship Preceding Suicide in Alcoholics

	Original Study ($N = 32$), Within		Present Study ($N = 50$), Within	
	1 Year	6 Weeks	1 Year	6 Weeks
Separated	9	7	15	9
Divorced	1	0	3	0
Widowed	1	0	0	0
Bereaved	1	0	10	3
Apart (other)	3	3	3	2
Total with affectional loss	15	10	25	13
Percentage affected[a]	47	31	50	26

[aa]In both the original and the present study, the observed number affected within 6 weeks of suicide significantly exceeds the number expected (χ^2 with Yates's correction, 1 df: 7.40 and 7.68, respectively; $P < 0.01$).

Note: From G. E. Murphy, J. W. Armstrong, S. L. Hermele, J. R. Fischer, and W. W. Clendenin. Suicide and Alcoholism. Interpersonal Loss Confirmed as a Predictor. *Arch. Gen. Psychiatry,* 1979, *36:*65–69. Copyright 1979, American Medical Association.

III

ALCOHOLICS WHO KILL THEMSELVES: CASE HISTORIES

4

Men with Onset of Alcoholism Before Age 25

Of 59 putative alcoholics regarding whom a primary informant was interviewed, 50 met the criteria then in use for a diagnosis of alcoholism. Forty-eight meet the diagnostic criteria of Feighner et al. (1972) for "definite" alcoholism and two for "probable" alcoholism. These are considerably more stringent criteria than those of DSM–III or of DSM-III-R, by either of which criteria all are either alcohol dependent or alcohol abusers. Our emphasis is on consequences of alcohol abuse, generally of a kind that will not occur in numbers until abusive drinking is well established. No attempt is made to distinguish addictive from abusive drinking, as no utility has been shown for the distinction, despite its recent introduction into our diagnostic nomenclature (APA, 1980).[1]

The life history of each subject, insofar as it was learned, is presented in this and the next three chapters. These histories contain all of the information we obtained. Except that the personal and social history is presented first, and the most recent events last, they largely follow the form of a conventional medical history. Each case history will be presented in exactly the same sequence: personal and social history followed by drinking history, then other psychiatric history, medical history, pertinent family history, and history of suicidal communication. The circumstances leading to the act will be summarized, followed by clinical diagnoses, toxicology, sources of information, and the informant's stated opinion of the reason(s) for the suicide. Finally, I present my own analysis of the factors most central to the suicide.

The form of presentation ensures that all issues are covered with as little redundancy as practical, while including both positive and relevant negative information. Particularly in matters of diagnosis, what is absent is often as important as what is present. Hence, a certain amount of repetition is inescapable. I have taken pains to show all that we learned. The reader is both enabled and invited to draw his/her own conclusions from the data. I wish we had obtained a physical description of our subjects to round out the behavioral picture, but, we didn't.

The numbering of the cases corresponds essentially to the sequence in which interviews were obtained, and has no other significance. Neither fictitious names nor assigned initials seemed appropriate to use because of the risk of a mistaken identification of a case by a reader. In presenting these case histories, I have employed those disguises that seemed necessary to protect the families of the deceased. They include deletions of names and distinctive sites of education or work, as well as blurring of high–profile families or occupations. These matters are not pertinent to our understanding of suicide in any event. Twenty years have elapsed since most of these suicides occurred. It is my intention that the data presented cannot prove embarrassing to anyone.

The cases are grouped here according to age and sex, but not age at death. Rather, they are arranged according to age of onset of problem drinking, insofar as that could be determined. That was done to see if there were informative differences between those with early versus later onset of problem drinking. When more than one subject had the same age of onset, the case histories are ordered according to their accession into the study. The case histories are segregated by sex because of the rather marked differences in the drinking careers of men and women. Alcoholism is far less frequent in women than in men—in a ratio of about 1:6. Suicide, in turn, is less frequent in women who are alcoholics than in men with the same diagnosis (see Table 7.1). Perhaps more important than either of these considerations is the fact that the drinking careers of women tend to be shorter and more fulminating. The order of presentation here will not prevent making other comparisons.

CASE HISTORIES

Case 46

Subject 46 was a 37–year-old single unemployed black male who died of hemorrhage secondary to laceration of both wrists, complicating a massive overdose of an antidepressant medication, while intoxicated. He was born and raised in the St. Louis metropolitan area and lived there with his Baptist parents for most of his life. His father was a factory worker, still employed. His mother was a homemaker. He had one brother, also living in St. Louis. He completed high school and worked sporadically in various factory and foundry jobs most of his adult life, apart from 3 years in military service in Korea from age 22 to 25. He served without problems and was honorably discharged without disability. It was reported that he was unhappy with himself ever since he left the service.

He was described as always high strung and sensitive to criticism but with no extreme personality traits. He never married. He reportedly had four or five good friends. So far as we know, there was no change in his social circumstances.

According to hospital records, he began to abuse alcohol in his mid–teens. He was a daily drinker by the time he was discharged from military service. It is uncertain when he began intravenous narcotic use, but at age 26 his father took him to the Federal Hospital at Lexington, Kentucky, where he underwent 3 months of treatment for heroin addiction. He decreased his drug use after discharge but increased his drinking. In addition to daily use of wine or liquor, he appears to have had episodes of several weeks to months of increased alcohol use: up to three quarts of fortified wine (Rosie O'Grady) or one and one-half fifths of gin per day. These were the circumstances that preceded his 6 admissions to a local public hospital in the last 6 years of his life. He typically entered with alcoholic hallucinosis (visual, auditory, and sometimes tactile), which cleared on detoxification. On two of these admissions he reported periods of abstinence preceding his binges. Alcoholic cirrhosis was his major medical problem, although alcoholic dementia was mentioned repeatedly in the hospital records. He attended the outpatient clinic of the hospital occasionally, but he declined formal treatment for his alcoholism.

His family and others thought he drank too much. He felt ashamed of himself and avoided his parents when drinking. He was disgusted with himself because he could not stop drinking, and he felt worthless because he could not support himself. He regularly drank in the morning to relieve tremulousness. On at least one occasion, while hospitalized, he was reported to have ingested shoe polish remover—as an alcohol substitute, not in a suicide attempt. He had hepatic cirrhosis, a history of binges and blackouts, and alcoholic hallucinosis on all but the last one of his six hospital admission. That one was to a general hospital where he had been taken after a severe beating with iron pipe by four assailants while he was drunk. His drug abuse history was known, but he consistently denied current use. On hospitalization 1 year before his death, "needle tracks" were noted on his arms. The beating occurred 3 months later. Was there a connection?

He had been arrested many times for public intoxication and held overnight in jail, but those were his only problems with the law. He had missed work from time to time because of his drinking, but according to the informant, he had not been fired or reprimanded. However, on one hospital admission it was recorded that he *had* been fired for drinking. For the last 10 months of his life, his drinking totally prevented him from working. While it was reported that he quit working, the same informant said that he was drawing unemployment compensation for the last 10 months, suggesting that he had either been fired or laid off.

The only record of any psychiatric condition or treatment other than his hospitalizations for alcohol and drug problems was from an outpatient visit 1 month after his last hospital discharge, 5 months before his suicide. At that time he was given amitriptyline (Elavil), a tricyclic antidepressant, for a depressive syndrome, as well as an antianxiety drug, and vitamins. His medication compliance was believed to be poor. He had low mood, weight loss, low energy, and fatigue over a 2–year period, had lost interest in movies, felt worthless, guilty, and a burden on his family. Oddly, inertia and indecision were denied, although he did little but drink for the last 10 months. He had not spoken of suicide for 7 years. He ate nothing for the last 3 days of his life

There was no family history of alcoholism, drug abuse, or suicide. The only relative with mental illness was a paternal grandmother who was admitted to a mental hospital in her old age for an unknown condition.

On only one occasion, 7 years prior to his death, did he make any comment about suicide. At that time he told his father he would be better off dead and wanted to die. He was reported to have been discouraged over his inability to quit drinking. He never again spoke of such thoughts. There was no suicide note.

Circumstances Leading to the Act

He had always lived with his parents and was ashamed of being dependent on them. His last hospital admission for alcoholism was 7 months earlier and his drinking had increased since then. He was weak and tremulous on the day of his death and his mother suggested he go to the hospital. He said it could wait one more day. He was having auditory and visual hallucinations at the time and had not eaten for 3 days. About 8:30 p.m. his father went across the street, leaving him alone for the first time that day, returning about a half hour later. He found the subject lying unconscious on his bed with both wrists slashed with a razor blade. A postmortem blood plasma level of 4.8 mg% of imipramine (Tofranil) (an antidepressant medication) was recorded (I rechecked the records to be sure it was not mistranscribed). It indicated a massive and potentially lethal overdose. The source of the imipramine was not discovered. Two hypodermic needles were found in a bottle at the scene. There was a tourniquet on his left upper arm. Was he shooting up at the same time he was bleeding out? Toxicological analysis for narcotics was not done.

Findings and Sources

Clinical Diagnosis: (1) Alcoholism, chronic; (2) probable secondary affective disorder; DSM–III–R: major depressive disorder; (3) alcoholic dementia; (4) narcotic addiction by history.
Toxicology: Blood alcohol concentration 0.268 g%; imipramine 4.8 mg%.
Primary Informant: Father, who saw him about daily.
Other Sources of Information: Coroner's death investigation report, hospital records.
Informant's Opinion of Reason for Suicide: Inability to stop drinking and get a job.

Comment

Most of this man's adult life seems to have revolved around drugs and alcohol, but there was no evidence that he was ever involved in drug dealing. He seems to have felt ashamed of his dependency on his parents but unable to take care of himself. His failure to even try to work in the last 10 months of his life is probably attributable to depression more than alcoholism, despite the informant's inability to confirm some symptoms of depression that seem almost certain to have been present. Depression had been diagnosed and therapy instituted in the city psychiatric outpatient department five months before his death. Without evidence of an acute precipitant, I nominate depression and alcoholism as the cause of his suicide. They have been found repeatedly here to be a lethal combination. Self-disgust was prominent.

Case 28

Subject 28 was a 52-year old married white protestant male, employed as a machinist at the time of his suicide by shotgun wound. He was born in southeastern Missouri. Whether he had siblings was not learned. Both parents were schoolteachers. His father deserted the family when he was 12 years old. He had no known school, legal, or psychological problems, and he had graduated from high school. He had a teaching certificate as well, but no details were available. He was married five times, the first time just before entering the Navy during World War II. While he was on active duty his wife obtained a divorce, had a child by another man, and then remarried him for a short time after the war. His third marriage, to a woman with three small children, lasted for less than a year and ended in divorce due to the wife's infidelity, as did a fourth marriage after 8 years. He had no children of his own, and had told his last wife that he was sterile. His last marriage, 8 years before his death, was stormy until the last year, owing to his abusiveness. "He lived in his own little world—work, hunting and fishing . . ." He was secretive and talked only when he was drinking. He had one friend, a deer hunting companion whom he saw about four times a year. He had worked as a machinist for a large manufacturing firm for the last 18 years of his life.

He began drinking at age 16 and drank in progressive amounts for his entire life, with no significant periods of abstinence except while hospitalized. He drank up to a case of beer or a fifth of hard liquor daily. "He would come home at 1:00 a.m. and drink beer until 5:00 a.m." His wife and stepson objected to his drinking. He had progressive absenteeism from work due to drinking or hangover; he was demoted from a supervisory position 6 months before his suicide. He was off work for the last several weeks of his life, presumably because of medical problems.

During periods of intoxication he became angry and combative. He had had physical fights with more than one of his wives while drunk. One year before his suicide he fractured his wife's arm when drunk. She fled the house. He continued drinking, then apparently fell asleep while smoking a cigarette, setting the bed afire. His eyes were thought to have been affected, as well as his skin. He was admitted to the St. Louis County hospital for treatment of his burns, and was transferred to a Veterans Administration hospital, where he had DTs. He was then transferred to a private hospital where he presumably received some psychiatric care. No details were available. Hospitalization lasted for several months. After that, he apparently ceased abusing his wife. For unclear reasons he feared return to a public or Veterans Administration hospital and said he would die first.

He had had one previous hospital admission for alcoholism 5 years earlier, culminating in several months in a nursing home. Whether he received any specific therapy for alcoholism or for any psychiatric condition was unknown, but he "took a lot of pills," including chlorpromazine. He had had one arrest for driving while intoxicated and was jailed overnight 5 years before his death. He was defensive about his drinking and hid bottles around the house. In the early years of their marriage, he frequently went alone on 3- to 4-day binges at his hunting cabin. He never lost any friends because he never had more than the one.

His personality was described as moody, sensitive, and socially isolated. He avoided crowds. He was described as high-strung and his feelings were easily hurt when he was drunk. He cried easily. During the last 6 months of life, he developed symptoms of depression including chronic low mood, anorexia and weight loss, insomnia, fatigue, loss of interest in activities, reduced sex drive, and psychomotor retardation. He was generally uncommunicative and was morose about his chronic health problems, his vision, and his demotion at work 6 months before his suicide. He gave up reading in the last month. Prior to that, "he was always reading." His wife said he took multiple drugs regularly, "one of which was Thorazine." She did not think he was addicted to drugs.

He was wounded in the back of the neck with shrapnel in World War II. It was reportedly an accident, not combat-related. He spent 2 years in military hospitals and was honorably discharged with a partial medical disability. He was described as being chronically in poor health and preoccupied with illness during his last years. Neck pain was one of his complaints. He had respiratory problems aggravated by heavy smoking, arteriosclerosis with "heart problems," and diabetes. He had been treated 10 years earlier for bursitis, and twice for alcoholism or related medical problems. He saw his family physician for treatment of diabetes and other conditions, the last visit having been 4 days before he ended his life.

There was no family history information available, other than the father's desertion of the family when the subject was 12 years old. "He never mentioned any relatives with mental illness or alcoholism."

He remarked to his wife several years before his death that he would be better off dead. He had frequently said, "I don't think it would be any worse if I were to blow the back of my head off." He had also said, a number of times, "I just wonder what is over on the other side when we leave this world." The last 3–4 weeks of his life his depression seemed to be worse, and he spoke of suicide several times.

Circumstances Leading to the Act

His mother had a stroke 2 or 3 weeks before his death. He drove to southern Missouri to see her in the hospital. The last few weeks he would sit alone in the dark most of the night, chain smoking, with periodic trips to the refrigerator for beer. He had seen his doctor on Friday and was too weak to walk home as he usually did. He stopped a taxicab and rode home. That evening, when he got up from the couch, he fell. His wife wanted to call the doctor, but he refused, so she helped him into bed. He was ill all weekend. He drank about as usual the day before his death, and he didn't go to work. He was unable to go to work on Tuesday, the day of his death. He did not drink that day.

He had taken a shotgun from his mother's home on a recent visit. Early in the afternoon he went outside "to put it in the trunk of the car." His wife thought his reason for going out with the gun did not make much sense. Ten minutes later she heard a shot and found him slumped against the car. An ambulance was called, and on arrival at the hospital he was pronounced dead of a 20-gauge shotgun wound below the left ear at the base of the skull. His wife said he used a hand-loaded shotgun shell with a slug (solid bullet) and "blew his head open and his brains out." He did not leave a suicide note.

Findings and Sources

Clinical Diagnosis: (1) Alcoholism, chronic; (2) secondary major depressive disorder.
Toxicology: Not done—presumably sober.
Primary Informant: Spouse, married 8 years.
Other Sources of Information: Stepson, coroner's death investigation record.
Informant's Opinion of Reason for Suicide: Feared he would be taken to a state or Veteran's Administration hospital (had said he would die first).

Comment

This was a remarkably isolated man. His stepson, who had known him from work before his last marriage, said he had no enemies, but no friends either, just one hunting companion. As described by his fourth wife, he hardly spoke at all, except when drinking. Then there were fights about his drinking. He had revealed almost nothing about himself in 8 years of marriage. His wife did know about his four previous marriages, and his belief that each of these women was unfaithful. For the last year, they had slept in separate rooms. He would drink beer most of the night. The picture that emerges is of a nearly silent household, with the nights punctuated by the occasional pop of a beer can being opened.

His demotion 6 months earlier and his mother's stroke, which was thought to be quite serious, were major recent losses. His wife seemed to have no clear idea of the depth of his feelings for his mother. Isolated, depressed, brooding about his demotion and his health problems, he apparently planned his suicide, having brought the lethal weapon from his mother's home a few weeks earlier. His strength failed him a few days before he took his life; he couldn't walk home from the doctor's office or get up to go to work. The cause of this weakness is obscure. His wife thought it was important in light of his expressed fear of having to go to a public or Veterans Administration hospital. Whether the depression or this new turn of events with his health should be considered more important is conjectural. The length of the evident planning leads me to nominate the depression as primary, with his and his mother's failing health as contributory.

Case 30

Subject 30 was a 41-year old divorced occupationally disabled white male who died by barbiturate overdose. He was born in St. Louis, the fourth in a Roman Catholic family of 11 children. His father was an alcoholic, often gone from the home. When his father worked, it was as a painter or paper hanger. He was physically abusive, neglected the family, and deserted them. They lost contact with him until the last 2 years. He died of carcinoma of the larynx 1 month before the subject's suicide. This subject spent 6 years in an orphanage, from age 3 to 9, together with the siblings alive at the time. He had no interest in school and was truant a great deal, finally quitting after sixth grade.

He served 3 years in the U.S. Navy during World War II and had a number of tattoos to show for it. He was honorably discharged. He worked in the Merchant Marine after World War II, then as a crewman on a river barge, and for the next 15 years at a number of blue-collar jobs, two dozen or more, according to a brother. His last and longest employment was for 4 years as an electrician. That job was ended by a disabling arm wound 10 months before his suicide.

At age 23, he married one of five sisters who were described as "party girls," three of them as prostitutes. His wife was 15 years old at the time. The marriage was stormy, with many fights and separations. Five children were born of this union. They were ultimately sent to the wife's mother when the final separation occurred. His wife had extramarital affairs. He frequently quizzed her about her relationships with other men and accused her of infidelity. On such an occasion, 13 months before his suicide, she left him and filed for divorce. The divorce became final 3 months before his death.

He began drinking "before age 17" and is described as a heavy drinker from then on, with no significant periods of abstinence. He generally drank beer, more than a six-pack a day and sometimes a case a day, plus unknown amounts of liquor. He went on drinking binges, suffered severe alcohol withdrawal, including shakes and DTs, had gastritis and a subtotal gastrectomy for peptic ulcer disease. He fought physically and verbally with his wife and had at least one arrest for assault on two police officers while drunk. Whether his many job changes were alcohol related was not known by the informants.

His drinking increased considerably in the last year of his life, after his wife left him. Although she and his family objected to his drinking, he did not believe he had a problem and never made any attempt to control or stop it. His wife told a social worker, about a year before he died, that he had driven away all of their friends. (Considering her propensity for extramarital affairs, if that was true, it may have been protective.) He had two psychiatric hospitalizations for alcoholism and related problems, 3 years, and 6 months prior to his suicide, with no detectable improvement. He took hypnotic medication every night for the last 3 years of his life.

Although suicide threats and attempts characterized his last two hospitalizations, he never received outpatient treatment for psychiatric or alcohol problems. Three years before his death he was intoxicated and scuffled with two police officers in an apparent attempt to obtain one officer's pistol, saying he wanted to die. He had just learned his wife was having "another" affair. He spent a week in a public hospital but received no subsequent psychiatric care. He did obtain a sedative from his medical doctor and used it regularly from that time on.

Depressive symptoms were aggravated when he was intoxicated. During the last 2–3 years of his life he made several suicide attempts with barbiturates, but apparently none resulted in hospitalization. Six months before his death, while intoxicated, he became suicidal and asked to be admitted to a private hospital. He was transferred to a state mental hospital because of a radiologic finding of lung lesions compatible with tuberculosis. He was discharged after 3 months, 2 months before his death. Discharge diagnoses were "tuberculosis of lung, minimal, quiescent," and "depressive neurosis." Three maternal aunts had died of tuberculosis. What treatment he received was undisclosed.

He was described as high-strung, with easily hurt feelings. He was periodically moody, with episodic outbursts of anger. During the last year he was greatly preoccupied with his wife's departure. He was constantly sad and joyless. Depressive symptoms included anorexia, weight loss, insomnia, social withdrawal, decreased activity and marked self-depreciation, as well as suicidal ideation. He was highly pessimistic about his future, particularly regarding the vocational implications of the impending amputation of his injured left arm.

He had a duodenal ulcer, treated by subtotal gastrectomy 8 years before his suicide. He continued to have epigastric complaints and probably a postgastrectomy dumping syndrome. Ten months before ending his life, he received a rifle bullet wound through his left humerus, producing a compound fracture. According to his brother, he was with his wife at the time of the occurrence. The brother believed his wife shot him, but he had no confirmation. "He told me a different story each time." The injury left him unable to work. There must have been extensive nerve damage, as his forearm was useless. He was to undergo amputation at the elbow in one week. His only other medical complaint was of frequent headaches.

His father was a definite alcoholic. Two sisters and two brothers were heavy drinkers or alcoholics. One of these brothers was also mentally slow and was hospitalized at least once, suicidally depressed. His mother had a "nervous breakdown" when he was 8 years old, but she recovered without hospitalization. A maternal aunt was hospitalized for "involutional paranoid state," with marked depressive features, auditory hallucinosis, and unsystematized delusions. His father's death of laryngeal carcinoma, less than a month before his suicide, was not thought by informants to have been particularly significant to him.

He began episodically expressing a desire to die about 3 years before taking his life, including trying to take a police officer's pistol and several overdoses of sedatives. When told his injured arm was to be amputated, he had stated to family members that he did not want to go on living if he could not return to work. He said he would be better off dead and spoke of taking his life. That was his last known expression of suicidal thoughts.

Circumstances Leading to the Act

He was devoted to his wife, despite her rather flagrant extramarital activities and a number of separations. He wouldn't say anything bad about her. When she left him for the last time, 13 months before his suicide, she placed the children with her mother and instituted divorce proceedings. He was distraught over being deserted by her. He lived alone in the apartment, became depressed, and increased his drinking. He was admitted to a private psychiatric hospital, where a diagnosis of "reactive depression, psychotic type" was made. He was released 2 months before his death. He ate little in the last 10 months unless his mother prepared him food and encouraged him to eat. "His clothes hung on him." He told his brother he couldn't stand the idea of an amputation. He saw no point in living if he couldn't work. A week before the scheduled surgery, he told family members he was going on a fishing trip with his former boss before the operation. Five days later a neighbor checked the apartment and found the entry door nailed shut. The apartment was entered and he was found dead. Present were two empty bottles that had each originally contained thrity 100-mg. secobarbital capsules.

He left three notes, two to his mother and one to his ex-wife. The first read.

To my Mother
Dear Mom.
I am going to try to die but please don't blame [wife's name] for [what] I do for she can't help it if she doesn't love me and don't let anyone hurt her. I ask this of all of you, please. If anything try to help her in every way you can for I love that woman with all my heart.
I don't care if she is the biggest pig in the world, she is a good mother to the kids
    Please forgive me if you can't read this for I am very sleepy. don't let them put me back ware [sic] I was, if God doesn't let me die   I just can't live this type of life.
"P.S. If God won't let me die please don't let them put me back in that ward. [nickname]

The second note:
To my Mother
Dear Mom.
    I am going to try to take my life but please do not blame (wife's name) for this. I love her and my kids very much but I can't have them for she is in love with some other man. Please don't let anyone hurt in any way [sic] for if they do they will just be hurting

me. Give her any thing that she wants for what I have is hers. My heart hurts when she hurts. [nickname]

And the third note:
Dear [wife's name]
    I love you to [sic] much to keep on going so I think I will make it this time. I told mom and my brother and you that I was going away for a week so no one can stop me. May God forgive me for what I am doing but I will never be no good to you or the kids the way I am and I know they can't fix my arm and I will not live with just one arm.
    All my love. [first name]
    I am getting to [sic] sleepy to write any more.

Findings and Sources

Clinical Diagnoses: (1) Alcoholism, chronic; (2) major depression (secondary).
Toxicology: Blood alcohol concentration 0.088 g%; barbiturate 3.2 mg% (secobarbital).
Primary Informant: Mother: saw him daily for last year.
Other Sources of Information: Brother, hospital records, coroner's death investigation report.
Informant's Opinion of Reason for Suicide: Fear of amputation.

Comment

This man made an unfortunate choice of a mate. Having been deserted by his father, he might well be expected to be sensitive to desertion, actual or implied. The discovery of his wife's having "another" affair drove him to an abortive suicide attempt. He didn't go off the deep end when she would leave him after their fights, however, or when she finally left him and filed for divorce. Why he did not might be a more important question to answer than why he finally did. (Not being depressed earlier is my leading hypothesis.) He did, somehow, get himself shot, costing him the use of his left arm. Then he became depressed. Shortly after the divorce became final he was hospitalized for the depression. It was recorded as both reactive and of psychotic proportions.

It was when he was told, 3 weeks before his suicide, that amputation of his forearm was indicated that he hit the skids. One supposes that he had nourished hopes of recovery of function. It is reasonable to assume that the amputation was to be the prelude to a prosthesis. However, he took it as signaling the end of his working life. That, he said, was intolerable, and that, in the end, sealed his doom. Alcoholism, plus depression, plus loss of status as a wage earner—a lethal combination!

Case 12

Subject 12 was a 69-year old white, Roman Catholic male, born near St. Louis in Illinois. His father was a huckster and his mother a housewife. The parental home was presumably intact. If he had siblings, we did not learn of it. Likewise, the extent of his education was not known by his second wife, our informant. He first married at age 27. His wife died of cancer 19 years later. His second marriage, at age 51, lasted 17½ years until his death. He had no children. He had been a crane operator for 19 years, then a shear operator for 8 years. Six years before his death he retired because of failing eyesight and received a social security pension. His wife believed he had held only three jobs in his entire working life. His wife arranged a move from a rural area back to St. Louis 1 week before his death. He would rather have waited until fall, when their garden would have become dormant, but she was insistent. After the move, he had virtually no social life.

He started drinking heavily at the age of 18. Its impact on his first marriage is unknown. Five years before his suicide, his second wife threatened to leave him because of his drinking, but she never carried out the threat. He drank daily, regularly had "the shakes" in the morning, and drank before breakfast. While his wife and some others thought he drank too much, he did not think so, or feel guilty about it. He experienced no legal or vocational problems. He drank approximately 1½ pints of hard liquor per day. He was able to abstain from drinking for 2 months about once a year. Following his retirement, and until 7 months before his death, he and his wife managed an apartment building in North St. Louis. They then moved to a small town in Illinois in order to have more space at a lower cost and for him to have a garden. There, he developed a drinking relationship with a nephew who lived nearby. His wife's insistence on moving back to the city was to break up that relationship, his only social life.

Apart from a complaint of fatigue of 3–4 months duration, a belief that he had stomach cancer, and a 3-month history of talk of dying, there was no information to support a diagnosis of depression.

He had two surgical operations 6 years before his death. One was for the removal of cataracts from both eyes and the other for a perforated appendix. He retired from his employment at that time. He had no other hospitalizations and had not been under medical care since that time. Nor was he known ever to have had psychiatric attention. During the last few months of his life he suffered from dyspnea and fatigue. He told his nephew he thought he had cancer of the stomach. His wife knew nothing about it until after his death. Family history was not obtainable.

Three months before his suicide, he stated to both his wife and his nephew that he would be better off dead. Around the same time he told his wife that he would never be a burden on her. He had told his nephew he didn't know why he had to suffer so much. These were his only reported communications on the matter.

Circumstances Leading to the Act

The move to an apartment in St. Louis 1 week before his death had been forced by his wife to break off the drinking relationship between the subject and his nephew. On the day of his death, he rose in apparently good spirits and went through the morning without incident. He consumed approximately a half-pint of whiskey. About midday he sat talking with his wife and smoking a cigarette at the kitchen table. Without giving any indication of his immediate intentions, he got up and went to the bedroom where he took his gun from the drawer. His wife heard him release the safety mechanism and went to the bedroom. She heard the shot and found him in the act of falling. He had shot himself in the head. He was taken to the hospital and underwent brain surgery, but he never regained consciousness and died 4 weeks later. He did not leave a suicide note.

Findings and Sources

Clinical Diagnosis: Alcoholism, chronic.
Toxicology: Not performed.
Primary Informant: Wife, married 17½ years, had known subject 22 years, saw him daily.
Other Sources of Information: Coroner's death investigation report, hospital records.
Informant's Opinion of Reason for Suicide: Thought he had cancer.

Comment

This subject's belief that he had stomach cancer, communicated only to his nephew–drinking companion, is puzzling. Was it a delusion, or simply an excuse to drink? It would most easily be understood as a mood–congruent delusion of depression, but other depressive symptoms were denied by the informant. He hadn't consulted a physician about his concern. This was a rather sparsely documented interview that leaves a lot to be desired, diagnostically. His concern about cancer does appear to coincide temporally with his communications about dying, so, at a minimum, it facilitated his decision. His wife's unilateral arrangement of the move suggests a level of domination not otherwise revealed. I counted his forced separation from his nephew as loss of a close interpersonal relationship. Handicapped visually, as he was, and deprived of his garden, life may have suddenly become very unrewarding for him. At 69 years of age, that may have been sufficient reason for his suicide.

Case 26

Subject 26 was a white male, 48 years old at the time of his suicide. He was born and raised in St. Louis, one of 14 children. The family was devout Roman Catholic. His father was a shipping clerk and part-time farmer, at least a heavy drinker all his life, who died of cancer when the subject was 33 years old. His mother was also a heavy alcohol user. She never worked outside of the home, being entirely occupied with running the household and raising 14 children. He had no school problems and seems to have been an average student. He fought with his brothers but was not involved in fights outside of the family, truancy or any other behavioral or legal problems. He completed the eighth grade and 5 years of machinist training in a technical school. He was drafted into the Army in World War II, but on the induction physical examination he was found to have chronic lung damage diagnosed initially as pulmonary tuberculosis and he was discharged without any significant military service. He then worked as a machinist for an electrical equipment manufacturer for 30 years, until 5 months before his death.

He was married at age 20 to a girl of 19, and they had five children, three girls and two boys. The children ranged in age from 12 to 26 years old at the time of his death. The marriage was stormy, owing to the subject's drinking and physical abuse of his wife. She threatened separation several times but never actually left him. During the last 5 years of their marriage, she worked evenings as a waitress to supplement their diminishing income. At the time of his death, they had been married for 28 years.

Earlier in his life, he had bowled and played golf and had been a Boy Scout leader. More recently he had played cards daily with fellow workers, but that ceased when he was fired 5 months before his death. He went to church when sober until the last 5 years of his life.

He began drinking heavily as a teenager and this pattern increased throughout his life. His wife regarded him as alcoholic for at least the last 18 years of his life. However, even during the first 10 years of the marriage he had frequent binges. Subsequently he began a pattern of daily drinking, at home or in his car, in amounts of a pint or more of liquor a day, and beer binges of up to a case a day. His heavy drinking increased after his father's death 15 years prior to the suicide. During the last ten years of his employment he missed up to 50% of his work time because of drinking but was spared termination for a long time through the influence of his brother, who was a union official. Shortly before being discharged he had signed a statement of understanding that this was his last chance. Finally his absenteeism did result in his being fired, 3 months before he ended his life. To the end he was regarded as an excellent worker when he was able to work. He then held four jobs for a week or two at a time, but in each case he was fired for drinking; finally he was unable to obtain work for the last month or two of his life.

He displayed nearly all of the symptoms of alcoholism, with daily shakes on arising, morning drinking, binges, blackouts, convulsions, and delusions associated with drinking. He hid liquor, got in fights while drunk, had auto accidents, and arrests for drunken driving, public intoxication, and disturbing the peace. He had job problems and terminations due to drinking, family and marital problems, and medical problems including hepatic cirrhosis, seizures, injuries due to falls, and malnutrition. Throughout all these difficulties he did not seem to consider himself alcoholic or feel guilty about drinking. Only after hospitalizations for medical problems did he say he should quit, and his resolve did not last long. He did manage to stay sober by taking disulfiram for 6 months, about 4 years before his suicide, but he discontinued that medication so he could drink to celebrate a wedding anniversary.

His wife described him as sweet and lovable when sober. When drunk, he behaved hatefully. On a number of occasions he broke up furniture in the home. He frequently threatened and at times did physically abuse family members. Three years before his death he threatened his wife and a daughter with a knife. On several occasions when drunk he would precipitate a family fight, then call the police, claiming that other family members had started the trouble. His wife thought he enjoyed the attention. During binges he would sleep or pass out during the day, then stay up at night and annoy his wife so she could not sleep, accusing her of neglecting him by working evenings. During the last 10 years of his life he became socially withdrawn, and friends began to avoid him. They would telephone his wife to learn how he was doing, but they didn't want to see him.

He had several hospitalizatons for alcoholism and malnutrition, the last one 3 years before his death. He was usually treated with antianxiety drugs, which he generally did not take after discharge. He never participated in any prolonged outpatient treatment and was not regarded as depressed except when drinking.

His personality was described as moody, hypersensitive, and high-strung. When drunk he was sad, depressed, joyless, and tearful. He was a compulsive worrier and frequent handwasher who compulsively checked locks and the gas stove. He did not abuse prescription drugs. Despite his being described as "depressed" after loss of his lifetime job, his wife could not cite symptoms that would justify a diagnosis of depressive disorder. Unquestionably, he was dysphoric during that time.

He had chronic bronchitis and shortness of breath during most of his adult life, probably due to pneumoconiosis secondary to occupational exposure to abrasive dust. (A military physician had originally diagnosed this condition as pulmonary tuberculosis.) He used cough syrup "by the bottle" according to his wife. She did not know what kind of cough syrup it was. He was reported to have been hospitalized about once a year during the last 10 years of his life for this condition. Hospital records we obtained suggest that may have been somewhat exaggerated. His medical condition was greatly aggravated by alcoholism, and he had hepatic cirrhosis. He had had a hemorrhoidectomy within the last 8 years.

Both of his parents were heavy drinkers and probably alcoholic. His mother was still drinking heavily on a daily basis at age 85 when he ended his life. "She used to laugh about having to drag him up the steps to bed when he was a teenager." He had 2 brothers and 3 sisters who were alcoholic. One brother burned down his own house and was described as a "homicidal maniac" by another family member. That brother had spent the last 15 years in a mental institution with an alcoholic dementia and seizure disorder. Two brothers were jailed, one for 3 years for a kidnapping threat and another for 1 ½ years for tire theft. His next younger sister stopped drinking after almost killing herself in an automobile accident. Family history of suicide and of suicide attempt were denied.

He first mentioned suicide to his wife 5 years before his demise, when he held a gun to this head while drunk. He spoke of suicide a year before his death, again when he was fired, 5 months before taking his life, and frequently thereafter. After being fired he expressed hopelessness. Three weeks before the end he told his priest he was considering suicide. He described the method he intended to use and said that both he and his family would be better off if he were dead. The priest did not mention any of this to his wife until the day after his death. During his last year he looked depressed, was disgusted with himself and the world, and was very angry when drunk.

Circumstances Leading to the Act

He was relatively sober on Thanksgiving Day, 3 days before his suicide. The next day he was drinking and told his wife he was going to withdraw all the money in their joint bank account. She prevented that by calling the bank and he obtained only $50, part of which he used to buy two bottles of liquor. He went to his son-in-law's service station, where his daughter offered to give him a ride home. When they got to the house he refused to get out of the car, so she proceeded toward the bank to deposit the day's receipts. He started hitting her and she stopped the car. A passing motorist came to her aid. The police were called and he was jailed overnight.

The next day he returned home sober. His wife told him to take the checkbook, pack his bags, and get out. According to the police investigation, she told him she was filing for divorce and telephoned an attorney. She had threatened divorce several times before but had never initiated action. She told the interviewer in this investigation that she called the attorney to arrange for the subject's commitment for alcoholism treatment. She thought he must have believed she was starting divorce proceedings, as I do.

He retrieved the liquor he had purchased the previous day and drank an entire bottle of it that morning, as he was packing his belongings. Later in the day his wife heard a gunshot and went into the bedroom. He said, "Get out of here and leave me alone." Then he said, "Goodbye, Dot," as she left the room. Shortly thereafter she heard a second shot. She returned to find him lying on the bed, snoring, but apparently uninjured. Only some time later did her son-in-law discover that he had shot himself in the right temple, the wound having been obscured by the position of his head. He was taken to a hospital where he died 7 hours after inflicting the fatal wound with a .22-caliber single shot firearm he had owned since he was 16 years old. His wife was surprised that there was still a gun in the house, as the police had removed both firearms and ammunition in the aftermath of an earlier family fracas. There was no suicide note.

Findings and Sources

Clinical Diagnosis: Alcoholism, chronic.
Toxicology: Not performed.
Primary Informant: Wife, married to him for 28 years; had known him 30 years; saw him daily.
Other Sources of Information: Daughter, hospital records, coroner's death investigation records.
Informant's Opinion of Reason for Suicide: He thought his wife was going to divorce him.

Comment

This man was born into a family in which alcohol was a way of life. Described as "lovable" when sober, his behavior turned ugly in his later years, when he drank. He harassed the family senselessly, seeming to take delight in making them uncomfortable. Coming from a sibship of 14, he may well have had concerns about lack of attention. He frequently accused his wife of neglecting him. Because of his behavior when drinking, he had driven away all of his friends. He had not only blown a good job after 30 years, he hadn't been able to keep any of several others, again owing to his drinking. He had been jailed less than 24 hours before his suicide for assaulting his daughter. His wife told him to pack and clear out, that she was going to get a divorce. While he was packing, she telephoned an attorney. It was then that he shot himself. Whether divorce or commitment, he was about to lose either his family or his freedom.

It may be that he wasn't depressed. His wife denied that he had the symptoms. He had certainly exhausted his options, short of "taking the pledge." What he had in mind in trying to withdraw all of the family's savings is a mystery. Since an actual separation had not occurred, this case was not included among those with recent loss of a close interpersonal relationship. The threat was as influential as an actual separation could have been.

Case 27

Subect 27 was a 42-year old Native American (Kodiak Indian) male, separated at the time of his death. He was born in Alaska and his mother, who had tuberculosis, died in childbirth. He had 2 older siblings, one of each sex. His father was a fisherman, "an alcoholic all his life" who died when the subject was 12 years old. He spent the next 6 years in an orphanage. He completed the eighth grade, without conduct or legal problems, but was "picked on" by other children. (He was physically small as an adult—probably also as a child.) He joined the Navy at age 18, during World War II, and served as a cook on shipboard in the Pacific. There were no problems other than heavy drinking during his military service and he was honorably discharged. He was an unskilled laborer and worked at construction jobs most of his life. During the last 10 years he held four jobs, leaving each because of inadequate pay or no work to do. He had been on his most recent job as a hod carrier for about 2 years at the time of his death, and he was earning the most money he ever had.

He married, at age 28, a woman he had known for 3 years. About 6 weeks prior to his suicide she left him after a beating, believing that he actually might kill her. She moved in with a mutual friend and was living with that man at the time of her husband's suicide. The couple had no children and few social contacts. His principal social life was in neighborhood bars. During his separation he had a few casual sexual contacts with women but no serious relationship. "He was dating seven women at one time. They all came to the funeral."

He was a heavy daily drinker, at least from age 18 on, with an increase during the last five years. He was not a binge drinker, but had a daily intake that reached two cases of beer a day. His only abstinent period was for 1 year at age 26, about the time he came to "the lower 48," and shortly after he first became acquainted with his wife. He suffered DTs and had medical problems that were not known in detail but that seemed to be aggravated by his drinking. He was frequently beaten and robbed while drunk. A year before he died he was hospitalized briefly for treatment of injuries sustained in that way.

Why it happened so often was unclear. His employer described him as "the nicest possible person," well liked by his co-workers, always smiling, very polite, and never causing trouble. He was a small man, "about 5'5" and 110 lbs." and quite dark skinned. He always felt inferior, and perhaps had an air of vulnerability about him, as he did have a history of being "picked on" in school. He did not have trouble with employment or the law as a consequence of his drinking. In fact, his last employer described him as a good worker, utterly dependable. It was his dependability that led to his body being discovered. The second day he failed to show up for work, his employer went to his apartment house looking for him.

His family and friends thought he drank excessively, but he did not seem to regard his drinking as a problem. The major difficulty related to drinking was his "crazy" assaultive behavior directed at his wife during the last 5 years of their 14-year marriage. His employer, a generous man, thought she was consistently unfaithful to him. She did not report that. She said that he frequently threatened and assaulted her while drunk. In the last year, on one occasion, he tried to hold her head in a gas oven. Another time he stabbed her. Once, in a drunken rage, he tried to suffocate her by obstructing her nose with "Vicks" salve.

He was never treated by a psychiatrist but was described as depressed for the last 5 years of his life. His personality was high-strung, sensitive, with outbursts of rage and crying spells. During the last year of his life he had fatigue, anorexia and weight loss, as well as self-reproach and feelings of worthlessness. He looked depressed, was sad and hopeless, with thoughts of suicide. He meets criteria for *probable* depression (DSM-III-R definite).

About 5 years before his suicide, he had been hospitalized for almost a year in a public hospital, but the details were not learned. Subsequently, he believed he had a serious, probably terminal illness and had told his wife that he had leukemia. He complained of nausea, stomach pain, chest pain, dyspnea, headache, dizziness, bladder trouble, and kidney trouble, but he had no consistent medical treatment. His wife knew of no medical confirmation of his somatic concerns. His only other hospitalization was after being beaten up by strangers a year before his death.

His father was alcoholic. His sister was said to have had a "nervous breakdown." Suicide or attempt in the family was denied.

Over the last five years of his life, when drunk, he would say to his wife that he wanted and expected to die. He spoke also of suicide from time to time. Two years before his death he made an attempt by hanging with a rope over the bathroom transom, and again 13 months before his suicide by putting his head in the gas oven. During the last few months, "He told me several times that he saw a little man sitting on the end of the bed, telling him that he was going to die before long." He said to his wife, "You would be better off if I were dead." Four months before his death he said, "I won't be here for my birthday." (He died 1 month before his birthday.) Just before the separation he said: "We might as well go together." He is said to have indicated his suicidal intention to his landlord as well, a short time before his death. He left two suicide notes, one to his wife and the other to friends at the tavern he frequented.

Circumstances Leading to the Act

Four to 6 weeks before his suicide, he beat his wife while drunk and told her to leave. She decided she had better do so, out of fear for her safety. Thereafter he was living alone. His daily drinking continued or increased, his depression progressed, and his physical ailments, whatever they were, caused him distress, but he continued to work daily. He was noted to be brooding over the loss of his wife. A day or two before his death he was beaten and robbed again. While alone in his apartment he hanged himself with a clothesline from the transom of the apartment door. His suicide note to his wife bespeaks his agony in that ambivalent relationship.

As a footnote to this narrative, his employer attended the funeral. He noted that the widow wept and cried copiously throughout. At the end of the ceremony, she dried her eyes and asked him, "Did I do all right?" She was living with another man from the day he threw her out.

Suicide note 1:   June 25, 1968
Dearest M_____

I guess you know what day this is! Number 13. I was hoping you would come around, but I guess my hopes were in vain. I love you very much honey although at times you wouldn't think so. I've been living in a world of hell since you've been gone, and I can't see any future in it. I just wish I knew where sis and Jr. were so I could say goodbye to them. When your [sic] receive this I will be resting in a world of peace and happiness. (Please don't blame yourself for this.) And live a good life. I want you to be happy, something that is not possible for me without you. Always remember that I love you honey and take care of yourself. I'll be thinking of you honey when I'm going. Time is growing short so I will say Goodbye darling. With all my love. Your loving husband. [nickname] I'm sorry!!

Note 2, written to bar acquaintances: 6/25/68 To J _____, M _____, H _____, & H _____ You have all made the past few Fridays and Saturday nights, nights that cannot be forgotten. Also G _____, P _____, B _____ and others that I've met. You're all (Wonderful people) H _____ tell F _____ I'm sorry we couldn't make that fishing trip. H _____ you've been a wonderful friend. Without your music and singing I don't think I'd have lasted this long. But I think it is time for me to go. You've been wonderful.

So to all of my friends there I will say goodbye & think of me, once in a while, B _____. As ever [full name].

Findings and Sources

Clinical Diagnoses: (1) Alcoholism, chronic; (2) probable secondary depression (DSM-III-R definite).
Toxicology: Not performed
Primary Informant: Spouse; known subject 17 years, married to him 14 years. (The interviewer commented that she seemed not very bright or observant.)
Other Sources of Information: Friend with whom widow had been living; employer; coroner's death investigation report.
Informant's Opinion of Reason for Suicide: "Not in his right mind or maybe down in the dumps."

Comment

Although this obviously tortured soul was a likeable, conscientious man, he nevertheless seemed to invite abuse. Not only was he repeatedly beaten and robbed when drunk, his wife was, in all likelihood, cheating on him. He seemed devoted to her and greatly troubled by her behavior. He abused her when he was drinking. He had had suicide on his mind for about 5 years—since a 1-year hospitalizaton about which his wife could give us no details. He reportedly thought he had leukemia, and he had a lot of physical complaints for which he didn't seek medical care. Probably a greater proximal impact was the domestic strife that resulted in marital separation 4–6 weeks before he took his life. In addition, he was depressed, meeting (on minimal information) criteria for probable major depressive disorder. His suicide note to his wife tells the tale. He was unwilling to go on living without her. The impact of his "recent loss of a close interpersonal relationship" is quite evident.

Case 29

Subject 29 was a 46-year-old married employed white male of no professed religion, whose life ended with a self-inflicted gunshot wound of the chest. The informant in this case was his brother-in-law, who had known him for just over 2 years but had lived with him for the first year. He probably had substantial biographical information from his wife, the subject's sister. (We didn't try to interview her because she was reportedly having a bad time with cancer.)

Their father, an alcoholic of unknown occupation, committed suicide by hanging when the subject was 6 years old. He lived with his grandmother for a year, then returned to his mother, who remarried. He had two full sisters and one half-brother. His mother worked as a nurse's aide. He had no known school, legal, or social problems, but he dropped out of school after tenth grade to help support the family. He enlisted in the Marine Corps at about age 19 and served for 3 years during World War II. He received a head injury in combat, for which he was hospitalized. While there, he was treated for "psychoneurosis" as well. He was decorated for combat, but whether with more than the Purple Heart is unknown. He was given a medical discharge (honorable) with partial disability and returned to his place of origin, where he married at age 22.

The marriage was stormy due to heavy drinking by both parties. His wife was given to taunting him. She reportedly would call him from a tavern to say she was drunk and having a good time with someone. He divorced her but continued to live with her. At age 24, when both had been drinking, he shot and killed her. He then attempted to kill himself by shooting himself in the chest, but he survived. He was tried and convicted of first-degree murder and sentenced to life imprisonment in the state where he grew up. In prison, he was initially irritable and rebellious. He drank and used stimulant drugs, and twice attempted suicide by sedative overdose. After a year or so he became "a model prisoner" although continuing amphetamine use for the next 8 years. He worked as chauffeur for the governor for an unknown length of time, living in the governor's mansion. He was paroled after 19 years, at age 43.

Upon leaving prison he lived with his mother for two months. He apparently resumed drinking almost at once, usually a fifth of liquor daily, occasionally up to two fifths plus a case of beer. His parole officer objected to the amount he drank, so he left the state and came to St. Louis to live with his sister and her husband. While there, he drank heavily and refused to seek employment. When out of money for alcohol he sold his blood in order to buy more. After a year, they threw him out. He soon married again, at age 45. He was living with his wife and her 7-year-old daughter at the time of his death. This second marriage, like the first, was badly affected by his drinking and related problems. Under family pressure he had obtained a job with a fence company where he worked off and on for 6 months until he was fired for frequent intoxication. His last job was with a furniture company, lasting a year until his death.

He had his first drink and his first episode of intoxication at age 16. By the time he entered the Marine Corps 3 years later he had a serious drinking problem. He went AWOL because of drinking, but escaped disciplinary action. Symptoms of alcoholism included morning drinking, inability to stop, blackouts, binges, DTs, drunk driving arrest, job problems, marital problems, acute medical problems, severe withdrawal reactions, and uxoricide committed while drunk, followed by a serious suicide attempt. He was not a sociable person and had no friends to lose. He seldom went out, but drank at home. Just a year before his death he was admitted to the St. Louis City Hospital with hematemesis and was subsequently transferred to the Veterans Administration Hospital with diagnoses of chronic alcoholism, alcoholic gastritis with hematemesis, and anemia secondary to blood loss. At that time, he was taking approximately eight aspirin tablets a day. The anticoagulant properties of aspirin no doubt contributed to the bleeding.

Following treatment for alcoholism at the Veterans Administration Hospital, he took disulfiram and was abstinent for 9 months. Then his stepfather, to whom he was close, died and he resumed drinking for the last 3 months of his life. He was last admitted to the city psychiatric hospital 7 weeks before his death, was treated for DTs, and was discharged 3 weeks later. He kept one followup appointment, missed a second one, and killed himself on the day of his next one. He had not been to work in 10 days, and was drinking continuously. His wife reported to the coroner's death investigator that he had been despondent for 2 weeks. (She was not available for our interview, having left the state.)

He was described as angry, resentful, high-strung, moody, sensitive, and easily moved to tears, chronically sad and indecisive. He shunned crowds. Depressive symptoms worsened after his stepfather's death. These included anorexia and weight loss, occasional insomnia, feelings of guilt and worthlessness, recurrent thoughts of death and suicide, and worsening of his chronic low mood. Other depressive symptoms may have been present as well. The informant simply didn't know.

He had recurrent headaches subsequent to his World War II head injury. They became worse in the last 2 years. He had been hospitalized for treatment of a gunshot wound of the chest following his first suicide attempt, at age 24. No other health problems were identified.

In addition to his father, who was alcoholic and a suicide at age 28, he had one sister who was alcoholic or a problem drinker. She was said to be nervous and moody, but was never hospitalized. The other sister had recurrent depression treated by medication and eventually by electroconvulsive therapy. She was suicidal and the electrotherapy was at her husband's insistence after she had asked him for a gun. His half-brother was described as nervous and spoiled by his mother. A paternal uncle had a "nervous breakdown" and may have committed suicide.

Frequently, when drunk, he spoke to anyone who was with him of committing suicide, of being better off dead, and of a desire to die. He had stated he was a burden to others. In addition to his suicide attempt after killing his wife, he made two suicide attempts while in prison, at least one by overdose.

Circumstances Leading to the Act

When he resumed drinking after his stepfather's death, 4 months before his own, this subject purchased a shotgun from his father-in-law. He had been drinking heavily and was unable to go to work for more than a week. On the night of his suicide he drank about a half-pint of whiskey and went to bed. He woke his wife at 3:00 a.m. complaining of pain in his chest and stomach. As he had done the previous night, he said he wanted to commit suicide and demanded that his wife give him his shotgun. She gave him the gun, without ammunition. He said, "You think you're so damn smart hiding the shells, but I've been saving these for 2 weeks. Now take the kid and get out." She took her daughter and went to a neighbor's home. A short time later he shot himself in the chest as in his attempt 21 years earlier; this time with immediately fatal result. He had been out of prison for only 3 years since the age of 24. There was no suicide note.

Findings and Sources

Clinical Diagnosis: (1) Alcoholism, chronic; (2) probable dysthymic disorder; (3) major depression a strong possibility.
Toxicology: Blood alcohol concentration 0.16 g%.
Primary Informant: Brother-in-law, had known the subject 2 years; saw him monthly in the last year.
Other Sources of Information: Medical records, wife's report to coroner's death investigator.
Informant's Opinion of Reason for Suicide: He feared having to return to the hospital.

Comment

With an alcoholic father who committed suicide at age 28 and an uncle with a "nervous breakdown," whose death was thought possibly a suicide, this subject had inauspicious antecedents. He somehow avoided school problems—perhaps because he had not started to drink until he left school at age 16. He might yet have avoided some of life's pitfalls, but he had the bad fortune to marry a woman who, herself, drank too much and provoked him sorely. He shot and killed her. It was his only known expression of violence until his suicide. Whether it was the structure provided by prison or the difficulty in obtaining alcohol it imposed, he became a model prisoner after a year of rebellion. Living in the governor's house, he surely could have obtained alcohol, so I favor the status of being a prisoner as the crucial factor. When he was paroled, he promptly recidivated.

Most depressive symptoms were denied by his brother-in-law, who may not have known, as he saw this very private person only monthly. The flavor, but not the known symptoms, argues for a major depression. Both the informant and the subject's wife reported him "despondent" after his stepfather's death. The fact that he did not go to work for the last 10 days of his life tends to support that opinion. His purchase of a shotgun shortly after his stepfather's death further supports the connection of that loss to the suicide. His relationship to his wife was not determined, but he had no other friends. Her passively handing him the shotgun and leaving without calling the police suggests that he may have worn out his welcome. The loss of his stepfather was the key factor in this suicide, as it destabilized him. That had occurred 4 months earlier and is thus not scorable under the recent loss category.

Case 34

Subject 34 was a white, married male of no professed religion. He was 45 years old at the time of his death by carbon monoxide poisoning. He was born in Illinois but had lived in the St. Louis area for 15 years. The parental home was intact. If there were siblings, it was not recorded. His father was in the insurance business and owned the home which the subject rented from him. After completing 2 years of college, he, too, went into the insurance business. He served overseas in the Army during World War II, from 1941 to 1945, and received an honorable discharge. He worked in the insurance business for 20 years, reaching the position of vice president of his company. He then went into a partnership in an investment company and had a financially disastrous episode with a real estate development. There was evidence of financial misdealings, but it was unclear whether he was a co-conspirator or an innocent victim. His last work was in his own investment company, which he formed 2 years before his death. At that time, lawsuits from the real estate fiasco and federal action concerning past income taxes were subjecting him to severe financial pressures. There is no direct evidence of drinking-related job problems, but he was drinking heavily while trying to conduct business matters.

He married soon after returning from military to civilian life. His first wife, a physician, objected to his drinking and abusiveness, and they were divorced after 7 years. He promptly remarried and that, too, was a stormy marriage due to drinking and fights. It, likewise, ended in divorce after 7 years, with mutual allegations of infidelity. (A hospital record of that time relates that his wife had left him for another man.) He was married a third time, to a woman described as a former prostitute and friend of gangsters. She ran around openly with other men. This marriage, in its sixth year, was about to end at the time of his suicide.

He had two sons from his first marriage, one of whom died of aplastic anemia at age 8. The other was 19 at the time of his death. A third son, from his second marriage, was then 12 years old. He was living with his third wife and her 16-year-old son when he died. He was reported to have entertained friends at home and to have gone with his wife or girlfriend to bars. The informant, his second ex-wife, didn't know whether that was still his pattern in the weeks before his death.

He was a problem drinker since his Army days, about age 20, and had a heavy daily alcohol intake for the last 4 years of his life. He knew he drank too much and was unable to stop. He felt guilty about his drinking, and particularly about causing the death of a young woman in an automobile accident while he was drunk, 15 years prior to his suicide. He had no other police trouble related to alcohol. His three marriages were adversely affected by his drinking. He was described as "abusive," but whether that extended beyond the verbal level was unclear. He drank before breakfast to relieve the shakes and had had withdrawal seizures and DTs as well. Concern about serious business problems, debts and back tax problems aggravated his drinking. Whether they were to some extent a result of drinking as well was not determined. He reportedly just sat in his office and drank for the last year or more. He seemed to have difficulty in conversation and trouble with recall during that time. He had been a regular user of sedatives for 8–9 years. There is no indication that he ever had a significant period of sobriety.

He was described as being chronically depressed, high-strung, moody and sensitive, easily hurt and moved to tears. Upon separation from his second wife he took an overdose of sedative medication in a suicide attempt and was hospitalized for medical treatment. A highly competent psychiatrist diagnosed depressive disorder, but he refused psychiatric treatment for either alcoholism or depression. Everyone, from his internist to his ex-wife, said he was depressed (or despondent) during the last year of his life. Constant low mood, guilt, and impaired memory and concentration, and weight loss are described. His nightly use of hypnotics documents insomnia. He had recurrent thoughts of suicide.

He was under medical care for diabetes and told his ex-wife in a letter that he had heart trouble. He had a medical and neurological hospitalization after two seizures which occurred 2 years before his suicide, while vacationing in Mexico. These were probably alcohol withdrawal seizures. His increasing daily drinking and depression caused concern about malnutrition. His hypnotic medication was prescribed by his family physician; he did not abuse it.

There was no family history of alcoholism, drug abuse, mental illness, or suicide. He made a suicide attempt 7 years earlier, after his second wife left him. He told her that someday he would kill himself. There was no other suicidal communication or attempt.

Circumstances Leading to the Act

He was drinking more heavily and was more depressed in the last year of his life. His secretary died of cancer about 8 months before his suicide and a close friend from cancer 4 months later. He had sustained heavy financial losses, was involved in major lawsuits, and was under unspecified pressure from the IRS over unpaid back taxes. He spent too much money and couldn't seem to stop it. He hadn't been taking his meals at home for some time, but spent $1200 a month at one of the city's more expensive restaurants. A month before his suicide his wife told him she would divorce him when school was out.

On the day of his death he and his wife returned home from a party and retired at 2:00 a.m. He got up, allegedly without waking his wife, went to the garage, attached a hose to the exhaust pipe of his automobile, started the engine, and sat in the car. He was wearing a terrycloth bath "sarong" and thongs. His wife said she awakened around 7:00 a.m. and found him there. She reported that she shut off the ignition, then, upon reentering the house, fainted and struck her head. An hour later, presumably when she revived, she called the police. He was pronounced dead of asphyxiation from carbon monoxide. It is of note that the second ex-wife, a police detective, and the subject's father believed the death was a homicide, but no charges were ever filed.

A note was given to the police by his wife. She said she found it on the kitchen table. It read approximately as follows: "My darling [or dearest], I am sorry, please forgive me." The informant said it was an old note, but how she knew that isn't recorded.

Findings and Sources

Clinical Diagnosis: (1) Alcoholism; (2) secondary affective disorder; (3) possible early alcoholic dementia.
Toxicology: Carbon monoxide saturation 85%; blood alcohol concentration, 0.36 g%.
Primary Informant: Second ex-wife; she saw him about once in 6 months.

Other Sources of Information: Police investigation report; coroner's death investigation report, hospital records.

Informant's Opinion of Reasons for Suicide: (1) Health bad; (2) Drinking; (3) Financial trouble; (4) Marital discord. (She also suspected the wife of homicide.)

Comment

It is not unusual for informants to be reluctant to accept suicide as the cause of death, even in the presence of overwhelming evidence. There is a suspicious element in this case, however. The victim's current wife reported that she discovered him in the car with the engine running, turned off the ignition, then fainted, striking her head and recovering an hour later to report it. The police report says the automobile engine was "very hot" when they arrived, which it should not have been if it had been off for an hour on a May morning. He was *very* intoxicated. I am not inclined to think he was led or carried to the automobile. Rather, I think it likely that his wife, discovering a suicide in progress, decided to be sure it ran its course. Why she would bother to report a time interval from discovery to reporting is not easy to explain under either theory—truth or guilt.

This subject had plenty to be upset about: major financial trouble and possibly major legal trouble as well. He was definitely depressed, his drinking was entirely out of control, and his wife had been threatening divorce for a month. He didn't handle that sort of thing well, as evidenced by a suicide attempt when his second wife left him. On balance, I nominate depression ahead of his financial/legal and marital troubles.

Case 24

Subject 24 was 37 years old, separated from his wife after 12 years of marriage and living alone at the time of his death. He was born in Chicago, into a middle-class Methodist home. He had a brother, 3 years his senior. His father was described as having manic episodes. After 40 years of marriage he abandoned the family, left the city, and was remarried 4 months later. He was again divorced after 7 years. The subject was 31 years old at the time his father left his mother. She died of a brain tumor 1 year later.

Nothing was learned of his childhood and youth, except that he accidentally set fire to a vacant lot at age 10 years. He saw combat in Korea during 2 years of service in the Army and was honorably discharged. He then entered a midwestern university, where his studies were interrupted by a major depressive illness. At age 25 he married a schoolteacher and they had two children, a daughter age 11 and a son age 9 at the time of his death. He attended and graduated from a university outside the United States. After graduation, he worked as a sales manager and troubleshooter for a large firm for three years. A dispute over his expense account led to a demotion, and he resigned. He next worked as a troubleshooter for a machinery manufacturing company for 6 years. He was fired as a result of a manic episode at the time of his move to St. Louis, 3 years before his suicide. He worked as a stockbroker for the last 3 years of his life. His income was higher than ever before, despite the increasing severity of his drinking problem. His social life was confined to bars or taverns for the last 6 months.

He began heavy drinking when he was in the Army in Korea (age 19–20), in association with a depressive episode. He had subsequent periods of both mania and depression. When manic, his alcohol tolerance was low and he was said to be unable to "hold" more than two drinks. During the last 4 months of his life, he was drinking more heavily than ever before, up to a case of beer or a pint of liquor daily.

One year before his death, he became intoxicated at an office party and while driving home he struck another auto head-on, then left the scene and "slept it off" on a side road over a mile away. He was arrested the following night and was sued by the other driver. The case was still in litigation at the time of his death.

Further symptoms of alcoholism included objections of family and friends, loss of friends, and fighting associated with drinking. He was threatening and physically assaultive to his wife when intoxicated. He never had counseling or treatment for alcoholism, nor did he attend Alcoholics Anonymous. He used sedatives for chronic insomnia during the last 3 years but was not known to abuse drugs.

His first depression occurred at age 19 while he was on active duty in the U.S. Army in Korea. In the course of it he began heavy drinking. He suffered another depressive episode at age 22 as a university student. At age 32 he had a full-blown manic episode, his first, accompanied by an alcoholic binge. His mania, apparently untreated, was followed by a depression. He was described by his wife as having marked mood swings. When depressed he was easily fatigued, cried easily, and was even more sensitive and easily hurt than usual. At these times he showed almost all of the vegetative symptoms of depression, including anorexia and weight loss, insomnia, social withdrawal, indecision, decreased energy and concentration, psychomotor retardation, and anhedonia. When manic, he was high-strung, had temper outbursts, wore brightly colored clothing, made rude remarks, and was hypersexual. After a manic episode he felt sinful or "dirty."

At 35, he and his family moved a great distance to the St. Louis area. Drinking the entire week of his move, he left all of the work to his wife. He climaxed that binge on a business trip with his boss, by appearing nearly nude and waving a pistol in the motel where he was staying, claiming that his wallet had been stolen. A local physician declined to treat him, being of the opinion that he was merely drunk. He was then brought by the police to a psychiatric hospital in the vicinity of St. Louis where he was seen for the first time by a psychiatrist and hospitalized for about 3 months. The psychiatrist diagnosed schizophrenic reaction, paranoid type, and alcoholism, while recording symptoms that would have led any user of modern diagnostic criteria to recognize bipolar affective disorder. He was treated with chlordiazepoxide (Librium) and chlorpromazine (Thorazine), and followed on an outpatient basis in a sporadic manner.

He had one 3-day hospitalization 4 months before his suicide, after his wife left him. On that occasion, the same psychiatrist rendered a diagnosis of "anxiety reaction." His last contact with his psychiatrist was about 6 weeks before his death, but only to leave a message. He saw a general practitioner for the first time 1 week before his suicide to obtain a sedative. Without recording a clinical history, the physician gave him a prescription he reported to me as pentobarbital (Nembutal) 100 mg, 10 capsules. The pharmacy's record showed a prescription for 50 such capsules, filled in that amount.

He was very self-centered, looked down on others, and was chronically worried about being poor. He was fearful of heights and frequently rechecked the house after leaving to be sure the door was locked, but these behaviors did not disrupt his life. A "drinking buddy" died suddenly while jogging several months before the subject's death and this upset him. He avoided all discussion of deaths of friends. During the year before his death he was chronically depressed, blamed himself for his marital and other problems, was angry and frustrated, and felt worthless, burdensome, and neglected. He accused his wife of running out on him when he needed her most. He does not appear to have had a personality disorder not explainable by his bipolar affective disorder.

He had amebic dysentery at age 25, but no other serious illness. Numerous physical complaints included chest pain and pain in the left arm for about the last 2 years of his life. He was said to be on a "health kick" with exercise and health foods. His only medical hospitalization was 5 years before his death for a "checkup," with no significant findings reported.

His father was described as having manic episodes but probably never received treatment. His paternal grandfather was alcoholic until age 45 when he married an 18-year-old Salvation Army worker and was "saved." His mother is reported to have had a nervous breakdown, but details were unknown to the informant. A paternal uncle had mood swings similar to his. His brother had an alcohol problem and behavior similar to his. This brother had four children, three of them boys with reading problems. Two of these boys were "drug addicts by age 16." The third was in a residential treatment center, "bright but wild." Family history of suicide and suicide attempt were denied.

His first expression of suicidal intent was to his wife at the end of a depressive episode 5 years before he took his life. He had placed a "suicide rider" on his life insurance policy 5 years earlier. He sometimes said that he would be better off dead, and that the family would also be better off in that event. Two years before his suicide he stated that he would kill himself rather than be hospitalized again. During the last 2 months of his life he frequently expressed the perception of "no hope" for the future and feeling that he was a burden to the family.

Circumstances Leading to the Act

He became jealous of his wife while she was away for 6 weeks at a summer teaching seminar, telephoning her late at night and early in the morning to check her whereabouts. He also threatened her on the phone. She suggested he see his psychiatrist, and he did spend one weekend in the hospital. After she returned home he told her he had had an extramarital affair while she was away. He subsequently alternated threats to her with protestations of love, all of the while drinking daily in large amounts.

His 10-year-old daughter was so frightened by his behavior that she remained in her room night and day to be able to call for help if needed. One day he twisted his wife's arm and threw a kitchen knife at her. His daughter locked herself in her room. He demanded that she come out, and when she did, he beat her. He then took some pills and passed out. (Was this a suicide attempt?) His wife took their two children and fled to a friend's home. The following day, 2 ½ months before his death, she left him and consulted an attorney. Two weeks later, she began divorce proceedings. Although she saw him weekly during the separation, he did not learn of the divorce action until papers were served on him 3–4 weeks before he took his life.

She offered him "nearly everything," but he would agree to nothing. They saw each other for the last time about a week before his death, when he visited her and was visibly shaken at the sight of a well-settled apartment. Their last telephone conversation was the next day, when he said he was in financial trouble. His assets had been frozen as a part of the divorce action. He asked for some frozen assets to be released, and she agreed, but her attorney refused. When she had not heard from him for several days she asked a neighbor to check the garage to determine if his car was there. Hearing that it was, she went to their home and found him dead in it. The ignition was on and the car had run out of fuel. Time of death was not determined, but he had last been in contact with his wife four days earlier. There was no suicide note.

Findings and Sources

Clinical Diagnoses: (1) Bipolar affective disorder. (2) alcoholism (secondary).
Toxicology: Not performed. No blood obtainable.
Primary Informant: Wife, married 12 years, had known him 13 years: saw him weekly in the last 2 ½ months.
Other Sources of Information: Psychiatrist, family physician (one visit only); coroner's death investigation report.
Informant's Opinion of Reason for Suicide: "The straw that broke the camel's back was my leaving him."

Comment

This man's wife stated that he became depressed after she left him, more so after he visited her in her well-settled apartment. There can be no question that he had bipolar affective disorder, with at least three hypomanic episodes and as many or more depressed episodes. It was in a hypomanic state that he abused and frightened his wife and drove her away. His alcohol abuse was not only secondary to his bipolar disorder in onset, but most of the negative consequences of his drinking were linked to mood swings. One seemed to feed the other.

I think his wife was correct in her assessment that the cause of his suicide was the fact of her leaving him. But that alone had not been enough. He became, as she said, depressed. Moreover, he was caught in a financial bind that neither he nor she could solve, and he was a man who worried a lot about lack of money. The combination of circumstances was overwhelming. Based on my study of other alcoholic suicides, the first two could have been sufficient, but the last event was the information that he could not get access to any of his money. His being served with divorce papers some 3–4 weeks before his suicide qualified him for inclusion in the threatened loss group, as the divorce had not yet occurred. As I see it, the visit to his wife's apartment a week before his suicide might have been enough. News that he couldn't get any money finalized it for him.

Case 9

Subject 9 was a 48-year old white twice-married male Protestant, born in a small town near St. Louis. He was thought not to have had siblings. His father, a laborer in the construction industry, was a heavy drinker but without known complicating problems. His mother died when he was 6 months old and he was raised by his grandmother and an aunt until adulthood. He either reached or completed the ninth grade. He was in military service between 1941 and 1945, served overseas in the Pacific arena, and received an honorable discharge. Subsequent to his military service, he had three jobs during his working life. He had worked for the last 21 years as a beer bottler and for the same employer for the last 18 years. He was first married at 31 and divorced at 38 because of his drinking and physical abuse. There was one child from this union, a son who was 19 years old at the time of his father's suicide. Three years later he married his second wife, 10 years his senior and previously married and divorced. He had known her for 17 years, having met her when she was a barmaid. He was physically abusive to her also when he was drinking heavily and struck her frequently during the earlier years of their marriage. He had ceased to do this in later years as she had fallen into poor health. His first wife lived a block away and he visited her when he got into arguments with his current wife. He had one close friend and his main social life occurred in bars or taverns. He was described as high-strung and moody. His feelings were hurt easily and he was given to outbursts of rage.

He was reported to have begun his drinking as "a little shaver," becoming intoxicated on home brew. He was a heavy drinker by the age of 20. His drinking and attendant brutality ended his first marriage and burdened the second one. In the last few months of his life, he was drinking excessively on the job (beer is freely available to beer bottlers during working hours) and consuming up to two fifths of whiskey a day in addition to beer at work. He had been warned that he would be fired if he continued this behavior, but he had not been fired or suspended. He had had driving trouble as a consequence of drinking, got into fights, and had a number of arrests and fines for peace disturbances, also drink-related. He drank before breakfast, thought he drank too much, felt guilty about his drinking, and lost friends on account of it. He experienced "shakes" but no other medical complications. He was not known to have had any medical attention for drinking and had no hospitalizations on account of it.

His wife had not noted any evidence of mental deterioration. However, for 6 months he had been carrying a pistol for "protection." He never specifically stated what he needed protection for or from, but he seemed somewhat fearful.

He had complained of fatigue for longer than 2 years, of inertia for about 2 years, and had expressed suicidal ideas from time to time over the last 2 years of his life. Other than feeling disgusted with himself and talking of suicide, he was not known to have had other depressive symptoms. During the last 6 months of his life, he had been taking an unknown amount of elixir of terpin hydrate (a cough suppressant containing 41% alcohol—i.e., 82 proof!). He said he was taking it for a sore throat and cough. A fellow worker told his wife that the subject thought he had cancer of the throat.

He had had attacks of dyspnea, palpitation, and cold sweats for 7 years. He consulted an osteopathic physician under the impression that he had "heart trouble" and was told that it was his "nerves." He had no other medical or psychiatric attention for that complaint. He had been hospitalized at age 21 for pneumonia and at 27 for "malaria" and a throat infection. No further medical history was reported.

The cause of his mother's death when he was 6 months old was not known to the informant. His father was reported to have been a heavy drinker, but without attendant consequences of it. No other family history was obtainable.

For 2 years, this subject had made oblique references to suicide. That behavior increased in the last 3–6 months of his life. He was quoted as saying, "I don't want to lay around to suffer. I would commit suicide and take you with me" (to his wife). (Consider this communication in relation to his fellow worker's statement that he believed he had cancer of the throat.) He had said, "I'd put a bullet in my head. That's the easiest way to go." Within 7–10 days of his suicide, he had talked about putting his affairs in order. He had never made a suicide attempt.

Circumstances Leading to the Act

On the day of his suicide, a Saturday, he was drinking heavily, as usual, and had several arguments with his wife. He flourished a .22-caliber revolver during an argument and his wife asked him to put it away. He left the house to visit his ex-wife and his wife locked him out. She wouldn't let him in until he put the gun away. Later, when he returned and sat down for a meal, an argument ensued over her preparation of the food. He took out his pistol and emptied it at his wife, striking her in the mouth and areas about the neck. Being out of cartridges he went out and obtained more, lay down beside his wife on the kitchen floor, and shot himself in the head. Both victims were taken to St. Louis City Hospital where he died almost 2 months later of a brain abscess secondary to self-inflicted gunshot wound. His wife made a good functional recovery and was our principal informant. There was no suicide note.

Findings and Sources

Clinical Diagnoses: (1) Alcoholism, chronic. (2) possible secondary affective disorder.
Toxicology: Not performed (subject known to have been drinking at the time of the act).
Primary Informant: Spouse, knew him for 24 years, married to him for last 7 years; saw him daily.
Other Sources of Information: Osteopathic physician, coroner's death investigation report, co-worker (on reason for suicide).
Informant's Opinion of Reason for Suicide: Went berserk because drink affected his mind. (Fellow worker's opinion: "He was worried about having cancer of the throat.")

Comment

Apart from a tendency to violence that had lessened in recent years, little was found to assist us in understanding this outcome. The subject seemed to have thought that he had cancer of the throat. Clear evidence of a depressive episode was not obtained, although dying and suicide had been on his mind for about 2 years. He was in trouble at work because of his abuse of alcohol, but he had not lost his job. He was drunk and flourishing a revolver. He became angry at his wife and emptied the pistol at her. The fact that he only wounded her and that he had to go out and buy more cartridges in order to shoot himself suggests to me a lack of premeditation. Having shot his wife with murderous intent, he likely saw no alternative to killing himself. His wife's assessment seems accurate: "He went berserk when he got mad this time from drinking." The only identifiable precipitants seem trivial.

I pondered long over the "interpersonal loss" implications of shooting one's wife. If he hadn't planned to kill her, but thought he had done so, he was confronted with a major interpersonal loss. The fact that she didn't die could hardly have been known to him. If he *had* intended to kill her, it was still a loss, but his suicide would likely have been planned in advance. I decided to err on the conservative side and not count this among the recent loss cases. It can be argued either way.

Case 13

Subject 13 was a 29-year-old single white male, born into comfortable circumstances. His father operated a service company. He had a sister, married at the time of his death, but whether she was older or younger was not learned. The family was intact. Little was learned of his earlier life, but by college age he was managing his life poorly. He tried three or four colleges, but probably didn't finish the second year. Apparently, this was owing to lack of application, rather than to lack of ability, as he seemed intelligent enough and considered that he had wasted his opportunity. The informant, who had known him casually for 21 years, and professionally for 6 months, regarded him as neither responsible nor truthful. He had worked as a semiskilled laborer for his father for some time after his college experience, but friction with his father led him to quit. He quit or was fired from his next job in the same industry after a fight with a coworker. He was not a steady worker until the last 8 months of his life, when he worked for a third employer in the office end of the industry. That man found his work entirely satisfactory and did not believe he had an alcohol problem. He lived alone in an efficiency apartment of good quality. His relationship with his father had been strained for years. They hardly spoke to one another.

He was a practicing homosexual who drank a lot and spent a lot on motel rooms for sex—sometimes with two different partners in a day. Thus, much of his social life was superficial. He was thought, however, to have had several close friends. He was ashamed of his homosexuality, his school failure, and his generally poor management of his life.

This young man had been drinking excessively since age 20 or 21. His psychiatrist thought he drank too much, as did his parents, but it was not known whether he thought so himself. He had been hospitalized for a gastrointestinal problem, thought to be secondary to his alcohol abuse, about a year before his death. He stopped drinking briefly after that. Whether any of his school troubles were secondary to alcohol abuse is uncertain, but the amount he spent on alcohol must have had a bearing on his need for extra money. No history was obtained of trouble with the police for fighting, disturbing the peace, or vehicular violations on account of his drinking. However, he was in major legal trouble because of embezzlement and passing bad checks; he was about to be taken into custody for this. He meets Feighner et al. (1972) criteria for "probable alcoholism."

The psychiatrist who was our informant regarded his patient as suffering from "a classical depression" of 7–8 months' duration. He thought the patient may have had the same problem 3–4 years earlier, for which he had been treated with psychotherapy at the Menninger Clinic in Topeka, Kansas. In addition to a sustained depressed mood, he had intermittent insomnia, a 30# to 40# weight gain, talked of suicide repeatedly, spoke of being "worthless" and "no good," and had made three suicide attempts. In the last week of his life, about the time of his last suicide attempt by overdose, he lost interest in all activities, did not go to work, withdrew from friends, felt profoundly guilty, said his family would be better off without him, and said his future was "nothing." (This assessment was not altogether unrealistic, in view of his impending legal troubles.)

In addition to recent major depression, he had a long history of pathological lying. He had written bad checks for years, which his parents would often cover. He had repeated school failures at the college level, for reasons not learned. Recently, he had been embezzling money from a trusting employer and was keeping a rented automobile beyond the contracted time without money to pay for it. Information is lacking on antisocial problems in adolescence.

He had one hospital admission, 8–12 months prior to his suicide, for gastritis, duodenitis or duodenal ulcer, probably related to his drinking.

His mother was described as "bizarre"—loud and overtalkative, and an abuser of amphetamine. His father was periodically depressed. No other family psychiatric history was known to the informant.

He had expressed suicidal thoughts to his parents, as well as to boyfriends, from time to time since the age of 20. More recently, he had expressed to his psychiatrist and to the psychiatrist's secretary the idea that he would be better off dead, and that his family would be better off without him. He took an overdose of unknown pills about a year before his suicide. He overdosed on pentobarbital (Nembutal) 6 months before his death and was hospitalized briefly. He overdosed with secobarbital (Seconal) and alcohol a week before ending his life.

Circumstances Leading to the Act

Over the last 6 months of his life, he had been embezzling money from his employer—perhaps as much as $5,000. He knew he was about to be confronted with this and couldn't cover the loss. Over the last 3 months, he had been writing bad checks again. His latest boyfriend had left him 4 weeks before his death and he was upset and depressed about it. At the time of his death he still had possession of a rented car several days beyond the term of the rental contract and expected trouble from that. On the day of his death, he visited his psychiatrist, who made arrangements for his hospital admission. He went home ostensibly to pack things he would need in the hospital but instead hanged himself, with a belt, in a closet. The psychiatrist said he left a note, but the parents wouldn't show it to anyone.

Findings and Sources

Clinical Diagnoses: (1) Probable alcoholism; DSM-III-R psychoactive substance abuse, mild. (2) major depressive disorder, second episode; (3) sexual disorder, not otherwise specified (DSM-III ego dystonic homosexuality). (4) personality disorder, unspecified.
Toxicology: Blood alcohol concentration 0.038 g%; barbiturates, narcotics, phenothiazines, antidepressants, neutral drugs all negative.
Primary Informant: Psychiatrist, who had known subject for 21 years, treated him for 6 months.
Other Sources of Information: Coroner's death investigation report.
Informant's Opinion of Reason for Suicide: "He was out of money, out of luck, and the police were closing in. He had no place to run—plus, he was classically depressed."

Comment

This subject meets criteria for "probable" alcoholism and for major depressive disorder. Weight gain, rather than loss, is not rare in depression, but it is not accounted for by the Washington University criteria used here. It is included in DSM-III-R under which the diagnosis is definite.

He had a great deal of character pathology, suggesting a diagnosis of antisocial personality disorder. He certainly exhibited antisocial traits in adulthood (lying, bad checks, fights, embezzlement). Lack of information regarding early symptoms leaves the diagnosis unsupported. Both alcohol as well as his driven sexual behavior, played a role in his final predicament. It is uncertain whether his parents would have bailed him out again, as they had in the past. He and his father were hardly on speaking terms. In his depressed state, he saw his situation as impossible. He hadn't conducted himself within the limits of the law for years, and perhaps felt himself unable to do so.

A boyfriend/lover left him 4 weeks before he ended his life. It would not be unreasonable to count him among those with interpersonal loss, but information was lacking as to the importance of that relationship to him. Much of his sex life was promiscuous, and he had undoubtedly lost boyfriends before. This time, however, he was both depressed and in serious legal trouble, as well as lacking family support. The combination proved lethal. Considering our limited knowledge of this young man's life, I chose not to count his interpersonal loss with the others, although it can be viewed either way.

Case 37

Subject 37 was a 50-year-old married white male, an unemployed manufacturing company executive who died of a drug overdose. He was born and raised in the Northeast, where his father was a research chemist and his mother a homemaker. The family was Roman Catholic. He had no known childhood or juvenile problems. Information was not obtained as to sibship. He graduated from high school and attended college for 3 years. He was in military service during World War II from age 22 to 26, and again during the Korean confilct, from age 31–32. Following his service in Korea, he received partial disability compensation for "nervousness." He married, at age 23, a girl he had known for 2 years. They had two children, a daughter, age 21, who was away at college and a son, age 17, living at home at the time of his death. The family had resided in St. Louis for 9 years, after moving from the East Coast.

After his military service during World War II he began a series of management jobs in manufacturing industries. He rose to a responsible position and typically would be recruited away from one company by another, rather than having to seek advancement. In his last job his drinking began to impair his effectiveness. Three months before his suicide he quarreled with management over a product price increase and left his job by mutual agreement. He was seeking employment through the services of an executive placement firm. He was described as having always been moody but generally productive and having a positive relationship with family and coworkers. Except for his wife and son, he seems to have been quite isolated socially in the last 3 months of his life. He never had any close friends.

He began to drink at about age 20 while in college and never had any control of his drinking from the beginning. He was a heavy drinker at the time of his marriage, but only on weekends. It was not possible for him to have just one or two drinks. If he drank, he always got drunk. He always felt guilty about it. He wanted to stop, his family wanted him to stop, and there was marital friction due to his drinking. In the last year of his life, when drinking, he would adhere stubbornly to untenable points of view when arguing with his wife. On two occasions, 7 and 6 months before his death, she found this so infuriating that she actually packed her bags to leave. Then she decided it was the alcohol talking. The next day, when sober, he would be quite pleasant and would tell her to disregard anything he had said. He was never abusive and rarely raised his voice during an argument. He had no legal or driving problems or medical condition attributable to drinking, and no withdrawal symptoms, or blackouts. He did sometimes drink in the morning after a weekend binge, but he missed work only 1 day with a hangover.

Eleven years before his suicide he began attending Alcoholics Anonymous and had a year of sobriety. Six years before his death, he was drinking up to 2 fifths a week; he then saw a psychiatrist for help. He asked to be given disulfiram (Antabuse), but his compliance with that medication was irregular—periods of several weeks of abstinence alternating with resumption of his previous pattern. His daughter refused to come home from college 2 years before his death because of his behavior while drinking. They would regularly argue at those times. During the last year of his life he was intoxicated at work several times, and at a business conference lasting several days he was obviously drinking every day. He quit his job 3 months before his death, then stopped drinking, except for three weekend binges. Four days before his suicide he began drinking steadily and was intoxicated at the time of his death.

He had a partial medical disability as a result of "nervousness" commencing during military service in Korea. His only psychiatric contacts were as an outpatient about 6 years before his suicide. At the time of his death he was taking chlordiazepoxide (Librium) and amobarbital (Tuinal). These had been prescribed earlier by his psychi-

opinionated and short tempered, and they felt unwelcome. He drank before breakfast, hid his whiskey bottles and drank surreptitiously the last 4–5 years of his life.

At age 51, 2½ years before his death, he had the first of three medical hospitalizations for complications of alcoholism. That and his second admission were for grand mal seizures. An electroencephalogram was "not definitely outside normal limits." He was found to have gouty arthritis of the great toe and was discharged on colchicine, phenylbutazone (Butazolidin) and phenytoin (Dilantin). He stopped drinking for 3–4 months and felt guilty on resuming it. It was his only attempt to stop. A year later, a fall, probably secondary to a grand mal seizure, led to his second hospital admission. He had stopped taking medication earlier. His third alcohol related admission was 8 months before his death, following 2–3 weeks of nausea and vomiting. His liver was enlarged and liver function studies were abnormal. The discharge diagnosis was "early nutritional cirrhosis of the liver." No specific therapy was given, although he was warned about the effects of drinking. That was his last medical contact. He never had inpatient treatment for alcoholism as such.

He had been passed over for promotion at work for at least 5 years, and as a result he "hated work" and talked of retiring "in 2 years." So far as is known, his job was not endangered. In those 5 years he was, according to his wife, "rarely drunk but never sober." His alcohol consumption did not vary noticeably in that period. He had been arrested briefly, 10 years before his death, in connection with an automobile accident. He had no other arrests or police trouble, and no convictions.

About a year before he died, he began sleeping more than usual and became "moody," slowed down, and joyless. He said, "It feels like I'm going nuts." His depression was slowly progressive, and by 6 months, he had lost interest in the house. Guilt about his drinking was of longer duration. In the last 2–3 months, he was clearly tired, physically slow, and looked depressed. He spoke of feeling sad, and of early retirement. He also complained of "back pain." On Christmas day, just over a month before his suicide, he stayed in his room alone and refused to join the family. That had never occurred before and didn't happen again. He never spoke of suicide and did not leave a note.

He had been hospitalized 10 years earlier for removal of a submaxillary salivary gland because of a stone in the duct. He had seen a physician for a complaint of "choking" (shortness of breath) about 8 months before his death and stopped smoking in the last two weeks because of it. Pulmonary emphysema seems likely, but the diagnosis was not learned.

His father was alcoholic. No other psychiatric history was known to informants. Suicide and suicide attempt were denied.

Circumstances Leading to the Act

His wife had no explanation for his suicide other than "he must have felt very badly." Neither informant nor examiners viewed the daughter's remarriage and moving out of the house as having had great significance for him. Apart from failure to be promoted at work, no other events of a potentially upsetting nature were identified within several years of his suicide. He had, however, become increasingly depressed over the last year.

On the day of the act he got up early and appeared cheerful and happy, not sad as he had for the previous several months. He dressed better than usual, went to see a chiropractor about his back pain and stopped to visit with his father, who lived nearby. He bought some cookies for his wife, which was unusual, as he had talked to her recently about how she ought to stop eating cookies and lose weight. He left home again for the afternoon shift but called in sick. He was seen by a neighbor to drive into his garage at 3:30 p.m. His wife and son-in-law found him at 4:00 a.m., dead, in the front seat of his car in the garage of his residence. The garage doors were closed and a hose extended from the exhaust pipe of the automobile through a rear window. The left front window of the automobile was open, and his legs protruded through it. The gasoline tank was half full, the ignition was turned on, and the ignition keys were in the glove compartment. The motor had stopped. A partially empty whiskey bottle was found on the garage floor.

Findings and Sources

Clinical Diagnoses: (1) Alcoholism, chronic. (2) probable secondary affective disorder. (DSM-III-R definite).
Toxicology: Blood alcohol concentration 0.158 g%; blood CO saturation, 62%.
Primary Informant: Wife, married 33 years; saw him daily.
Other Sources of Information: Coroner's death investigation report, hospital records.
Informant's Opinion of Reason for Suicide: "He must have felt very badly."

Comment

There seems to have been very little change in this man's recent life, and that which occurred did not appear to have troubled him. His alcoholism antedated his depression by many years. This suicide is similar to that seen in primary, uncomplicated depression that ends in suicide. Nothing much had happened. The depression got the best of him. His suicide was in response to internal, not external cues.

Case 15

Subject 15 was a 44-year-old, married employed white Protestant male factory worker, born in southeastern Missouri. His father was a farmer, his mother, a housewife. He had at least two brothers, one of whom was also an alcoholic and committed suicide 4 months before this subject did, somewhere outside of our search area. He completed the eighth grade of school, married at age 21, and moved to the St. Louis area shortly thereafter. The couple had 4 children. A son, aged 21, was married and out of the house. He was living with his wife and sons 17 and 7 and a daughter 3 years old at the time of his death. He had been a "lead man" for an unknown length of time at the manufacturing plant where he had worked for 17 years. He blamed his increased drinking on "pressure at work." Sometime during the last year of his life he requested and received demotion from lead man back to laborer, with a consequent decrease in pay. That change did not reduce his drinking or prove beneficial in any way. He had no close friends. His only social life was in bars or taverns.

He was reported to have been "a drinker" all of his married life—since age 21—consuming a pint of liquor about 2 times a week without abusiveness or complications. That pattern changed to daily drinking about 3 years before his demise, and his wife thought he had lost control of his drinking only in the last 6–12 months. (One hospital record puts it nearer to 2 years.) However, she also said he had stopped drinking altogether about 10 years earlier, then resumed it after 6 months abstinence. Thus, at a minimum, he had had 11 years of problem drinking. He had outbursts of rage when drinking, throughout his married life. Despite his rages, he was described as not happy unless he was drinking. In the last 3 years of his life, with the increased drinking, he became physically abusive of his wife, and on one occasion threatened to kill her. On another occasion he broke one or more of her finger bones. She left him several times for a week or so after he beat her, but they were not separated at the time of his death.

He thought he drank too much, felt guilty about it, and tried a number of times to stop but was unable to maintain sobriety. His wife unquestionably objected to his drinking. His brother and his doctor also thought he drank too much. Owing to his wife's objection to his drinking, he would slip out of the house to taverns or drink in the garage. He drank before breakfast for at least the last 3 years of his life. He was reported by his wife to have been hospitalized more than once for DTs, although we found no record of it. He certainly had been hospitalized with gastritis and malnutrition 15 months before his death, as well as for detoxification 6 and 10 months later. On the second hospitalization laboratory evidence of early Laennec's cirrhosis was found, along with borderline diabetes. He went on benders, lasting from 2 days to 1½ weeks, and had been reprimanded on more than one occasion for his absenteeism. Although he had no record of alcohol-related arrests, he had struck a parked car while driving drunk.

Some 5–6 months before his suicide he had to sell their home and automobile and move the family to a smaller apartment when his hospital bills, other debts, and alcohol expenses, along with lost pay from lost time from work had made it impossible for him to keep up payments on the house. In the 2 months before his last hospitalization he drank more than usual.

He had been moody and highly strung for as long as the informant could remember. He chain-smoked and picked his fingernails constantly. He stopped taking his wife out to the movies 8 years before his suicide. They had previously gone twice a week. His appetite had been poor for the last 5 years. During the last year of his life he became markedly depressed, and wouldn't take his son fishing. He was hospitalized for depression 3–4 months before his suicide and received 15 electroconvulsive (ECT) treatments. He was still considerably confused upon discharge 2 weeks before he took his life. He was also still depressed, saying he was worse off than he had ever been. He slept little, sat around doing nothing, and spoke hardly at all. He said he could not and did not want to return to work. Because of his poor appetite he lost the weight he had gained in the hospital. He felt ashamed about causing the family problems and losing his house and car and referred to their apartment as a "slum." He had missed 6 months' work in the last year of his life due to his alcoholism and hospitalizations.

His mother had died 1 year before he did and his alcoholic brother committed suicide 8 months later, by overdose of sleeping tablets. He was reportedly saddened by these events but did not seem unduly upset.

He had begun to speak of suicide about 3 years before the event, around the time he increased his drinking. In the last year he told his wife and others several times that he would shoot himself, that he would be better off dead, that he was a burden, and that the family would be better off without him. He also spoke of a desire to die. In the last 2 weeks he expressed all of these ideas to his wife and to his brother and sister-in-law. He advised his wife to take out more life insurance on him, because he was going to kill himself. She thought he was trying to scare her with suicide threats. Since he had threatened so many times, she ignored him after awhile. About 3 months before his death, he wrote three notes expressing his feelings of worthlessness. Copies were not obtainable.

Circumstances Leading to the Act

He was immensely upset and disgusted with himself over losing the house and automobile. He considered their less commodious apartment "a slum" and himself a failure. His hospitalization for depression, following shortly on this move, coincided closely with his brother's suicide. He received 15 ECT treatments. Since his release, 2 weeks before his death, he was confused and suffered from a loss of memory, symptoms not uncommon following a long course of ECT. Less typically, he seemed to have become more depressed. He just sat: sometimes he looked at TV. To his wife's knowledge, he did not drink at all. He rarely spoke in the last week. He told his wife he was "worse off" after his hospital stay and did appear to be so. She threatened to return him to the hospital, which he hated.

He was expected to return to work in a week but felt entirely incapable of doing his assigned job. The day before his suicide, he became disoriented and confused and did not recognize his children. The doctor had advised that someone stay with him constantly and his 17-year-old son was keeping a watch on him. On the morning of his suicide, he sent his son out to get some cigarettes for him. When the son returned, he found his father dead, having shot himself in the chest with a .410 caliber shotgun. A suicide note read:

> [Wife's first name] I know this is not right, but maybe you will be better off with me gone. I know it is my fault I don't think I can hold down a job now. I haven't done as much wrong ase [sic] you think I have. After this is all over, why don't you get these kids out of this slums [sic] because they will end like me.
> I always thought I made you a living if you care, keep those two little babies from seeing this.
> I wish you would take them to [his hometown] until they grow up where it is quiet.
> I don't know if I will get anything from [employer's] Insurance, but if I do let [name of unidentified person] you I and [first names of sons and daughter] at home [sic] but one thing I didn't know was that you wanted to have everything your way, but you run out on everything and I know I can never get it back. Those men are still working 7 days a week and I can't stand the loss as I don't care to work I am a hell of a lot worse off now than I was before I went to the hospital.
> [Full name, street address]

Findings and Sources

Clinical Diagnoses: (1) Alcoholism, chronic; (2) major depressive disorder (probably secondary); (3) diabetes mellitus, diet controlled.
Toxicology: Not performed.
Primary Informant: Wife, married 23 years; saw him daily.
Other Sources of Information: Hospital records, coroner's death investigation report.
Informant's Opinion of Reason of Suicide: Humiliation, defeat.

Comment

There seems to have been a cavalcade of upsetting events in the last year of this man's life: his mother's death, his brother's suicide, his voluntary demotion. His repeated hospitalizations and consequent job absenteeism had both reduced and overtaxed his earning capacity to the extent of greatly compromising the family's standard of living, and that distressed him greatly. On his last hospitalization, 3–4 months before his suicide, he received what might ordinarily be a quite adequate course of ECT, but his depression was not improved. His wife had threatened to have him rehospitalized, a prospect that he hated. His post-ECT amnesia seems to have been quite marked and may have contributed to the decompensation of brain function (delirium) that characterized his last day alive.

His world was certainly crashing down around him. He was to have been under constant surveillance because of his expressed suicidal thoughts. He craftily secured the necessary moments of freedom to do himself in by sending his 17-year-old son to the store for cigarettes. His hopelessness about his ability to provide for his family seems to have been the chief motivation for his suicide. It was intensified by his self-disgust and his fear of rehospitalization. Delirium may have contributed to the outcome, but only in hastening it. His course was already set. He is one of only two subjects in this study who was not drinking right up to the time of their suicide.

Case 18

This 35-year-old single white male construction worker was born in a small Arkansas town. His father was a carpenter and his mother a homemaker. He had one brother. He went to work in the construction trade after his third year of high school. Raised as a Baptist, he was not a churchgoer. His family moved from Arkansas to St. Louis when he was 8, briefly to central Missouri when he was 25, then back to St. Louis. They moved to southeast Missouri 2 years before his death. Except for 2–3 years of honorable service in the Army during the Korean conflict, he lived with his parents all of his life, whether in Arkansas, in St. Louis, or elsewhere, when not working, and whenever work did not take him away. Work was seasonal and irregular. Having found no steady employment in 3 months, he came to St. Louis to look for work 3 weeks before his death.

He had two close friends, a male drinking partner and a married woman who moved to California with her husband 4 years before his suicide. Before moving away, the woman periodically left her husband to be with him. When they were together he drank less, took better care of his appearance and tried to lose weight. At those times he liked to bowl, play cards, and attend baseball games. After she left, he gradually lost interest in those activities. He still liked reading, hunting, fishing and seeing friends at the tavern. He was described as a moody person. Often outgoing, he might isolate himself in his room or speak little for hours or days, unrelated to alcohol consumption. This became more pronounced in the last year of his life.

Previously a normal drinker, while in the Army at age 21–23, he began to drink more heavily. He was experiencing negative consequences of it at least 12 years before his death. He had stated that he thought he drank too much and felt guilty about it. It is uncertain whether he made efforts to stop, but once started, he drank until the bar closed. His family objected to his drinking, as did the informant. In the last year, when drinking, "he went into himself and resented being talked to. He was persistently depressed when drinking." For most of his working life he confined his drinking to weekends while working and drank little when between jobs. Previously a reliable worker, in recent years he adopted a pattern of working until he had some money, then he would quit and drink. As a consequence, he became recognized as a less desirable employee and was laid off earlier and hired later than others. He had had little employment for the last year; almost none in the last 3 months.

He had several automobile accidents and 4–5 speeding tickets over the last 12 years of his life. Two years before his death he was arrested for speeding and a vehicular collision related to drinking. His driver's license was revoked for 1 year as a consequence. About that time he stopped drinking altogether for 6 months and was "like he used to be—nice, sweet, easy going." Also about that time he filed for bankruptcy. The reason was not learned. His brother said he looked depressed at times but denied knowledge of all but one symptom of a depressive syndrome: a progressive loss of interest in previous activities in the last 4 years of his life.

He was never hospitalized and had last seen a doctor about 4 years before his death, concerning a desire to lose weight.

A maternal aunt reportedly drank a lot, as did her husband. The family history was otherwise reported as negative for psychiatric illness, including alcoholism, suicide and suicide attempt.

On one occasion, about 2 years before his death, his mother was trying to get him to cut down on his drinking. He became angry and said that he would end it all. He may have communicated similarly to his grandmother at about that time as well. No more recent communication was known to the informant.

Circumstances Leading to the Act

A year before he took his life, a bartender at the bar he frequented committed suicide. He wondered aloud how anyone could or would want to take his life. He had not worked steadily for the final year. He had gone through his small savings and came to St. Louis to look for work 3 weeks before his suicide. He lived alone in a transient hotel and was last seen by the informant one week before his death. He had been drinking but did not seem to be depressed. On the night of his suicide 2 unidentified men took him home drunk from the neighborhood bar. He shot himself in the right frontal area of the head with a .25-caliber pistol that night. He did not leave a note.

Findings and Sources

Clinical Diagnosis: Alcoholism, chronic.
Toxicology: Not performed.
Primary Informant: Brother, who had little contact with him for the last 3 years until 3 weeks before his suicide when he came to St. Louis to look for work. Seen 2–3 times in last 3 weeks.
Other Sources of Information: Coroner's death investigation report.
Informant's opinion of reason for suicide: (1) Out of money and out of a job; (2) drunk; (3) impulsive act.

Comment

This man was largely a loner, with one male friend and a woman friend who used to periodically leave her husband and live with him. When she and her husband moved to California, 4 years before his death, he began to drink more. That affected his desirability as an employee in a typically episodic industry. His search for work in St. Louis was apparently fruitless. He had always lived with his parents except when work took him away. Alone and unemployed, he had only limited contact with his brother, who had not observed the symptoms of a depressive syndrome. We are left with the conclusion that being alone, unemployed and drunk comprised the lethal combination of circumstances for a man with a rather aimless existence.

Case 19

This 35-year-old white separated male was born in Arkansas and had spent 16 or 17 years in St. Louis. His father was a farmer, his mother a homemaker. He had a brother who was a secondary informant. We didn't learn if he had other siblings. His parental home was intact. He quit school in or at the end of seventh grade. He was married at the age of 19 and had 2 children, a daughter aged 16 and a son aged 13 at the time of his death. His religion was Pentecostal and he had wanted to be a preacher. He had done all of the necessary work for it, but his wife wouldn't allow it. Three years before taking his life this would-be minister of the gospel left his wife and children, rented an apartment, and lived with his childhood sweetheart until the day before his death. His wife had refused to give him a divorce.

His working life was 18 years but no information was obtained concerning his employment previous to leaving his wife. He had held five jobs during the last 2½ years. Reportedly, he was a good worker, liked by his employers, who were always reluctant to lose him. For a year he was a policeman. He quit that job after getting drunk, arguing with his wife, and pulling a gun on her. For the next year he was self-employed as a tavern owner (he held half-interest and his girlfriend held half). Six months before ending his life he sold his interest to his brother because he got bored. He similarly became bored and quit a job as a taxi driver and a simultaneous job as clerk in an all night grocery after 2 months. The last 4 months of his life he worked nights in a meat packing plant. He was lonely working the night shift, saying it was "dreary." He wanted to change jobs, although he was earning the most money he had ever made.

He and his wife owed $2,000 to a loan company that was continuously after him. His wife called frequently, wanting her child support money, which on one occasion she "blew" on a trip with another man. It troubled him that, with child support payments, he was unable to give his paramour the material things he would have liked to.

He began to drink heavily at the age of 23 or 24. His general pattern involved getting drunk, arguing, and fighting. According to his girlfriend, his drinking worsened in the last 3 years, to the point of his consuming a case of 8-ounce beers in 24 hours. Apparently, buying cases of 8-ounce bottles was his way of trying to control his drinking; however, he didn't stop drinking until it was all gone. In the final 3 months of his life he reportedly had experienced decreased tolerance for alcohol. He would get very drunk on 24 ounces of beer and could not handle whiskey at all. He thought he drank too much and felt guilty about it. His family and others thought he drank too much, too.

His brother said people liked him; "He had hundreds of close friends," except when he was drinking. People tended to leave him alone then. His girlfriend described him as a loner. His social life occurred mainly in taverns. A good worker when sober, he quit jobs when drunk, apparently by not showing up for work. "Bosses always wanted him back," but he never returned to a former employer.

When drinking, he was exceedingly jealous of his girlfriend. He fought constantly with her, threw dishes and ash trays at her, and blackened her eyes repeatedly. In the last months, he often hung around outside of her tavern, peeping in windows to see whom she was talking to. Since his stint as a policeman he always carried a pistol; when angry, he would put it to her head and threaten to kill her. He would also threaten suicide by putting the gun to his own head. He was depressed when his girlfriend was not around but cheered up when she was. He had experienced no loss of interest in sex.

Six or 7 months before his suicide, in a fit of anger, he tried to burn down the tavern (of which he had recently sold his half-interest to his brother) by placing a lighted candle next to a can of gasoline at the establishment. The arrangement was unlikely to have been successful, but he seemed to have expected it to be. He had no known arrests. Hospitalized for abdominal pain 16 months before his demise, he received a diagnosis of acute gastroenteritis. The record showed that he had a hospitalization 1–2 years earlier and was diagnosed as having a "liver ailment." He had seen a doctor 6 months before his death for reasons probably associated with alcoholism—"If he drank a lot his liver would swell and he would double up with stomach pains and chew his fingers. This would last until he sobered up." He went on benders and had shakes but never had DTs. Morning drinking was denied.

Over the last 3 years of his life he was high-strung, moody, sensitive, and cried easily—symptoms connected with his drinking. The duration may have been much longer, but that was how long the informant had known him. He often said to his girlfriend that he had done something terrible and that when he got "real old" he would tell her about it. He sometimes dwelt on this when drunk. He had outbursts of rage and talked constantly about his own death and killing his girlfriend during those final 3 years.

There was no record of his having psychiatric treatment. While living with his wife he took "nerve pills" daily and said he couldn't live without them. He took none after leaving her. He was troubled by insomnia at intervals and took over-the-counter drugs for it. Three weeks before his death, a male friend from the tavern died and he was very concerned about that.

An automobile wreck about 3 years before his death, for which he refused hospitalization, left him with headaches. Often the glands in his neck (at the base of the mandible) would swell and his neck would get red and hot.

The family had no history of alcoholism, psychiatric illness, or suicide.

Two years before ending his life, when his wife pressed him for money, he told her he would kill himself. For the last 6 months he had talked with his girlfriend about suicide almost nightly (or whenever drunk). He frequently said, "Come and lay down beside me and I'll kill us both now; lay close and I'll kill us both and it'll be over with." Then he would cry. He believed that his daughter would be better off without him because she would get his life insurance money. He called her the night before his suicide, after his girlfriend left him, and said he would kill himself. He never talked to his brother about suicide.

Circumstances Leading to the Act

His brother said that the subject had wanted to go back to his wife but she would not have him. Now she was divorcing him. The divorce, which would have been final in 2 weeks, gave him custody of their 15-year-old daughter and he was going to have to move to St. Charles, a town 20 miles distant from St. Louis, *the next day,* into a house near her high school so she could finish her schooling there. He would be alone during the day while she was at school and would work at night. His brother thought he could not face the added responsibility, or the idea of being alone. "He couldn't stand being alone."

During the last 3 years of his life, he had drunk more heavily, had been physically abusive toward his girlfriend, and threatened suicide frequently. For about the last 4 months he had been acting "funny" and had been unusually jealous and "mean." She had told him she would leave him if he hit her again. He did and she did, the day before his suicide. She told him they were finished, packed her clothes, and moved out of their apartment after an argument which resulted in her receiving two black eyes. He said, "Without you, my life is over." Although this was one of many arguments accompanied by physical abuse and brief separation, he reportedly told another bar customer after she left, "She's really gone this time."

The next evening, he was in the tavern she co-owned with his brother. He danced with other women and she became angry. She then danced with another man and he became outraged (as usual). He bloodied her nose and pushed her to the floor. When she asked why he could dance with others and she couldn't, he hit her once more. He said that it was all right for him to do so but not acceptable for her. They and the subject's brother went to a nearby cafe where the argument resumed; the girlfriend began to cry and asked his brother to take her home. He took her to her car, which was at the tavern, and the subject followed them. He tried to pin her car against the wall. She was able to get away, however, and he followed her ("he rode my bumper") to her sister's house. She parked and got out. He got out, pulled his pistol ("he had done this a million times before"), ran up to her, and said, "If it's all over between us, it's all over for me." She said, "Oh, [his name], don't talk like that." He put the pistol to his head and pulled the trigger. She thinks it was an accident and that he thought the safety was on.

Findings and Sources

Clinical Diagnosis: Alcoholism, chronic.
Toxicology: Blood alcohol concentration 0.15 g%.
Primary Informant: Girlfriend, a "childhood sweetheart," who had lived with him for the last 3 years, and saw him daily.
Other Sources of Information: Subject's brother, hospital records, coroner's death investigation report.
Informant's Opinion of Reason for Suicide: Girlfriend: accident; Brother: couldn't face the responsibility of caring for his daughter or being alone.

Comment

If one believes in "love addiction," this might serve as an example. This subject was obsessed with the woman he had left his wife for and had lived with for 3 years. The attraction was mutual and intense, surviving much psychic pain (his) and physical abuse (his of her). She packed her clothes and left him, as she had threatened to do, the morning after he blacked both of her eyes in an argument. That night, her dancing with another man brought down the full force of his jealousy on her and further physical assault. After further argument at a nearby cafe, he confronted her once again, in front of her sister's home. Holding his pistol to his head, he pulled the trigger. The agony of this relationship is evidenced by his having repeatedly proposed to kill both her and himself—a denouement she repeatedly declined to share.

The brother thought the subject was still in love with his wife and wanted to go back to her. She, however, after holding out for 3 years, was finally divorcing him. The divorce was to be final in 2 weeks. Remarkably, *he* was to have custody of their 15-year-old daughter. (The circumstances that could result in a drunken, deserting father receiving custody of a teenage daughter stretch one's imagination. Sadly, the details are lacking.) That custody was to begin the next day and required him to live outside of St. Louis, in what is now a bedroom suburb of the city but was then the boondocks. Hating his work, frightened of responsibility for his daughter, rejected by both of the women to whom he was (or had been) attached, fearful of living alone, drunk, he found the solution he had contemplated for months, albeit alone, not with his paramour. Depression seems not to have been a factor, though how he could have escaped it is puzzling. He qualifies for "recent loss."

Case 21

Subject 21 was a divorced white male, 47 years old at the time of his suicide by hanging. He was born in New York City. His father was a tinsmith, a periodic heavy drinker, who got very friendly and loved everyone when he was drinking. He died of cancer 8 years before the subject's death. His mother was a homemaker, and there was one sibling, a brother. Other than the father's periodic drinking, the home was not described as unusual. Both parents were Roman Catholic. He was nonobservant as an adult. As a child he attended a parochial school, where he was chronically unhappy. He complained that his mother always believed the Sisters (nuns) rather than him. It was not known if there were major school problems, but he dropped out after completing the 10th grade and went to work. In 1941, at age 20, he enlisted in the Navy and served for 4 years in World War II. He saw action and received decorations, the nature of which were unknown to the informant. There was no record of disciplinary action or other problems. He was medically discharged with a 10% psychiatric disability and a diagnosis of "anxiety reaction."

He married his first wife at age 24, about the time of his discharge. They had one child, a girl born when he was 26. They came to St. Louis when he was 28 and he remained here until his death, 20 years later. The marriage was unhappy and ended in divorce when he was 31. His second marriage, at age 32, was stormy. There were three boys born of that union, aged 15, 13, and 6 years when he died. His wife described him as moody, angry, verbally and sometimes physically abusive, hostile to others, emotionally distant from his family, and with few friends except drinking partners. She and their three sons had left him on several occasions for up to a week or 2, only to return. They were finally separated 13 months before his suicide and divorced 5 months later. After the separation, he lived "one place and another" for 5 months, then lived in a trailer for 6 months before taking a live-in job as janitor of an apartment building. His only social life was in taverns, where he was largely unwelcome.

He was believed to have commenced heavy drinking while in military service (age 20–24), although it could have begun earlier. He attended AA for a short time after his discharge from the Navy. His first marriage, from age 24 to 31, was marked by his heavy drinking and physical abuse of his wife. Through most of the 15 years of his second marriage he was a heavy weekend drinker, occasionally physically abusive, with no social life except at taverns. He blamed his wife for his drinking, which became daily in the last few years. He frequently had fights in taverns and ultimately was barred from several due to his disruptiveness.

His employment record was erratic. He had a total of 15 jobs during the last 20 years of his life; the longest lasted 5 years from age 41 to 46. He was discharged for drinking at age 30 and threatened with discharge for drinking before work or on the job about 2 years before his suicide. He worked generally as a welder, with many periods of employment of a few weeks to 6 months. Having little seniority, he was vulnerable to temporary layoffs. He characteristically failed to return for reemployment on callback after being laid off. His last job was a part-time one as a janitor. He had held it for 1 week.

Binge drinking occurred throughout the marriage, and he sometimes drank before breakfast. He denied concern about his drinking but had periods of 3–6 months of abstinence occasionally during the second marriage. He was abstinent for nearly 2 years when he was about 40, commencing around the time his father died. He did not talk of suicide during that entire period of sobriety. Then he resumed his drinking, which progressed in severity. His wife, mother, neighbors, even his drinking partners agreed that he drank too much. He was reported to have had visual hallucinations ("The Japs are coming!") when drunk, beginning before his longest period of sobriety.

He frequently drove while drunk and was arrested for speeding and running a red light at age 34. Although intoxicated at the time, he was not charged with driving while intoxicated. A DWI citation 2 or 3 years before his death cost him $100. He was arrested for public intoxication 5 months before his suicide and fined $25. Following his separation he drank more heavily than usual. He telephoned his wife and threatened to kill her, "if anything happens to the kids." Three years before his death he presented for admission at the Veterans Administration Hospital with "inability to control excessive intake of alcohol". After an 8-day hospital stay, he was discharged on "mild chemotherapy" (chlordiazepoxide), with a diagnosis of "psychoneurosis, anxiety reaction, in good partial remission." He abused or misused prescribed chlordiazepoxide after that. Five months before his death—3 months after his second divorce—he had a 1-day admission to St. Louis State Hospital, after stating that he intended to hang himself. He was intoxicated with alcohol on admission.

His last psychiatric admission was 6 weeks before his death, when he returned to the Veterans' Administration Hospital with complaints of depression and insomnia. He gave a history of drinking a pint of whiskey a day plus unknown amounts of beer. He was poorly nourished, had a worried expression, and complained of being "bothered by everything," especially by noise in his place of work. Typically for that time, neither the presence nor absence of key depressive symptoms was recorded. He reportedly denied suicidal thoughts, had good contact with reality but poor judgment. His intellectual abilities appeared to be reduced. He participated in an alcoholism treatment program and was on chlorpromazine 300 mg, four times a day "for restlessness."

After about 2 weeks in the hospital, he was given a 14-day leave. He returned unexpectedly after 2 days, stating that he had wanted to hang himself and showing physical evidence of a wire mark and bruise on the left side of his neck. One week later, he discharged himself against medical advice. At that time he was tense, depressed, and stated that his only problem was drinking, which he needed to stop in order to support his family. Two days after signing out of the hospital, he was arrested for shoplifting at a shopping center. In a separate episode the same day, he was arrested for breaking into his second ex-wife's home. For that he was charged with illegal entry, destruction of property, disturbing the peace, resisting arrest, and using abusive and vulgar language. He spent 9 days in jail and was fined $100 for each of the two episodes. That same day he secured a janitorial job and a room in an apartment building. This last move was to avoid creditors. (He owed a rather substantial amount to one department store.) The judge suspended his sentence a week before his suicide "because he was a sick man." Nineteen days after leaving the hospital, he was dead.

He had been hospitalized for a medical condition 9 months before his suicide, at the Veterans Administration Hospital. He gave a 10-month history of progressive symptoms of rheumatoid arthritis. Physical and laboratory findings were altogether consistent with the diagnosis, and he was treated with gold injections and phenylbutazone (Butazolidine) during a 2-month hospitalization. There were no other significant medical problems known. Although malnutrition, weight loss, and anemia were noted, these signs were attributed to his heavy drinking.

His father was an episodic heavy drinker. A grandfather and two maternal uncles were alcoholic. One of the latter died of renal failure, supposedly secondary to alcoholism. There was no other history of mental illness, and no record of suicide or suicide attempt in the family.

In his second marriage, this subject frequently expressed an intention to commit suicide in a very specific manner: by hanging. As a teenager, he had learned of the suicide by hanging of a man he did not know. His brother had described seeing the shadow of the man hanging from a door. This stayed on his mind and he spoke of it often to his second wife. Over the last 7–8 years he would taunt his wife by asking, "How would you like it for the kids to wake up and see me hanging on the door?" Beginning around 2 years before his suicide, he threatened on several occasions to kill his wife before taking his own life. Subsequent to the final marital separation, he called her on more than one occasion "at about 3:00 a.m." to say he hated her and the world and that he intended to make a name for himself before he left this world. On the day before his suicide, he telephoned his *first* wife and said he was going to hang himself.

Circumstances Leading to the Act

After separation from his second wife, 13 months before his suicide, he increased his drinking to daily and lived one place and another. On leave from his last Veterans' Administration hospital admission, he started to commit suicide by hanging. A week later, he signed himself out against medical advice.

He probably resumed drinking heavily almost immediately, as judged by his arrest 2 days later for shoplifting and separately for breaking into his second wife's home. That led to his being jailed for the next 9 days. On release from jail he obtained a room and janitorial duties in an apartment building, "to avoid creditors." Five days later his landlord entered his apartment and found his body hanging from a door, with a cord around his neck, running over the top of the door and tied to the doorknob. A cup with powdered coffee was on the stove and a pan of water had boiled dry. No suicide note was found. He had taken his life on his second son's birthday, a fact gleaned from the record but not commented on by his second wife. She did not think that alcoholism, per se, was the cause of his suicide. "He wore alcoholism as a badge. 'We're different as a group. You people don't understand us'," she quoted him as saying.

Findings and Sources

Clinical Diagnosis: (1) Alcoholism, chronic; (2) probable major depression (DSM-III-R definite). (3) rheumatoid arthritis.
Toxicology: Blood alcohol content 0.00%.
Primary Informant: Second ex-wife, who had known him at least 17 years. She rarely saw him, but they talked by telephone weekly.
Other Sources of Information: Hospital records, coroner's death investigation report.
Informants's Opinion of Reason for Suicide: Accident. "He was only trying to taunt me."

Comment

This man had been preoccupied with suicide by hanging since sometime in his teens. Over the years he had incurred all but a few of the consequences of alcohol abuse that constitute our criterion symptoms. Despite rather early onset of problems, he was not known to have harmed his health importantly. He had, however, alienated two wives and all of his friends. One is entitled to wonder that he did not take his life when his second wife left him—but he didn't. He kept in touch by calling her weekly up to the end. What changed?

He was recently out of the psychiatric hospital (against medical advice), was in debt and without a job (unless one considers his custodial duties that), had gotten himself in trouble with the law, and he was probably clinically depressed. The fact that his ex-wife had not seen him recently, except to have him arrested, left her uninformed about a number of the symptoms needed for a confident diagnosis of depression. Nevertheless, there were enough for a diagnosis of "probable" major depression of several months duration. Surprisingly, he was not drinking on the day he took his life. He was preparing a cup of coffee, but interrupted that and hung himself. Alone, friendless, jobless, in debt, depressed, he may not have had the wherewithal to buy a bottle. Impulse? Not altogether. He told his first wife a day earlier what he intended doing. I think he realized he had "come to the end of his rope."

Case 33

Subject 33 was a 50-year old single unemployed white Roman Catholic male, living alone at the time of his death by gunshot wound of the head. He was a native of the St. Louis area and lived there all of his life except for his time in the Navy. He had no unusual problems in childhood and the parental home was not thought to have been unusual or chaotic. His father was a civil court employee and his mother a homemaker. Two sisters were still living in the St. Louis area at the time of his death. He dropped out of high school after 2 or 3 years and worked at unknown blue collar jobs until entering the Navy during World War II. He reportedly served overseas and was honorably discharged. Dates were not known to the informant.

After returning to civilian life he worked as a pipefitter for 15 years until a year before his death and was active in union affairs. Two informants thought that he might have been involved in extralegal activities. They reported that at one point he had been indicted along with several other union officials. One informant described him as "a labor racketeer, drawing a big salary but not working at all." Whatever the nature of his actual work, he was usually employed and drawing a handsome paycheck, but going from one job to another, in part because of the nature of the work. He was fired several times. The last firing, a year before his suicide, was for absenteeism.

He was never interested in marriage and is reported to have become uncomfortable when the subject was raised. (Our primary informant became obviously uncomfortable when asked if there had been a change in his sex drive.) He had lived with one sister and his mother, but fought with them. His sister left the home 18 months prior to his suicide, tired of the fighting. She telephoned him daily and visited him two or three times a week. Two months before his death, "he drove his mother out." He lived alone from then until his death. He had few interests and his only social life was with other customers at bars.

He began heavy drinking in his early 20s, when he was in the Navy, and had progressive daily drinking until his death. Estimates of his liquor consumption vary with informants, ranging from a pint to well over a fifth of liquor a day. He had blackouts, benders, morning drinking, severe withdrawal symptoms including DTs, an accident while driving drunk, and arrests for disturbing the peace. He was fired "many times." At least some of these were alcohol related. His binges were at home:

he tended to withdraw from others when drinking and not be seen outside of the house for weeks at a time. He felt guilty about his drinking and thought he drank too much, as did his family. He also abused medications, particularly sedatives. He had serious medical problems aggravated by drinking and had been told several years before he died that he had hepatic cirrhosis and would die in 6 months.

He had been abstinent for about a year at some point, but thereafter was unable to control his drinking. He underwent a personality change when drinking, becoming moody, high-strung, sensitive, easily moved to tears, and given to outbursts of rage and fights with family members. During the last 5 years of his life he was hospitalized for alcoholism and medical problems approximately 10 times, without effect on his drinking pattern. On one hospitalization, a diagnosis of organic brain syndrome was made because of evidence of memory impairment and confabulation. He was said to have been drinking even more heavily than usual during the last 1–2 months of his life.

He was preoccupied with his health, which had been poor for at least 10 years. Social withdrawal also characterized his last years. There is no indication that he ever received any formal psychiatric treatment or that he was given any medication other than sedatives. He appeared to the informant to have had low mood and sadness for an unspecified length of time. Other depressive symptoms reported included anorexia, fatigue, low self-esteem and disgust with himself, and a loss of interest. This last symptom was present for about 5 years. Insomnia was denied, but he regularly took prescription medication for sleep. His anorexia was episodic and related to drinking. He was obese and his weight tended to fluctuate downward with his bouts of heavy drinking.

He had diabetes mellitus, which was poorly controlled. He had had several toes amputated as a result of diabetic vasculopathy. He had recurrent staphylococcal infections, a rectal fistula, and diabetic leg ulcers, leading to multiple hospitalizations. A diagnosis of alcoholic cirrhosis had been confirmed by liver biopsy. Just before his death his family was trying to get him to enter the hospital again but he refused.

There was no family history of suicide, attempted suicide, alcoholism or drug abuse, and the only relative with any reported emotional problems was a sister who became "nervous" after the death of her 7-year-old son.

He never mentioned suicide and did not communicate in any way that was suggestive of suicidal preoccupation. His family was surprised by the act and one informant did not believe that he intended to kill himself.

Circumstances Leading to the Act

He was living alone for the last 2 months of his life, having driven his mother out of the house. Neighbors said he was drinking more heavily than ever at the approach of the Christmas season, and keeping very much to himself. His mother was vacationing in Florida since he drove her away. He had told his sisters he wanted to be alone and didn't want them to phone or visit. That was not unusual for him. He was seen last by a sister and brother-in-law on Christmas day, when they stopped to leave presents for him. He was so drunk he couldn't get out of bed. An in-law of the informant died the same day and the family was preoccupied with that until 3 days after Christmas. When the family became concerned at failure of repeated attempts to reach him by telephone, his brother-in-law entered the house and found him lying in bed, in his underwear, dead of a gunshot wound of the head. The house was filled with "an unbearable odor," suggesting that he had been dead for 2–3 days. There is no suggestion that the in-law's death was known to the subject or had any influence on him. There were many empty liquor bottles around the house. The .38-caliber revolver with which he had shot himself was lying on the floor beside the bed. No note was found.

Findings and Sources

Clinical Diagnosis: (1) Alcoholism, chronic; (2) secondary depression; (3) probable mild alcoholic dementia; (4) diabetes mellitus; (5) hepatic cirrhosis.
Toxicology: No toxicologic analysis was performed.
Primary Informant: Sister who saw him several times a week and spoke with him daily.
Other Sources of Information: Police investigation report; coroner's investigation report. (His internist refused permission to release hospital records without his mother's signature. She was unavailable and had not been informed of the manner of his death.)
Informant's Opinion of Reason for Suicide: "He was disgusted with himself. He couldn't face responsibility."

Comment

An alcoholic of nearly 30 years standing, this man had accumulated most of the negative consequences of this behavior that we systematically look at. He had serious health problems, most importantly those secondary to diabetes. Despite being fired several times on account of his drinking, he was thought to still be drawing $500 a week from the reputedly hoodlum-ridden Pipefitter's Union. He was reported to have had most of the symptoms of a depressive syndrome for about the last 5 years of his life, perhaps worse toward the end. He had driven his sister away with his ugly behavior, then his mother, so that he was living alone for the last 2 months of his life. He drank more and more, never spoke of suicide, but did himself in without warning. Depressed, living alone, and sick, with some degree of alcoholic dementia—all of these factors likely played a role in his demise. His mother's departure, 2 months before his death, does not qualify as a loss within 6 weeks.

Case 3

Subject 3 was a 35-year old white married Baptist male, born in St. Louis. His father was a grocery store butcher; his mother, a housewife who sold cosmetics door-to-door part time. The parental home was intact. The whole family was described by the informant as "excessively nervous, high strung, and easily angered." He graduated from high school, served 4 years in the Air Force between the ages of 18 and 22, had no disciplinary actions, and received an honorable discharge. He was married at the age of 19 while in military service and had three children, sons aged 14 and 4 years and a daughter aged 13 years at the time of his death.

Upon leaving military service, he obtained the best paying job he ever had, as a bread salesman. He started drinking at about that time (age 23), at first because he liked it and later because he felt it helped him to maintain his long hours as a bread salesman. He rapidly attained a daily consumption of a fifth of hard liquor. Within 3–4 years of his beginning drinking, his family was becoming impoverished because of the money he spent on drink. He was fired at the age of 27 because of drinking. As a consequence, he also lost the house he had been purchasing. He continued to drink heavily, while working as an insurance salesman. After about 2 years, he was involved in an automobile accident while drunk and was hospitalized for 6 months in a Veterans Administration hospital for treatment of his alcoholism. He resumed drinking shortly after his release. His last job was clerical and the second best paying job he ever had. He had held it for 6 years until his death. Five months before his took his life, he and his family had moved to better housing than they had previously occupied.

He had a second psychiatric hospitalization for alcoholism at age 32. He had about 10 arrests related to drinking, all in the last 3 years of his life. These were for traffic violations, fighting, disturbing the peace, and drunkenness. About 2 years before his demise, his drinking pattern shifted from daily to episodic. He would drink heavily the first 2 weeks of the month, then stop for the last 2 weeks because of lack of money. He was reported to have had hallucinations when drunk during the last year to 18 months of his life. Fifteen months before his death, he was drunk while attending a job-related refresher course. He was suspended for a week and put on probation for 6 months.

About six months before his suicide his tolerance for alcohol appeared to decrease. Around that time he joined AA, saw a psychiatrist periodically, and took disulfiram (Antabuse). He must not have been consistently abstinent, however, as he suffered an epileptic seizure 4 months before his death. He was hospitalized for 10 days and was prescribed phenytoin (Dilantin) and phenobarbital as prophylaxis against further seizures. His supervisor said that "he just wasn't what he used to be" after his seizure. His last visit to the psychiatrist was 5 weeks before his suicide. He stopped taking disulfiram and resumed drinking episodically in relation to his pay periods. When sober, he was described as courteous and kind; when drunk, he was both physically and verbally abusive for the last two years of his life. As a result, the marital relationship was severely strained. He displayed this aggressiveness not only toward his family, but to strangers as well. He had only one close friend and his only social life was in taverns.

There is no indication of early episodes of depression. About 7 months before his suicide, he became depressed, slashed his arm with a razor blade, and was briefly admitted to a psychiatric hospital. Within a month, he repeated that act and was again briefly hospitalized. On both admissions he was described as depressed. It is not known whether he received any antidepressant medication, as hospital records were not obtained. His wife failed to sign the necessary releases. Following his epileptic seizure, he looked depressed and sad, experienced a 20-pound weight loss, complained of fatigue, expressed guilt feelings repeatedly, was indecisive and lost social and general interest. While he had been impotent for about 18 months, he lost interest in sex only in the last 4 months. He had complained of insomnia throughout his adult life, and it is not known if there had been a recent change. A diagnosis of secondary affective disorder is justified on the basis of these symptoms.

In the grand mal convulsive seizure he experienced about 4 months before his death, he fell hard and hurt his head. Neurological workup in the City Hospital turned up no specific findings. Whether he took the prescribed phenytoin and phenobarbital was not known, but he had no further seizures. Thereafter, he seemed not to have been himself, complaining of headaches, dizziness, fatigue, diplopia, and poor memory. He said he felt like he was losing his mind. He had no other known chronic or severe medical illnesses.

There was no family history of suicide, suicide attempt, alcoholism, or psychiatric illness.

For about the last year of his life, at times when he was drunk, he spoke of killing himself. Over the last 7 months, he had said several times to his wife that he thought she and the family would be better off if he were dead. He said it only when he was drunk. When sober, he said he didn't want to die.

Circumstances Leading to the Act

During the last 2 years of his life, he had become aggressive, used foul language, and complained that his family and friends didn't like him. He was at times physically abusive when drunk. When he became abusive, his wife would leave with the children for a few hours or overnight. She had never previously left for longer periods. He became depressed about 7 months before his death and made two suicide attempts. His depression worsened considerably in the last 4 months, following the epileptic seizure. Thirty-six hours before his suicide, because he was drunk and abusive to the family, his wife took their children to a relative's home, called police, and went with them to try to talk him into going to a psychiatric hospital. He talked them out of it and stayed at home alone while his wife stayed with the children. He talked with his aunt and with his psychiatrist by telephone on the day his wife left and on the day of his suicide, but he is not known to have mentioned suicide. The second morning after leaving, his wife returned with the children to fetch some school clothes and to again urge him to accept hospitalization. She found him dead of exsanguination, having slashed his left arm, opposite the elbow, with a razor blade. He did not leave a note.

His wife had not specifically told him of her intent to separate from him but had never been away from him so long before. *She told the death investigator that she was not intending to return to live with him.*

Findings and Sources

Clinical Diagnosis: (1) Alcoholism, chronic. (2) secondary affective disorder.
Toxicology: Blood alcohol concentration 0.09 g%.
Primary Informant: Spouse, who had known him and lived with him for at least 16 years.
Other Sources of Information: Attending psychiatrist, coroner's death investigation report.
Informant's Opinion of Reason for Suicide: (1) Unable to control drinking; (2) felt family, including children, had turned against him; (3) depressed because he'd spent all of his money, depriving family.

Comment

Twelve years of progressive worsening of his alcoholism led to his becoming physically abusive of his wife in the last 2 years. Within the last year he became clinically depressed for the first time. His wife had left him for a few hours or overnight on a number of occasions when he was abusive. What was different on the last occasion, 36 hours before she found him dead, was that this time she did not intend to return to him. Although she said she had not specifically told him this, the likelihood is great that she had somehow communicated her intent. He had one close friend and his only social life was in taverns. I counted this as a case of recent loss of a close interpersonal relationship because of his wife's leaving and her admitted intent to separate.

Case 4

Subject 4 was a 52-year old, white, married male of no professed religion. He was born and raised in Chicago and lived in St. Louis the last 28 years of his life. His father was a carpet layer and an alcoholic. His mother's occupation, if any, was not learned. His parents separated and were divorced when he was 8 years old. Who raised him after that was not learned, but in later years he was said to have "hated the sight of" his mother. He completed the 10th grade in school. He was first married at the age of 21 and divorced 2 years later, allegedly because his wife was unfaithful. He married a second time at age 24 and remained married to and living with his second wife until the time of his death. They had four daughters of whom the oldest was killed in an automobile accident when she was 14 years of age. The others were age 21, 15, and 13 at the time of his death. He served 4 years in military service during World War II and 4 months during the Korean War without being exposed to combat. He had no disciplinary actions and received honorable discharges.

He held a job as a paint foreman full-time for the last 28 years of his life. That job was never in danger as far as is known. He had been fired by a previous employer for sleeping on the job. Seven months before his death he needed extra money in order to purchase a new car. He asked his employer for extra work and was refused. He found a part-time job working 3 nights a week in a service station, where he regularly consumed a 6-pack of beer during his shift. His social life was confined to on-the-job contacts and bar or tavern visits.

He was already a heavy drinker at the age of 24 when he married his second wife, 28 years before his suicide. Although he promised her he would stop drinking if she married him, he claimed inability to do so. He regularly drank a half-case of beer a day, increasing to a case per day when he was feeling depressed or upset. Since his wife would not let him drink at home, he did his drinking in taverns and outside. Whether he increased his consumption shortly before his death is not known. He thought he drank too much but gave no evidence of feeling guilty about it. He experienced morning tremulousness but no other physical symptoms were reported.

Eleven years prior to his suicide, he had a head-on automobile collision while drinking. His eldest daughter was killed. The other two daughters in the car were less seriously injured. From that time on, his wife called him "murderer." Two to three weeks before his suicide, again while drinking, he was the driver in a hit-and-run accident. He had been charged with this offense. Following that accident, he said he would stop drinking, but "couldn't."

He had been a transvestite since before marrying his second wife. She would not allow him to cross-dress at home, but he sometimes wore women's garments under his clothes at work. He had periods of low mood, believed to have antedated the second marriage. These episodes were variable in duration and severity but became worse 11 years before his death, shortly before the automobile accident in which his daughter was killed. For about the last year of his life, he had exhibited anorexia, insomnia, indecisiveness, a general loss of interest, and was continuously sad. No change was noted in his customarily low interest in sex. He had complained of failing memory and feelings of worthlessness for about 3 years.

He saw a psychiatrist once, about 2½ weeks before his death, at his wife's insistence. She cited marital difficulties occasioned by his drinking, depression, and transvestism. What leverage she may have used to bring about this consultation and its outcome was not learned. His part-time employer thought he seemed more depressed after that, but it was also the period following his hit-and-run accident.

This subject had annual physical examinations by the company physician, with no abnormal findings. Several years before his death, he had seen an internist, who gave him "pep pills." He continued to take these, but neither the amount nor the frequency is known. His only other known medical attention was after the automobile accident in which his daughter was killed. He was hospitalized with multiple rib fractures, a lacerated lung, and other lacerations and contusions. At that time he gave a history of a cervical fracture 3 years earlier. No further details were obtained.

His father and a paternal uncle were described as alcoholic. No other family history of psychiatric illness was obtained. Suicide and suicide attempt were denied.

About 30 years before he took his life, he had jumped in the river after having been fired for sleeping on the job. He spoke with a friend about his suicidal thoughts at that time, and had talked intermittently of wanting to die since then. He had spoken directly to his wife of suicide off and on for 10 or more years. For about 5 years, he had periodically said he would be better off dead and that the family would be better off if he were dead. To his part-time employer of the last 7 months of his life, he had said on several occasions, "I don't see why I keep on living." No change in frequency or pattern of these communications was reported.

Circumstances Leading to the Act

Following the automobile collision in which their daughter was killed, his previously sweet wife became bitter toward him and repeatedly called him a murderer. "She never let him forget it." This unpleasant relationship continued for 11 years until his death. For the last 3 years he had said (with probable justification) that his wife hated him. Three months before he ended his life his mother died. He reportedly "hated the sight of her." At that time, he and his father had a verbal argument over the subject's refusal to visit him. The nature of their relationship was not further described. About the time he was involved in a hit-and-run accident, he learned that his oldest daughter, who was in college, was pregnant out of wedlock. He was much upset by that news. He was concerned about his children's college education and had set up a trust fund for each of them to secure it.

On the night of his suicide he reported to work at his part-time job as usual. At 10:55 p.m., he telephoned his wife and told her where their car was parked, then hung up. He was found the next morning in the garage of the service station, where one automobile's engine was still running and another was "on" and out of gasoline. He was to have been in court the following morning on the hit-and-run charge.

He left a suicide note saying "Virginia—thanks for nothing." [first name signed].

Findings and Sources

Clinical Diagnoses: (1) Alcoholism, chronic; (2) major depressive disorder, uncertain if primary or secondary; (3) transvestism.
Toxicology: Blood alcohol concentration 0.020 g %. Blood CO saturation 75%.
Primary Informant: Wife, married 28 years; saw him daily.
Other Sources of Information: Employer on part-time job, coroner's death investigation report, hospital records.
Informant's Opinion of Reason for Suicide: (1) Anxiety about his transvestism; (2) periodic low mood; (3) prospect of court appearance.

Comment

This man's home life was dominated by an angry and vindictive wife. Her refusal to allow him to drink at home or to cross-dress are perhaps within normal limits. However, she never let him forget that he was driving under the influence of alcohol 11 years earlier, when their daughter was killed. She repeatedly called him a murderer. He was devoted to his daughters, and the recent news of the out-of-wedlock pregnancy of one of them can only have increased his distress. He had episodic depressions that had begun before his second marriage. Whether depression antedated his alcoholism or the reverse is unknown. His drinking increased when he was depressed, as he was shortly before his daughter was killed. He was also in an episode of depression of about a year's duration when he killed himself. He was to go to court on a hit-and-run vehicular accident charge on the day after his body was found. His bitter note to his wife attests to the hostility he lived with. Beyond that, he was substantially without friends. Depression, shame, and the prospect of jail seem to have been more than he could tolerate.

Case 11

Subject 11 was a 50-year-old white married Protestant male, born and raised in Missouri. His father, a railroad worker, was alcoholic most of his life, but the parental home remained intact. With no siblings, he was "coddled" as a child and allowed to do as he pleased. In his mother's eyes he could do no wrong. He had no school problems, was popular at school, and was elected class president. Following graduation from high school he worked first driving an oil delivery truck, then as a grocery store clerk. He was employed as a railroad switchman for the last 27 years of his life. He married at 22, with his mother disapproving of the marriage. She continued her disapproval throughout the marriage. They had three children, daughters aged 27 and 19, and a son aged 17 years when he died. In the marriage, he never admitted he was wrong. He served in the military occupation of Japan for 18 months and received an honorable discharge, then returned to his switchman's job.

He started to drink heavily at age 24. There was a 3-week marital separation when he was 31, nine years into the marriage, because of his drinking. He was reported to have first lost control at the age of 41, the year of his first hospitalization for alcoholism. He was subsequently hospitalized at least five times. He stopped drinking altogether about 4 years prior to his suicide with the help of AA. This change was precipitated by his wife leaving him. She returned to him in 2 weeks. After 2 years of sobriety, he resumed his bibulous ways for unknown reasons. About a year before his death he accepted hospitalization for treatment after his two younger children confronted him with their intention to leave home if he did not stop drinking. His sobriety didn't last, however, and he resumed drinking daily. He had been arrested several times over a period of 20 years for disturbing the peace, as a consequence of assaulting his wife when drunk. Following the last such fracas, 3 weeks before his suicide, she caused a peace bond to be issued. One week later they separated by mutual consent and he moved to a motel.

He thought he drank too much but was not known to have felt guilty about his inability to control it. His wife and others objected to his drinking and he lost friends because of it. He experienced blackouts, tremulousness, seizures, and DTs. He sometimes drank before breakfast and went on benders. For 3–4 years he had been rather preoccupied with his inability to perform sexually. He had previously regarded sex as the most important part of marriage. In his last year his memory deteriorated. He would forget where he put the car and leave his things at work. Sometime in the last year, he was warned at work to stop drinking or be fired. The subject's wife said that he was a different person when he drank. When sober he was considerate, had different friends, and a social life. He was involved in Boy Scouts and church functions. When drunk and sobering, he was depressed and hostile, and his associates were other barflies.

He, like many others in this study, was described as "high strung" all his life. He was known to have had outbursts of rage from his early 20s, probably antedating his alcohol problems. During a hospitalization 4 months before his death, he was diagnosed as suffering from a "depressive reaction" as well as chronic alcoholism. In the last few months of his life he lost interest in things, was joyless, was generally less active, looked depressed, and performed poorly on his job. He expressed feelings of worthlessness and complained of fatigue. During that time, he continued to talk of suicide. He had always been indecisive, and it is not known whether that worsened. Insomnia had been an intermittent problem for years. For about a year he had been slower in his movements and his memory had deteriorated noticeably. He clearly met criteria for a major depressive episode. He may have had an early alcoholic dementia as well. On his last two hospitalizations he was noted to have an enlarged liver. He had no other known major illness.

His father was alcoholic most of his life. Family history of suicide or suicide attempt was denied.

From almost the beginning of the marriage he intermittently told his wife that he would kill himself. She regarded this as a ploy to get his own way. His threats of suicide were more pronounced when he was "drying out." For 10 years he had said on these occasions that both he and the family would be better off if he were dead. Five years before his suicide he was observed by neighbors to be sitting in his car holding a gun. The police were called and took the gun away. He spoke repeatedly of wanting to die in the last 15 months.

Circumstances of the Act

In the last 6 months he had gradually become depressed and lost interest in things generally. During a hospitalization for alcoholism 4 months before his death, "depressive reaction" was diagnosed. Two weeks before he took his life, his wife asked him to leave their home because of his continued drinking and unpleasant behavior. He moved into a motel. On the day of his suicide, he took a taxi from his motel to his home and shot himself outside the home with a 20-gauge shotgun he had purchased that afternoon. There was no one home at the time. His wife was in a hospital for reasons and duration that were not learned. The children were staying with a neighbor. His son stopped by the house later that same day to check on the family animals on the way to visit his mother in the hospital. He found his father dead. No suicide note was found.

Findings and Sources

Clinical Diagnosis: (1) Alcoholism, chronic; (2) major depressive disorder secondary to alcoholism; (3) possible early alcoholic dementia.
Toxicology: Blood alcohol concentration, 0.35 g%.
Primary Informant: Spouse, married 28 years, had known subject about 33 years, saw him daily until last 2 weeks.
Other Informants: Coroner's death investigation report, hospital records.
Informant's Opinion of Reason for Suicide: (1) Inability to control drinking which caused family disruption; (2) threatened with firing.

Comment

In his long drinking career, this subject incurred all but a very few of the negative consequences of drinking that constitute our criteria for the diagnosis of alcoholism. His physical abuse of his wife resulted in two marital separations, one at age 31 and one 2 weeks before his suicide. The interviewer in this case did not record much detail about the circumstances of the final separation. Was divorce threatened? Was the separation to be permanent? We don't know.

His wife had had a peace bond issued a week before the separation, after a fight in which he beat her. The reason for her being in a hospital at the time of his death was not recorded. Given the time sequence, it seems unlikely to have been a result of his abuse. Although he had been threatened with firing from his job, there was no history of action on the matter. He had developed a clear-cut depression in the last few months, perhaps for the first time in his life. He had been drinking heavily and steadily for a year or more, and as a consequence he had no social support system other than tavern companions. The marital separation, occurring in the context of a major depressive episode, appears to have been the crucial factor. He is numbered among those with recent loss of a close relationship.

Case 31

Subject 31 was a divorced white male attorney who had been unable to work for 8 years at the time of his suicide by gunshot wound at age 57. He was born in Missouri and lived in the state most of his life. His father was an alcoholic construction worker who divorced his wife when the subject was 8 years old and died a short time later, cause unreported. He was nominally Roman Catholic. He was raised by his mother and his aunt, who had been after him for years to return to the church. His mother worked as a legal secretary until she died as a result of burns sustained in an apartment fire when he was 52. He had progressed through law school without difficulties, and graduated at age 23. He practiced law for about 7 years until World War II, then entered the Army for 2 years. He served overseas, was decorated, and was honorably discharged as a lieutenant.

He had excellent opportunities as an attorney in New York and Chicago after leaving military service but his mother and aunt "staged scenes" to dissuade him from leaving. They frustrated any attempts at independence. "They ran his life. He wasn't man enough to defy them." He worked in a specialized field of law but had performance problems due to drinking, was fired frequently, and finally was unable to obtain any type of legal job. He tried unsuccessfully to sell insurance. For the last 8 years of his life, he was unemployable, had no money, and depended on his mother and subsequently his aunt for handouts. He had few friends. He was described as high-strung, avoiding crowds, and moody. He never showed any outbursts of emotion, and was "always a gentleman, drunk or sober."

He married during the war but was divorced 3 years later and never remarried. The marriage was childless and he considered it "cold." His mother and aunt "wrecked it." For the remainder of his life he lived with these two women until his mother's death 5 years before his, and then with his aunt, who became progressively senile and deaf. They were living in a one-room efficiency apartment at the time of his death. Two months before he died his aunt became ill and reportedly was given "2 months to live." She was hospitalized in a terminal state 2 weeks before his suicide, leaving him alone in the apartment.

A hospital record notes that he reported he was an alcoholic by age 24, about the time he graduated from law school. He did not experience loss of control until he was 43. He became a daily drinker of at least a pint of liquor with periodic overnight binges. His mother and aunt strongly objected, so he never drank in the home, but hid bottles and drank outside the building or disappeared overnight to drink. For the last 8 years of his life, he was unemployable secondary to organic mental changes. Psychological testing on hospitalization 7 years before his death showed "definite organicity." Two years later he was noted to confabulate. In the last year he had problems with simple arithmetic and comprehension. He had withdrawal seizures on two occasions, 9 and 5 years before his death, had had DTs and more frequently, shakes, nausea, and vomiting. In a sense, he drank before breakfast, in that he never ate breakfast.

He was hospitalized for treatment of alcoholism at age 45 and again at about age 49 in a private hospital. After that, he remained sober for nearly 2 years. During that hiatus he had a girlfriend. He then relapsed and had three admissions to a public hospital within a 2-year period, but he continued to drink. He had no legal problems. During the last 2 weeks of his life, with his aunt hospitalized, he drank at home. At the time of his first public hospital admission 7 years before his suicide, he reported that he had been using elixir of terpin hydrate with codeine daily for 2 years. He also was a regular sedative user. Despite the informant's belief that this behavior continued, no medication bottles of any sort were found after his death.

His depressive symptoms appear to have been of many years' duration but worse in the last 3 years of his life. He did not receive treatment for any condition other than his alcoholism. He was anorexic, lost considerable weight, and had chronic insomnia with nightly sedative use, anhedonia, loss of interest in everything but reading, low energy, and indecision. He had had gastroenteritis related to his alcoholism, and one hospital record noted early emphysematous changes in the lungs and recurrent urinary tract infections, but his health was generally adequate. His only medical hospitalizations were for a hemorrhoidectomy and bilateral inguinal herniorrhaphy. He had not seen a physician on any regular basis during the last few years of his life, and it is not known how he obtained sedatives.

His father was alcoholic but there was no other alcoholism known in the family. A maternal aunt was described as "hysteric" but there seems to be no history of mental illness requiring hospitalization.

He mentioned suicide on only 2 known occasions, about 2 weeks before his death and once several months earlier. He said he would be better off dead. When his aunt was hospitalized, he said if he had a .38 he would shoot himself.

Circumstances Leading to the Act

He had been alone for the 2 weeks since his aunt was hospitalized, terminally ill. He began drinking at home for the first time, since no one was there to object, and became more despondent. He obtained a .38-caliber revolver and shot himself in the bathtub. A family friend (the primary informant) had been talking to him on the telephone daily, and after being unable to reach him for 4 days, she had the apartment checked. He was found having been dead for several days. There was no suicide note, but notes found around the apartment begged his aunt to turn the radio down so he could sleep. (She was quite deaf.)

Findings and Sources

Clinical Diagnosis: (1) Alcoholism; (2) alcoholic dementia; (3) secondary depression versus organic mood syndrome, depressed.
Toxicology: No analysis performed.
Primary Informant: A long-time friend of the family who saw him every 2–3 weeks.
Other Sources of Information: Hospital records, coroner's death investigation report.
Informant's Opinion of Reason for Suicide: (1) "He wasn't allowed to live his own life"; (2) "he was unhappy."

Comment

This unfortunate man's life was entirely dominated by his mother and his aunt. They made virtually all of his decisions for him, except about drinking. He rebelled twice, once by marrying over their objections and later by having a girlfriend for 2 years. His promising career in the law was blighted by these women's determination to keep him at home. Alcohol was his principal sedative, although he abused elixir of terpin hydrate with codeine, and perhaps other sedative drugs as well.

He wasn't allowed to drink in the home, so he drank surreptitiously outside and in the garage. He was not a barfly and seemingly had no companions. His drinking damaged his brain—there had been clear evidence of it for at least 7 years—and he was unable to take care of himself. He was depressed as well. He was unemployable and totally dependent on his senile aunt for sustenance. This must have been a miserable existence, as she was extremely deaf. There cannot have been much communication—or much love between them. When she was taken to the hospital with terminal cancer he spoke of suicide. He lived alone for 2 weeks, then bought a pistol and shot himself in the head. He had been rendered totally helpless, first by maternal domination, later by his alcoholic dementia. Lacking both the experience and the mental capacity for self-care, he had no other choice than to end his blighted life. I counted loss of his aunt among recent loss cases because she was gone and he was alone, and he had been told not to expect her to survive. (She didn't.)

DISCUSSION

Early onset is one of the characteristic features of alcoholism in males. This first grouping was chosen to highlight that phenomenon. The range of survival time of these early-onset alcoholics *as alcoholics* until their suicide is surprisingly wide—from 9 to 51 years, with a mean of 24.8 ± 9.4 years. Mean age at death was 45.6 ± 8.99 years.

A familial aspect of alcoholism has been recognized since antiquity (Goodwin, 1979). Carrying the matter a step further, based on his Danish adoption study, Goodwin observed that individual cases of alcoholism may be classified as either familial or nonfamilial. The familial type is characterized by a family history of severe alcoholism, an early onset, and a severe course.

Cross-fostering studies have contributed further to our understanding of both genetic and environmental influences on the disorder (Boman, Sigvardsson, & Cloninger, 1981; Cloninger, Boman, & Sigvardsson, 1981). Such studies capitalize on the extensive and careful parish registries of the Scandinavian countries that go back more than 100 years. From these, it has been possible to identify individuals of both alcoholic and nonalcoholic parentage who have been adopted into nonrelated families very early in life. By tracing these individuals' records into adulthood, the outcome regarding alcoholism in those with and without an alcoholic natural parent, raised by either non-alcoholic or alcoholic adoptive parents, has been learned. Large numbers of these unplanned experiments have been found.

Table 4.1 Background Characteristics: Men with Onset Before Age 25, by Age of Onset

Patient Number	Age at Suicide	Parental Home[a]	Family History	Education yr	Civil State
46	37	intact	paternal grandmother: PH when elderly	12	s
28	52	father: deserted (12 yo)	NI	12	m
30	41	father: frequently absent; subject: orphanage (3–9 yo)	father: alcoholic; 2 sisters, 2 brothers: alcoholic or heavy drinkers	6	div
12	69	NI	NI	DK	m
26	48	intact	father, mother: alcoholic; 2 brothers, 3 sisters: alcoholic	14	m
27	42	mother: died (birth); father: died (12 yo)	father: heavy drinker; sister: NBD	8	sep
29	46	father: suicide (6 yo) stepfather	father: alcoholic, suicide; sister: drinker?; sister: depressed, ECT paternal uncle: NBD?	10	m
34	45	intact	negative	14	m
24	37	intact	father: manic episodes; brother, paternal grandfather: alcoholic; paternal uncle: mood swings	16	sep 2-1/2 mo
9	48	mother: died (6 mo) grandmother, aunt: raised subject	father: heavy drinker	9	m
13	29	intact	father: depressed	13	s
37	50	intact	maternal uncle: alcoholic	15	m
2	54	intact	father: alcoholic	9	m
15	44	intact	brother: alcoholic, suicide	8	m
18	35	intact	maternal aunt: heavy drinker	11	s
19	35	intact	negative	7	sep 3 yr
21	47	intact	father, grandfather, 2 uncles: alcoholic	10	div 8 mo
33	50	intact	sister: "nervous" after 7 yo son died	10 or 11	s
3	35	intact	negative	12	m
4	52	sep/div (8yr)	father, paternal uncle: alcoholic	10	m
11	50	intact	father: alcoholic	12	sep 2 wk
31	57	parents div (8 yo)	father: alcoholic; maternal aunt: "hysteric"	18	div

Key: 0 = none; apt = apartment, div = divorced; DK = don't know; ECT = electroconvulsive therapy; m = married; mo = month(s); NBD = nervous breakdown: NI = no information; PH = psychiatric hospital; s = single; sep = separated; wk = week(s); yo = years old; yr = year(s).

[a]Age given in parentheses is that of the subject at the time of the occurrence.

Number of Marriages/ Duration (yr)	Age and Sex of Progeny	Living Circumstances	Drinking Locale	Social Support
0	0	parents	home	some
5/2, 1, 1, 8, 8	0	wife, stepson	home	0
1/17	17♂, 15♂, 13♀, 10♀, 4♂	*alone* 13 mo	taverns	0
2/19, 17-1/2	0	wife	with friends, home	0 lost 1, 1 wk
1/28	26♀, 24♀, 23♂, 21♀, 12♂	wife 3 children	home, auto	0
1/14	0	*alone*	taverns	taverns
2/1, 1, yr	0	wife, stepdaughter	home	almost 0
3/7, 7, 6	died at 8♂, 19♂, 12♂	wife, stepson	tavern, home, office	presumably good
1/12	11♀, 9♂	*alone* 2½ mo	bar/tavern	tavern
2/7, 6	19♂	wife	bars	angry with spouse, tavern, friend
0	0	*alone* 2 yr	bars, apt	0, 1 wk
1/27	21♀, 17♂	wife, son	home	wife, son; possibly OK
1/33	25♀	wife	on job, home	work only, wife ±
1/23	21♂, 17♂, 7♂, 3♀	wife, 3 children	home, bar/tavern	bar/tavern, family distant
0	0	*alone* 3 wk	tavern, 1 friend	0, 3 wk except tavern
1/15	15♀, 12♂	*alone* 1 day	bar/tavern	tavern
2/7, 15	22♀, 15♂ 13♂, 6♂	*alone* 13 mo	taverns	0
0	0	*alone* 2 mo	home, bars	bars only
1/14	14♂, 13♀ 4♂	*alone* 2 days	bar/tavern, home	tavern, abused wife
2/2, 28	died at 14♀, 21♀ 15♀, 13♀	wife, 2 minor children	job, tavern	tavern, co-workers, abused wife
1/27	27♀, 19♀, 17♂	*alone* motel	tavern,	tavern
1/3	0	*alone* 2 wk	alone	0

Table 4.2 Alcohol-Related History: Men with Onset Before Age 25, by Age of Onset

Patient Number	Age at Suicide	Drink Onset/ Duration (yr)	Fights[a]	Arrests[b]	Abusive[c]	Serious Health Problems[d]
46	37	15/22	0	P	0	cirrhosis, dementia
28	52	16/36	+	V	P	diabetes
30	41	17/24	A	F	P	DU, TB
12	69	18/51	0	0	0	[0, thought stomach cancer]
26	48	18/30	A	F, P, V	P	pneumoconiosis, cirrhosis
27	42	18/24	+	0	P	[DK, thought leukemia]
29	46	18/28	+	V	H	0
34	45	20/25	0	0	P+	diabetes
24	37	19/18	+	V	P	0
9	48	20/28	A	F	P	[0, thought throat cancer]
13	29	20/9	0	0	0	DU
37	50	20/30	0	0	0	0
2	54	21/33	0	V	0	cirrhosis, seizure disorder [gout]
15	44	21/23	+	0	P	cirrhosis
18	35	23/12	0	0	0	0
19	35	23/12	+	0	P	liver
21	47	23/24	+	V	P	[rheumatoid arthritis]
33	50	23/27	A (V)	F	V	diabetes, PVD, cirrhosis
3	35	24/11	A	F	P	seizure disorder
4	52	<24/28+	0	V	abused	0
11	50	24/26	A	F	P	cirrhosis, mild dementia
31	57	24/33	0	0	0	dementia

[a]A = arrest; + indicates fights without arrests; 0 = none.
[b]P = peace disturbance; V = vehicular offense; F = fighting; 0 = none.
[c]P = physical; V = verbal; 0 = none.
[d]DK = don't know; DU = duodenal ulcer; PVD = peripheral vascular disease; TB = pulmonary tuberculosis; 0 = none.
[e]ECT = electroconvulsive therapy; MAD = major affective disorder; S/A = suicide attempt; 0 = none.
[f]0 = none, 1° = primary; 2° = secondary; AD = affective disorder; BAD = bipolar affective disorder; MAD = major affective disorder; prob = probable.

Last Hospital Treatment[e]	Employment	Other Diagnoses[f]	Other Substance Abuse	Suicide Attempts
7 mo, head trauma, DTs	unemployed 10 mo	prob 2° AD	narcotics	0
1 yr, burns, DTs	employed 0 × 3 wk	2° AD	past only	+
2 mo, TB	unemployed × 10 mo	2° AD	0	+ several
6 yr, not alcoholism	retired 6 yr	0	0	0
5 mo, asthma	unemployed	0	cough syrup	0
5 yr, medical	employed 0 × 1 day	prob 2° AD	0	+(2)
1 mo, DTs	employed 0 × 10 day	0	amphetamines	+(3)
2 yr, seizure	employed (self)	2° AD	prescriptions only	+
4 mo, "anxiety"	employed	BAD	0	0
21 yr, "malaria"	employed	0	elixir terpine hydrate	0
6 mo, S/A	employed 0 × 1 wk	prob 2° AD	0	+(3)
0	unemployed 3 mo	prob 2° AD	prescriptions only	0
8 mo, gastritis	employed 0 × 1 day	2° AD	0	0
3 wk, MAD-ECT	employed 0 × 4 mo	2° AD	0	0
0	unemployed 3 mo	0	0	0
18 mo, gastritis	employed 0 × 1 day	0	"nerve pills" in past	0
19 days, depression	part time	prob 2° AD	chlordiazepoxide prescriptions	+
<1 yr, diabetes	unemployed 1 yr	2° AD	sedatives	0
4 mo, seizure	prob not but DK	2° AD	Librium	+(2)
0	employed	MAD 1° vs. 2° AD	"pep pill"	+
4 mo, alcoholism, depression	employed abs × ?	2° AD	0	threat
5 yr, alcoholism	unemployed × 8 yr	2° AD	elixir terpine hydrate, sed	0

97

Type 2 versus Type 1 Alcoholics

Based on the study of those "experiments," Cloninger (1987) has proposed that early onset alcoholism—that is, in the teens and early 20's—is more characteristic of males than of females and exhibits certain distinctive features. Among them are an alcoholic father, spontaneous alcohol seeking (daily drinking), greater likelihood of fighting, arrests for fighting, and vehicular offenses, and likelihood of serious health problems. Cloninger referred to this as Type 2, or "male pattern alcoholism." Adolescent onset, severe alcohol problems, extensive treatment and criminal activity in the *fathers* were found to be associated with Type 2 alcoholism in the sons. This both supports and extends Goodwin's concept of familial alcoholism (Goodwin, 1979). The adopted away offspring of such fathers had an equally elevated rate of developing alcoholism whether they had been raised by drinking or nondrinking adoptive parents. Personality characteristics said to be typical of Type 2 alcoholics include high novelty–seeking behaviors (impulsive, exploratory), low harm avoidance (considerable risk taking) and low reward dependence (lack of concern for the approval of others) (Cloninger, 1987).[2]

Cloninger's Type 1 alcoholic has onset after age 25 and exhibits loss of control (benders and inability to stop drinking appear to bear on this issue) and guilt and fear about alcohol dependence (guilt about drinking). Inability to abstain (daily drinking) is said to be infrequent, as is a history of fighting and arrests. Type 1 alcoholics are characterized as "milieu–limited," because the rather low risk of developing the clinical syndrome is doubled when the adopted-away individual with an alcoholic biological parent is exposed to alcohol abuse in the cross-fostering parents (an alcoholic milieu). Adult onset alcoholism in either father or mother, little treatment, and no criminality were characteristic of the biological background of Type 1 alcoholics. They are described as anxious, with low impulsivity, high harm avoidance and high reward dependence—in other words, passive and cautious, sensitive to the opinions of others (Cloninger, 1987).

I have arranged the case histories and most of the tables chronologically from earliest to latest age of onset of problem drinking to allow the reader to make a different age break, if he or she so wishes. Twenty-two of the male suicides in the present study were identified as experiencing onset of alcohol problems before their 25th birthday. Table 4.1 briefly summarizes various historical features of these subjects. At a minimum, 12 (57% of those with information) had a family history of alcoholism, eight in the father. Two additional fathers were identified as heavy drinkers. Our informants, usually spouses, were often poorly informed concerning the victim's antecedents. Consequently, not only is the family history of alcoholism a minimum figure, we were unable to obtain enough knowledge of behavior problems before age 16 to make a diagnosis of antisocial personality disorder (ASPD) in any case. Nor do we have the data for strict comparisons regarding past violence or antisocial behavior in the fathers. Family histories that were obtained confirm the expectation of considerable family loading on alcoholism. All but four of the early onset alcoholics were daily drinkers. There were 13 (59%) with a history of fighting, but only six (27%) were known to have been arrested for it. In all, 12 (55%) had a history of one or more arrests, nine (41%) for vehicular offenses.

Despite the considerable duration of alcohol abuse, only 59% had what I considered to be serious medical problems (see Table 4.2 for details). Cirrhosis (in one case

MEN WITH ONSET OF ALCOHOLISM BEFORE AGE 25

simply characterized as "liver disease" by the attending physician) was reported in 8 cases (36%), duodenal ulcer in 2, diabetes mellitus in 3. Three others without recent medical examination had confided to someone a belief that they suffered from a malignancy. Eighteen (82%) had had at least a psychiatric consultation regarding their alcoholism. Fifteen (68%) had had one or more alcohol-related hospitalizations.

Addictive drinking was identified by a history of benders and/or inability to stop drinking. Benders were reported in 15 (83%) of the 18 with pertinent information. Inability to stop drinking characterized 16 (84% of 19 with information). One or both of these features were found in 20 cases. Information was lacking in one case. This represents a prevalence of 95% of addictionlike behavior among those early onset alcoholics in whom there was information. That feature has not been thought to be characteristic of Type 2 alcoholics. Of the 22 with early onset alcoholism, 11 (50%) (cases 2, 3, 4, 9, 11, 26, 28, 29, 30, 31, 33) had at least 3 of the suggested six criterion characteristics (early onset, father alcoholic, daily drinking, fighting arrests, vehicular arrests, serious health problems) and so might be considered Type 2 alcoholics. Six of them (cases 4, 11, 26, 29, 30, 31) were reportedly untroubled by guilt. On the other hand, none of these was reportedly free of evidence of loss of control.

Table 4.2 brings together the alcohol-related aspects of their careers. Note that 13, or 72% of those ever married, were reported to have been physically abusive of one or more spouses. Surprisingly, 14 (64%) came from intact homes. In at least 5 of these, as well as at least 5 others, the subject had been exposed to the behavior of a heavily drinking or alcoholic father. More broadly, the family history was positive for alcoholism in 11, half of the early onset cases, and 65% of those with any information. If reported heavy drinking is included, the number increases to 14, or 82% of families with information on this matter.

Of the 22 early onset alcoholics, 4 (18%) had never married. An additional 7 (32%) were either divorced or separated at the time of their death. Of those 11 currently married and together, 6 had had one or more previous marriages. Only 5 were still in their first marriage—for a mean of 25 years. Social support was very thin in at least 4 of these cases. All but 2 of the 18 ever married had had 1 or more marital disruptions such as divorce or separation (Table 4.1). Sixteen (73%) had an accompanying affective disorder, primary in two case histories. This is essentially the same rate of depression found in the entire material. The question of Type 1 versus Type 2 alcoholism is further discussed following presentation of the cases of men with alcoholism onset between age 25 and 55 (Chapter 5).

5

Men with Onset of Alcoholism from Age 25 to 44

In this group of men with onset of alcoholism from age 25 through 44, the mean age at onset (31.1 years) and median (30 years) are skewed toward the younger side. That is not particularly surprising, as the onset of alcoholism tends to be in the young adult years. One subject is included here in whom we had no way of estimating the age at which he began abusive drinking. Inasmuch as he died at age 35, it is certain that he does not belong in the group with late onset. Nothing particularly distinguishes this group either diagnostically or with respect to duration of alcoholism (Table 5.1). The mean age at death (50.1 + 9.1 years) is about 5 years higher and the duration of alcohol abuse (18.9 + 7.1 years) about 5 years less than is the case with alcoholics with earlier onset.

CASE HISTORIES

Case 1

Subject 1 was a 50-year-old married white man of nominally Lutheran faith. He was born in St. Louis. His father was a laborer, also born in St. Louis. His mother ran off when he was 6 months old and his father divorced her. Nothing further is known of her. He was raised by his paternal grandmother, also divorced. He stayed intermittently with his father, who remarried, but lived mainly with the grandmother. He completed the 10th grade and went to work, leaving his grandmother's home permanently when he entered military service in July, 1942. He married for the first and only time in September of the same year. He received an honorable discharge from the military service 1 year later for reasons we did not learn. He had held a clerical civil service job for 26 years, the last 12 years at the same grade, earning $13,000–$14,000 a year. He had one child, a son, 16, still living at home. His only friends were in the tavern, and he had an unknown amount of contact with relatives.

He began drinking in his late teens, and his first inebriation occurred shortly thereafter. In his mid-20s he began to drink to relieve tension, as when confronted with added responsibilities. (I consider this the onset of his problem drinking.) In his early 30s he was stopping every night at a bar on his way home from work. For more than 10 years he had been uncomfortable in groups of people. This gradually worsened until he "had to have some drinks to go places." In his early 40s he was a binge drinker. Some binges lasted as long as 2 weeks. They tended to coincide with his low moods. At times he would stay dry for a month. For the 4–5 years prior to his suicide he had been a steady daily drinker with shakes in the morning, avid drinking, seclusive drinking, taking bottles to work, and seeing his friends less. He was hospitalized twice, chiefly because of his drinking, but never received inpatient treatment specifically for his alcoholism.

His wife said he never admitted having a problem with alcohol, although he did express guilt about his drinking. She thought he drank too much, as did his supervisor, and he lost friends because of it. It is not known whether he made efforts to limit his drinking. He drank before breakfast and at all times of the day. Eight weeks before his suicide, he was fired from the civil service job he had held for 26 years. The firing was, at least in part, alcohol related. He never fought or threatened anyone and was never arrested. During the last weeks he was drinking a fifth of wine and 6–12 bottles of beer daily.

He was described by his wife as always a moody person, often brooding about his work. Early in the marriage he had periods of time when he "felt great." At other times he felt the whole world was against him. The periods of feeling down became progressively longer and deeper and outweighed by far his good moods. He tended to be preoccupied and would not talk about what was on his mind. He was described as having "an inferiority complex" and being perfectionistic with regard to his personal grooming and perhaps with respect to his work as well. He bathed daily. His clothes had to be very neat and his shoes shined. For about 3 years before his death he occasionally expressed the belief that "a person" was following him and that he needed protection. He started to carry a gun in the car with him. He would not say who the "person" was. Increasingly, when driving his car he looked back as though he thought someone might be following him.

Beginning about 3 years before his death, his wife noticed progressive impotence. Six months later she learned that he was seeing another woman and confronted him. She told him she was thinking of leaving him. In the wake of that confrontation he had an automobile accident with alleged head injury. He was not hospitalized, but from that time on his memory was not as good as before, and he seemed a bit mixed up and forgetful. He couldn't tolerate noise, became irritable, and had trouble controlling his temper. He complained of tinnitus and thought he heard a song repeatedly.

For the last year of his life he had disturbed sleep throughout the night, complained of fatigue, found it more of an effort to get up and go to work, and was slow in his movements. He was indecisive, had lost interest in things, and appeared sad and joyless. Since his firing he appeared depressed, disgusted with himself and the world; he felt worthless, blaming himself for his and his family's troubles and professing himself a burden to others. He had lost 15 pounds over about a 2-year period and had exhibited increasing anorexia for 6–8 months, most pronounced in the last month.

He had gouty arthritis of the knees and ankles for about 8 years. His first significant hospitalization was a little over 2½ years before his death, ostensibly for evaluation of left pectoral chest pain, which had occurred on two occasions several months earlier.

His liver was enlarged, with abnormal liver function tests, and he had a tremor. History obtained from his wife at that time showed "the patient has also expressed paranoid ideas and has been depressed. There has also been a sex problem." Psychiatric consultation did not further illuminate any of these issues. The psychiatric diagnosis given was "anxiety reaction with symptomatic alcoholism." The medical diagnosis was "gout; liver dysfunction probably due to fatty infiltration." He saw the psychiatrist for about 2 months after that, receiving "a green and black capsule."

The second hospitalization, 4 months before his suicide, was for the same ostensible complaint of chest pain, although his doctor reported that he hospitalized him to get him off alcohol. Provisional diagnoses of hepatic cirrhosis and myocardial involvement were not substantiated by further study. The final clinical diagnosis was "gouty arthritis responsive to Benemid and cortisone." Most of the time he took colchicine for it and followed a low-purine diet. The drinking history was noted but was not a part of the discharge diagnosis.

So far as the wife knew, the family history was negative for alcoholism and affective disorder.

In the last 3 years of his life he spoke intermittently to his wife of wanting to die, of feeling that he would be better off dead, and of committing suicide.

Circumstances Leading to the Act

Two and one half years prior to his suicide he was involved in an automobile accident and supposedly sustained a head injury, although he was not hospitalized. Whether the accident was alcohol related was not learned. He subsequently had a slight memory deficit, was very irritable, couldn't tolerate noise, and had trouble controlling his temper.

His drinking increased, his job performance suffered, and 3–4 months before his suicide he was asked by his supervisor for a letter of resignation. His response was, "That would be like signing my death certificate" (or words to that effect). He did not submit the letter and was fired 8 weeks before his suicide, after 26 years in civil service. He failed to find another job in St. Louis and went to Miami to seek employment. He was also unsuccessful there. According to his wife, that appeared to be the last straw; his mood plummeted. His drinking had increased after he was fired, but 2 days before his death he stopped drinking and complained of feeling cold. He exhibited some tremor. On the day of his death he complained of feeling bad and his wife offered to stay home with him. He declined the offer. When his 16-year-old son returned home from school at about 2:45 p.m. he found him in the bedroom, with a gunshot wound of the head from a .32-caliber revolver. He was breathing stertorously and expired shortly thereafter.

He left the following suicide note:

> 'Closed casket' 'No visitors except family'. No flowers—return all. Don't spend a nickel/not necessary. Get Bob to start and let him and Dad go from there. The retirement can be used as you wish—buy the house Not sell it? See Betty M., AVCOM.
> This is going to be a blow for [son's name] but this sometimes is the price to pay. I Tried.
> The whole matter evolves around the in-capability of people to understand what is in fact truth. I could name several but I will not. All I ask is to remain (BLAH).

There is still an outstanding check $75.00?
Just remember that I have never done a thing that would out [*sic*] YOU, or the GOVERNMENT, or our family position in a situation of being compromised. I have been beaten, I have had a attempted bribery, telephone calls yet I still remain within the bounds of what is to be and I will not sell out."
[subject's initials]

Findings and Sources

Clinical Diagnosis: (1) Alcoholism, chronic; (2) major depressive disorder, secondary to alcoholism.
Toxicology: Not performed.
Primary Informant: Wife, married 25 ½ years; saw him daily.
Other Sources of Information: Coroner's death investigation report, hospital records, attending physician.
Informant's Opinion of Reason for Suicide: He was depressed over his inability to find work and over his alcoholism.

Comment

Although his drinking and first intoxication began in his late teens, it is unclear when this man first encountered problems from his drinking. He was using alcohol as a sedative by his mid-20s and had become a binge drinker by his mid-40s. Job performance must have suffered longer than that, as he had remained in the same civil service grade for the last 12 years. An auto accident in which he allegedly sustained a head injury occurred immediately after his wife confronted him with her knowledge of his extramarital affair and her thoughts of leaving him. She didn't leave, but his memory worsened and he became progressively more depressed. It appears that he had a full-blown retarded depression for the last year. Asked to resign from his job, he refused and was fired 2 months before his suicide. His inability to find other work was the final blow. His job seems to have been his sole source of self-esteem, and that was gone. He had no friends, no work, a troubled marriage, and a major depression. Even alcohol didn't help. He probably didn't drink at all for the last 2 days.

Case 17

Subject 17 was a 30-year-old white married male, born and largely raised in St. Louis. He had no siblings. His father was a farmer in rural Missouri, who died when the subject was 16. He was generally a loner, but sociable when drinking. He had been married for 7 years and had three children, a son age 5 and daughters 3 and 2 years old at the time of his death. He was reportedly raised to believe that "money would solve all of his problems." He spent money impulsively, often to buy gifts for his wife after arguments, and then worried about his ability to pay the bills. He borrowed money from his mother on several occasions and never paid any of it back. She stopped lending him money after his wife told her she would see none of it if anything happened to him. Raised Roman Catholic, he was observant of his religion. "He never missed a Sunday."

He held a doctoral degree in the health care field and had been self-employed for a little over 5 years after completing his professional training. His income was rather modest for the profession he was in. He worried about people not being satisfied with his work, and as a result found the pursuit of his profession increasingly stressful. These problems were thought to have given rise to his drinking, which became progressively worse. His wife described him as "sort of a loner," but he did have at least three male friends, two of them professionals, whom he met daily in a bar during the last 1½ years of his life.

He held some drinking parties in his teens, but was never out of line. According to his wife, 2 years before his suicide his friends teased him about the birth of his third child, 10 months after the second child. This joshing upset him quite a bit. Almost immediately he began to drink heavily. (The history given by the psychiatrist who treated him was that he began drinking excessively shortly after commencing his private practice 5 years before taking his life.) He never drank while working or worked when he felt drunk; however, his standards in this regard are unknown. He drank daily until drunk, except when working, and he sometimes missed work as a result. In the last year of his life he worked only 3 days a week, spending the remaining time drinking. At that point he earned only a little less than his maximum.

He stopped interacting with the family. His wife became embittered about his behavior and his frequent promises to quit drinking. Although mostly depressed, he occasionally became happy. In that state he impulsively bought a boat, then a lot on a lake. He sold his wife's car to help meet the payments on the lot. He had eight minor automobile accidents as a result of drinking in the last year of his life and received a DWI citation, which he beat in court. He was abstinent for 1 month after that and was "like his old self." He saw a physician specializing in treatment of alcoholism twice during that time, stopping when he learned he was being given placebo medication.

After resuming drinking he became careless about his language to the point that others complained about his crude remarks. One year before taking his life he was drunk in a bar and became loud. His wife asked him to be quiet and he threw her against a wall. Three months before his death, while drunk, he wanted to talk to his son, who was asleep. His wife wouldn't allow it, and he slapped her. These behaviors were otherwise foreign to him. It is not known how much he drank, because nearly all of his drinking was done in taverns. He had blackouts and morning tremulousness, but no other physical problems with alcohol. He acknowledged that he drank too much and felt guilty about it but could not control it. Not only his wife, but others objected to his drinking so much.

He was described as always tense, and dealing with people upset him. Just over 3 years before his death he first consulted a psychiatrist. He had been under the care of a general practitioner before that, receiving amitriptyline (Elavil) and chlordiazepoxide (Librium) for depression. He was markedly depressed, lacking in interest, lethargic, anorexic, with a 15-pound weight loss, complained of insomnia, stopped work for 1 month and stayed in bed. The psychiatrist diagnosed him as schizoid, with an obsessive-compulsive personality, and depressed as well, seemingly on the basis of interpretation of the Minnesota Multiphasic Personality Inventory (MMPI).

He did well at first with treatment but then began to drink more. When the psychiatrist wished to hospitalize him, about 14 months before his demise, he refused and stopped attending. He received no further psychiatric attention although he continued to exhibit fatigue, anorexia, disinterest, inertia, slower thinking, and low self-esteem as well as depressed mood most of the time. Apparently he had received open prescriptions because he continued to take chlordiazepoxide, up to twelve 25-mg capsules a day until his death. He had brief periods of heightened feelings of well-being. His interest in sex returned in the last year. He uncharacteristically bought a few sex magazines and made inappropriate sexual remarks to women.

Thirteen months prior to his suicide he complained of stomach pains and thought he had a peptic ulcer. He consulted an osteopathic physician, who found no radiologic evidence of an ulcer. The doctor urged him to stop drinking, but the advice went unheeded. He had no other medical or surgical problems.

His mother was said to have been depressed often and to have had one bad depressive episode. His father, a farmer, was depressed the last year of his life. He took the horses and wagon to the field one day, and they returned without him. He was found dead in the field—the wagon having run over his head. The subject always believed his father had killed himself in that manner. This stayed on his mind, especially during the last 2 years. Other family members regarded the father's death as an accident.

Eleven months before his suicide, his wife left him for 2 days. He was very upset and called her to say she would be "really sorry" if she didn't come back. She did (and she was). In the last year of his life he said on several occasions he was no good and his wife would be better off without him. On the day of his suicide he asked his wife to help him control his drinking. She expressed disinterest and he said, "I don't know what I'll do." No more direct communication was reported.

Circumstances Leading to the Act

The evening before he took his life he seemed solemn and told his wife there was something on his mind that he wanted to discuss with her. He did not discuss anything. Later he went out with a male friend. He told him, too, there was something he wanted to discuss, but he never got around to it. They stopped by the subject's office and he made a "vulgar comment" in front of an 18-year-old cleaning girl. She became frightened and called the owner of the building, who called the subject's wife. She, in turn, located him by telephone and asked him to be more careful about what he said in front of others or he might be misunderstood and find himself in trouble. That led to an argument. He and his friend spent the evening at the friend's home playing cards and drinking. Around midnight the friend called the informant and told her the subject would stay at his house that night because he had been drinking and should not drive.

When he returned home early the next morning he asked his wife to call his office assistant to cancel his morning appointments, as he felt too sick to work. She refused, saying, "You're always too sick to work but you're never too sick to drink." Another argument ensued. He made the call to his office assistant. He then went to bed and "slept better than he had in months." He awoke about noon and they discussed his drinking and financial problems. He said he would try to stop drinking and she said she had heard that promise before. He told her that he would "take care of those problems today" and would see her that afternoon. He left for his office, crying, and prepared to see his afternoon patients. His assistant left the office for lunch. On returning, she found a note on the door advising her not to be surprised at what she saw.

His body was in one of the rooms of the office suite, with a gunshot wound of the head. On the desk was a handwritten "last will and testament." Either as a part of this or separately he acknowledged his alcohol problem and stated he was despondent over increased debt. He expressed sorrow about causing his wife so much trouble and being a burden to her. The note included advice not to marry anyone who drinks and the wish for her to have his attorney friend (and drinking partner) handle the estate. We did not obtain a copy of the note(s). In his wallet was a funeral remembrance card memorializing his father's death 12 years earlier.

Findings and Sources

Clinical Diagnosis: (1) Alcoholism, chronic; (2) major affective disorder, probably secondary, possibly bipolar II.
Toxicology: Blood alcohol concentration 0.25 g%.
Primary Informant: Wife, married 7 years; saw him daily.
Other Sources of Information: Coroner's death investigation report, police investigation report, psychiatrist who had treated him.
Informant's Opinion of Reason for Suicide: Marital problems, self-disgust, and inability to cope with life.

Comment

This man had extreme anxiety concerning his adequacy in the practice of his profession from the very beginning, 5 years before he took his life. That anxiety seems to have been the basis for his excessive drinking. His sensitivity to disapproval was further challenged when friends teased him about having a third child 10 months after the second one. He not only increased his drinking; he also became clinically depressed and consulted a psychiatrist about that time. He responded initially to treatment, but then relapsed, refused hospitalization, and terminated his psychiatric contact. Both depression and alcohol abuse became intractable. He seemed to become quite phobic about his practice, reducing it to 3 days a week and drinking the rest of the time. Meanwhile, his relationship with his wife was deteriorating. She had become fed up with his drinking and his neglect of her and his practice. Just before his suicide, she refused to cover for him or to help him cover for himself. He had lost the last bulwark between himself and his anxiety-provoking practice. Depressed, with his drinking out of control, he had no place to hide.

Case 38

Subject 38 was a 42-year-old unemployed married white male, a native of the St. Louis area. He lived there all his life except for a period of military service. His father was a mechanic who had divorced his wife when the subject was about 15 years old. He was raised in the Roman Catholic faith. He was frequently in fights as a child and was believed to have been truant from school as well. He left school after the eighth grade and entered military service at age 17, after the end of World War II. He was honorably discharged after 2 years in service.

He was married at 20 and remained so for nearly 22 years, until his death. The couple had seven children, ages from 3 to 21 years at the time of his demise. He had worked steadily as a laborer for a railroad for 22 years, beginning after he left school, and interrupted by his military service. He was finally fired for drinking. He then worked as a security guard, as a mortuary employee, and for a local hospital, often holding more than one job at a time. Five years before his death he became self-employed doing landscaping and yard work, and was considered very good at it, "a perfectionist." For the last 7 or 8 months of his life he would leave his sons on a job and go off to do errands or drink. At the end he was not able to function adequately in running the business.

He began drinking while in military service and drank heavily from age 25, with progressive loss of control. His wife described him as a "plateau drinker" throughout their marriage. Three years before his suicide she finally confronted the fact that she was married to an alcoholic and began to attend Alanon. A year later, he, in turn, began attending Alcoholics Anonymous, but he continued to drink. His last attendance was on the night before his suicide. During the last year of his life he had five hospitalizations for alcoholism, four at public hospitals and one at a VA hospital, but was unable to remain sober. On one of these occasions, he was discharged for "violent behavior." He drank daily, in amounts up to a fifth of vodka a day, plus "all the beer he could hold." He had many alcohol-related job problems, including three formal reprimands while working for the railroad. He was fired at least three times because of his drinking and its attendant misbehavior. During the last 6–8 months of his life he was frequently unable to work.

When drunk, he was irrational, angry, verbally and physically abusive, and seemed to provoke arguments. He had physically assaulted his wife three times, had fought with his two older sons several times in the last year, and had struck a daughter. He threw a wrench at his son and once threatened his family with a gun. He got into fights in bars. He took pleasure in such things as deliberately jamming his car horn so it would honk continuously and pretending it was stuck, to annoy his neighbors. He quite justifiably thought his neighbors were "out to get him." They or family members called the police several times. He had become progressively isolated socially as his drinking became worse, and he had had no social life for years, if ever.

He did not suffer withdrawal symptoms or medical complications of alcoholism, but he had blackouts and drank in the morning. During the last 6 months of his life he was drinking less, but that was attributed mainly to his frequent hospitalizations. Because of both his drinking and his absences, his income had become inadequate, and he had applied for welfare support 4 months before his death. The children's needs were secondary to his alcohol habit. He was not described as a drug abuser, yet 10 days before his suicide he was discharged from his last hospital admission for smoking marijuana in the hospital. On the night of his suicide his wife had him arrested and jailed.

He experienced anorexia, weight loss, and insomnia when drinking, but he did not seem to have a depressive syndrome. He was always considered unusually sensitive, and his feelings were hurt easily. He had been uncomfortable in crowds for the last 10 years. During the last 5 years of his life he became more moody, isolated from friends, and irritable, losing interest in activities. When last seen by a physician at a public hospital clinic he asked for a tranquilizer to deal with his temper and was given chlordiazepoxide (Librium). He had hoped to be readmitted to the hospital but was refused, at least in part because of the marijuana incident mentioned previously. He was hospitalized once for a foot injury which required surgery. His other hospitalizations were for alcoholism, and no significant medical condition was found on any admission.

There was no family history of mental illness, alcoholism, or suicide.

He had lost interest in most activities. He said that he had done everything he wanted to do and had nothing left to do. Two months before the end of his life he told his wife that perhaps she should think about leaving him as she would be better off without him. There was no other communication that could be considered suicidal, and no known previous attempts or plans.

Circumstances Leading to the Act

In the last year of his life he was unable to do the heavier landscaping work, and thus was more dependent on his sons for help. He had two acquaintances who had died of alcoholism within the month before his own death. He was not close to either of them. Two weeks before taking his life, he had been discharged from alcoholism treatment for smoking marijuana. Three days before his suicide he saw a doctor in the St. Louis County Hospital outpatient clinic and was discouraged from seeking readmission. He was described as "getting out on the wrong side of bed" on the day of his death. He asked his 17-year-old son to go with him to cut grass. His son refused and a minor argument ensued. Then he went off alone to do yard work and to "get tanked." Returning home drunk, he was still angry about his son's refusal to help. He said he would wait for his son and "cut him with a knife." When his son had not returned home at midnight, he began making a disturbance, in part by turning up the volume on the TV to its maximum and refusing to lower it. His wife then called the police. He was taken to jail and placed in a detention cell, where he was found hanging with his knotted undershirt a few hours later. There was no suicide note.

Findings and Sources

Clinical Diagnosis: Alcoholism, chronic.
Toxicology: Blood alcohol concentration 0.201 mg%, with negative barbiturate and salicylate levels.
Primary Informant: Wife, married 21½ years, had known subject 23 years; saw him daily.
Other Sources of Information: Coroner's death investigation report, hospital records.
Informant's Opinion of Reason for Suicide: (1) Saw he was unable to work as well as before ("the last straw"); (2) alcoholic, couldn't stop drinking.

Comment

This man's alcohol habit was of about 16 years' duration, but his interpersonal behavior seems to have become a problem only in the last 5 years, after he lost his railroad job. Then he became exceedingly difficult. He alienated nearly everyone, including his own family, by his provocative and bellicose behavior. As his alcohol abuse encroached more and more on his ability to work, he became more dependent on his sons for help in his landscaping business. When his 17-year-old son refused to help him one day, he was confronted with the loss of his ability to command the services of his children. His solution was to assault his son, but he was jailed instead. It was his first experience with involuntary detention.

Our informant thought depressive symptoms were confined to his drinking episodes. To be sure, he was drinking heavily before and on the day of his death, but a depressive syndrome was not identifiable with any degree of assurance in this case. I think his jailing brought home to him the true extent of his loss of control, both of himself and of his family. He could no longer maintain his self-esteem by pushing others around. He had already concluded that he had done everything he wanted to do. There was nothing left to keep him going.

Case 40

Subject 40 was a 56-year-old unemployed single white male who died in a public hospital several hours after lacerating his left wrist. He was born in North Carolina and his father was killed in a logging accident when the subject was 5 years old. Very little is known of his childhood, but he was raised by one of his three sisters from the age of 12. Religious affiliation was unknown and seems unlikely. He had lived in the St. Louis area all of his adult life except during military service in World War II from 1941 to 1945, receiving an honorable discharge. He worked on farms during the first few years of his working life, then as a laborer until about 5 years before his death, when his failing health prevented working.

He never married, had few friends, and lived on social security disability and VA benefits in a rooming house. The informant, who drank six to eight beers during the interview, said he had known him for 25 years and saw him daily. His main social life seems to have been either in bars or drinking with his landlord.

He was thought to have begun drinking around age 25, perhaps during his military service. He was always a binge drinker. Twice or once a month, when he received money, he would drink for about 5 days until his money was gone. He had mild withdrawal tremors and morning drinking. Others objected to the amount he drank, and he felt guilty about it. He had been fired four or five times for drinking on the job. He was argumentative and combative when drunk and involved in many fights. He seemed to think he could whip anyone and often chose his co-combatants unwisely. As a result, he was often beaten up. One such fracas, 7 years before his suicide, sent him to the St. Louis City Hospital with a linear fracture of the skull in the temporo-parietal area and a remote subdural hematoma. That left him with a seizure disorder and a poor memory. He gradually lost the ability to put in a day's work. He had been working out of the union hall on a day-to-day basis for several years. His last job had been on a loading dock. In the last 5 years of his life he was unemployable.

Some 5 or 6 months before his death he had attacked the informant with a knife while drinking. He had been arrested and jailed overnight on two occasions for intoxication and disturbing the peace. His last arrest was 2 months before his death. He had hepatic cirrhosis resulting from his alcoholism, as well as hypertension. He had been treated several times at VA hospitals and city hospitals for intoxication or alcoholism. There was no evidence that he received any more treatment than drying out. His last hospital admission occurred 4 months before his death. He had complained that he thought he was dying. He was discharged within 24 hours.

He had had two outpatient visits to the city's public psychiatric hospital for depression, his last a week before his suicide. Treatment was not recorded in the materials available to me and there was no mention of alcoholism in the chart. He does not appear to have been hospitalized for depression. He was described as always solemn, speaking little except when drunk, and never laughing. He was high-strung and given to outbursts of rage, generally when drunk. Following his skull fracture his memory became poor and he had trouble thinking, but he was described as oriented to place and time and able to understand things as well as before. (There is reason to doubt the validity of this report by our bibulous informant.) After he became unable to work, he had chronic low mood, fatigue, insomnia, anorexia, weight loss, decreased activity, feelings of worthlessness and guilt, and made repeated references to suicide. He became impotent after onset of his depression and was especially sensitive about it in the last 2 years. He would become angry when friends spoke of sexual matters. In the last year he spoke of feeling sad.

Nothing is known of his family except that he had three sisters, all living where they grew up. Our informant had no further knowledge of the family.

By the time he had become too impaired physically to work, this subject began to speak of being no good, that he would be better off dead, and that he was going to cut his throat. These statements were generally made while drinking.

Circumstances Leading to the Act

He had been drinking all day in a bar near his place of residence and was thrown out because he had become abusive and may have gotten into a fight. He went to a drugstore to buy liquor and laid $2.00 on the counter. When he turned to get the liquor, his money had "disappeared" and he received nothing. He left, cursing, returned to the rooming house, and complained angrily to his landlord. The landlord advised him to return to the drugstore and explain things to the owner. Instead, he went across the street to a filling station for a few minutes, where he apparently cut his wrist with a knife, severing tendons and his left radial artery. Then he returned and sat on the front steps of the rooming house. After some time it was noticed that he was bleeding profusely. He was taken to a public hospital where he died about 8 hours later. He did not leave a note.

Findings and Sources

Clinical Diagnosis: (1) Alcoholism, chronic; (2) secondary depression; (3) probable posttraumatic dementia.
Toxicology: Blood alcohol concentration 0.15g%.
Primary Informant: Landlord, had known subject for 25 years.
Other Sources of Information: Coroner's death investigation report, hospital records (perused but not copied).
Informant's Opinion of Reason for Suicide: He felt worthless because he couldn't work.

Comment

This solemn, joyless laborer was pugnacious when drunk and got his skull cracked 7 years before his death as a result. There was thought to be brain damage, but the report is conflicting, in that he was said to have had trouble with both thinking and memory but to be oriented and able to understand. The head injury led to job disability, and when he became unable to work he felt worthless. He developed most, if not all of the criterion symptoms of depression at that time. If the depression worsened subsequently, it was not reported. His suicide seems to have been impulsive, rather than planned, although he had spoken of suicide on a number of occasions when drunk. Depressed, drunk, and humiliated by the loss of his drinking money, he took the fatal step. The fact that he died in a hospital 8 hours later suggests that he may have reopened a repaired wound, although hypovolemic shock alone could account for the outcome. A report of his final hours was not obtainable.

Case 6

Subject 6 was a 49-year-old separated, employed white male nonobserving Protestant. Born in Texas, he lived in St. Louis the last 11 years of his life. His father was a lifelong alcoholic whose occupation was not learned; his mother was a schoolteacher. He had no siblings. His parents were divorced when he was 8 years old. He was raised by his maternal grandparents after that. He worked his way through college prior to World War II, joining the Marine Corps Reserve during that time. He served on active duty from the beginning of the war until after its end, rising from enlisted status to officer's rank. He was honorably discharged and received a 70% disability pension for unspecified "service-connected" disability, possibly renal disease. While in the service, at age 25, he married for the first and only time. A son, born of that union within the year, had gone on to college and was out of the home but in the city.

After obtaining a master's degree, he worked for one company for the remainder of his life. He became a division manager, a job that required considerable travel. He was never fired, but 8 months before his suicide, he was put on probation because of his drinking. He worked only 1 day in the last 3½ weeks of his life.

In a brief retrospective account of his drinking history, written while attending AA in the last year of his life, he recorded that he took his first drink in his late teens and was drunk several times on gin and home brew before entering college. Attending college in a dry town, he brewed his own beer and drank to achieve a glow but not drunkenness. As an enlisted man in the Marine Corps, he drank only beer, but upon becoming an officer he drank rum and scotch. He recorded that he got drunk "good" only three or four times while in the Marines. "Post war days back to beer to keep from getting drunk." He was described by his wife as a steady but reasonable drinker in his 20s and early 30s. By age 35 he had developed a pattern of binge drinking. (At age 49 he gave a physician a history of having consumed a fifth of gin or bourbon daily without exception for 20 years. I date his problems with control to age 27 or 28.) In the course of traveling for his employer he went on benders lasting 2 to 7 days at a time. He was a seclusive, solitary drinker. He claimed to have lost control of his drinking only after hospitalization for a nephrectomy 2 ½ years before his suicide.

His first psychiatric hospitalization for alcoholism occurred 27 months before his death, following a grand mal seizure. No evidence of liver damage was found. He had a second psychiatric hospitalization 6 months later, for alcohol withdrawal syndrome accompanied by another grand mal seizure. He was put on probation at work less than a year before he died. Seven months before he ended his life he joined AA, took disulfiram (Antabuse) and stayed sober for 4 months. Then he drank almost constantly until his suicide. He was loud and verbally abusive, causing his wife to leave him 30 days before his suicide. He worked only 1 day in the last 3 ½ weeks of his life and was aware that he had lost control of his drinking. He had never had a vehicular accident or police contact.

He was described as having outbursts of rage all of his life, not restricted to times when he was drinking but worse when he was. He had no symptoms of affective disorder. He never had any close friends and had almost no social life, although he associated with business contacts at times. He had taken hypnotics and sedatives daily for years. These included Sominex and Nytol (over-the-counter drugs containing diphenhydramine), chlordiazepoxide (Librium) by prescription, and "animal drugs" (veterinary preparations). Both he and his wife thought he took too many drugs, but there was no evidence of addiction. In the last 6 months his memory had become poor. He had trouble thinking and organizing his thoughts. He was sometimes uncertain about the date and he did not read or understand things as well as before. He complained of slowed thinking and impaired memory.

He had suffered from recurrent bilateral renal calculi (kidney stones) for about 25 years, with several surgical removals. He had bilateral chronic pyelonephritis for 15 years as a result of the stones. Ten years before his death, a right nephrectomy had been attempted but abandoned because of adhesions and bleeding. Postoperative wound infection left him with periodic purulent drainage from multiple sinuses in the right flank. Preoperatively, he was noted to have hypertension, cardiomegaly, and electrocardiographic evidence of two old, healed myocardial infarctions. The removal of the kidney was finally accomplished 3 years before his death. He continued regular medical outpatient consultation for his renal disease. He had had diminished interest in sex for 15 years, attributing it to his kidney disease. It did not seem to disturb him.

His father was a lifelong alcoholic. No other family history concerning psychiatric illness was obtainable.

Circumstances Leading to the Act

During his period of sobriety, beginning 7 months before he ended his life, he gave an AA talk at a hospital and became aware of patients who were committed for custodial care in advanced stages of central nervous system degeneration due to alcoholism. He became apprehensive that he might end up that way if he began drinking again. When he did resume drinking, 3 months before his suicide, he became loud and verbally abusive. Because of that, his wife left him 30 days before his death and he then lived alone in their duplex dwelling. She remained in almost daily contact with him by telephone. He expressed both to her and to a neighbor his fear of being committed to a psychiatric hospital. His wife and son had an appointment to see him on the day of his suicide, to have him sign income tax forms. He expressed fear that they were coming to have him committed. His son found him in an upstairs bedroom, dead of a

.38-caliber pistol wound of the head. He had never spoken of suicide and left no suicide note. Of jottings he made during his period of sobriety and participation in AA, the last note is poignant: "It really feels good to be sober, think clearly, and am finding happiness within myself."

Findings and Sources

Clinical Diagnosis: (1) Alcoholism, chronic; (2) chronic pyelonephritis; (3) renal hypertension; (4) arteriosclerotic cardiovascular disease; (5) mild mental deterioration.
Toxicology: Blood alcohol concentration 0.30 g%.
Primary Informant: Wife, married to subject for 24 years; saw daily or talked by telephone.
Other Sources of Information: Subject's notes on his drinking history, neighbor, hospital records, coroner's death investigation report.
Informant's Opinion of Reason for Suicide: (1) Loss of control of drinking; (2) fear of hospital commitment.

Comment

No evidence of a depressive syndrome was elicited in this case. He was a loner and a solitary drinker. His wife left him 30 days before his suicide but stayed in almost daily contact by telephone. She reported that the separation was by mutual agreement. It was her opinion that fear of being committed to a psychiatric hospital for long-term care was the precipitant of his suicide. In support of this opinion are (1) her report that he had become disturbed at seeing patients with alcoholic dementia in a psychiatric hospital a few months before his suicide; (2) both his supervisor and a next-door neighbor had said he feared being committed; and (3) her report of his statement of that fear. While the timing of these communications is uncertain, their import is clear. In addition, he had totally lost control of his drinking, so that he had been unable to report to work for all but 1 day in the last 3 weeks of his life. He took his life within hours of an expected visit by his wife and grown son, to secure his signature on an income tax form. He was thoroughly drunk (BAC 0.30 g%) when he shot himself, as he had perhaps been for days.

Although I judged the marital separation as less important than his fear of rehospitalization and his inability to get control of himself, that event qualifies him for the category of recent loss of a close relationship.

Case 8

Subject 8 was a 57-year-old white married Protestant male, born in Denver but living in St. Louis since age 7. He and his younger brother were raised by both parents together. His father was a manufacturer's representative and his mother, a homemaker. After he graduated from high school, he obtained additional course credits from trade schools and night schools. He married for the first and only time at the age of 21, 36 years before his suicide by gunshot. There were two children, a daughter aged 31 and a son aged 30 at the time of his death. Some 4½ months before taking his life he told a psychiatrist that his wife had refused to have sex with him for 10 years, (I assume this was related to his drinking), characterizing her as "vindictive" as well as "strong willed" and saying she "has always run things."

It is not clear why he did not serve in the armed forces during World War II. He had worked for the same employer for 23 years until he was fired, 7 months before his death. He had achieved a well-paying job in sales. He and his son then established a janitorial contracting business, which was just beginning to attract customers. When he resumed drinking a month before his death, he considered himself a failure. He had two close friends who visited in his home.

He started drinking in his 20s, during World War II, "to calm his nerves," as a result of increased responsibility. His early drinking was in binges. He had become a steady, heavy drinker by the age of 30 and in his later years claimed to consume up to two fifths of vodka per day. He told doctors he didn't know why he drank. He mostly drank alone, at home, and did not frequent bars or taverns. He had 25 or more hospitalizations, often related to drinking or its complications. He had outbursts of rage only when drinking. Eighteen years before his death, he remained abstinent for a year, then resumed drinking as usual. He had had alcoholic hallucinosis in the past, as well as frequent morning "shakes," but not DTs. At times he drank before breakfast.

His wife noted that his memory and mental activity were declining over the last 1½ years. In late years his work performance began to deteriorate and after being given a leave of absence to "get himself squared away," which he failed to accomplish, he was fired. About the same time his wife left him, planning a divorce. He briefly attended AA meetings. Two months later he was arrested and fined for driving while intoxicated. Four months before his death, following one of his many hospitalizations, he reestablished abstinence and persuaded his wife to return to live with him. One month before he died, he started drinking again and promptly got himself admitted to a psychiatric hospital for drying out. He was discharged 3 weeks before his suicide and remained sober for 2½ weeks, then resumed drinking. He was sharply aware of his inability to control his drinking, thought he drank too much and reportedly lost friends because of it.

Over the years, he had seen a number of psychiatrists and was told he had "manic-depressive disease." His wife described him as "up for two weeks then down for two weeks" but "more down than up" in the last 2 years. Some of his hospitalizations were for depression, the last one possibly 3 years before his death. He had been treated at times with antidepressants but had refused electroconvulsive therapy. He had taken both "pep pills" daily and hypnotics nightly for many years. His wife thought he took too many. For most of the last year of his life, he had appeared depressed, disgusted with himself and the world, and he felt worthless and a burden. In the last 2 months he had increased insomnia, fatigue, indecisiveness, and an increase in suicidal communication.

For 2 years he seemed to have had increasing trouble thinking. His memory had become poor in the last 1½ years. Although he was oriented for time and place, he couldn't read or understand things as well in the last year as previously.

He had laboratory evidence of liver dysfunction at least 6 years before his death. He was radiologically diagnosed 2½ years before his death as having an active duodenal ulcer with bleeding. An asymptomatic duodenal deformity had been noted radiologically 4 years earlier. He had mild hypertension and no other medical disease.

Neither parent was known to have had psychiatric illness but his younger brother had been an alcoholic for 10 years at the time of the subject's death. A maternal uncle and subsequently the uncle's daughter both committed suicide. No other family history of psychiatric illness was obtained.

Intermittently over the last 10 years of his life, when drinking, he spoke of committing suicide, claiming he would be better off dead and that he would die before his spouse. Two years before his suicide he spoke of wanting to die and also told his wife he would kill her and then himself. One year later he said the family would be better off if he were dead. Two months before his death, when buying a suit, he said to his wife, "I won't live long enough to wear this suit out. I will be buried in it." On the day of his suicide he implied suicidal intent for the last time. He had never made a suicide attempt except for the fatal act.

Circumstances Leading to the Act

His wife held a full-time job and was very much "the boss" at home. In the year before his death, she inherited some money. At about the time he lost his job, she left him and was planning divorce. She reportedly lost 30 pounds in 3 months following the separation. (Did the separation have this effect on her, or was it in preparation for her freedom?) He voiced the opinion that she would not have left him had she not come into some money. However, he persuaded her to come back 4 months before his death, claiming that he had achieved sobriety. One month before he died, he began to drink again, got himself hospitalized, and was again sober until the last 4 days, when he resumed drinking. The day before he took his life, he admitted to his wife and son that he had let them down and said that he was "a failure." On the day of his suicide he implied suicidal intent, and his wife took a gun away from him. He went out of the house and returned in an hour. His wife talked with him about being hospitalized at a state psychiatric facility. While she was calling to arrange for his admission, he shot himself in the head with a .22-caliber pistol. He did not leave a note.

Findings and Sources

Clinical Diagnoses: (1) Alcoholism, chronic; (2) secondary affective disorder; (3) duodenal ulcer; (4) hepatocellular disease; (5) mild mental deterioration.
Toxicology: Not performed.
Primary Informant: Spouse, who knew him for at least 36 years.
Other Sources of Information: Hospital records, coroner's death investigation report.
Informant's Opinion of Reason for Suicide: Disappointed, discouraged, despondent about inability to control his drinking.

Comment

This subject had been unable to control his drinking for any extended period of time. Having lost a good job, he was blowing away a new business venture. His wife was out of patience with him, had achieved a degree of financial independence, and had already left him once because of his drinking. She dominated him, by his account. She intended to have him rehospitalized because of his drinking and was making the arrangements by telephone when he shot himself. Why he did not take his life when his wife left him is puzzling. He had just lost, or was about to lose, a good, steady job of 23 years duration at that time, his drinking was out of control, and he had an arrest for driving while intoxicated. A psychiatric hospital admission 4 weeks before his suicide was apparently on his own initiative. An unusually detailed admission history made no mention of depression, yet he appears to have developed a clear-cut depression about 2 months before his suicide. Perhaps that was the crucial factor—the necessary but not sufficient ingredient, to which was added the loss of autonomy in his wife's unilateral action in arranging for his rehospitalization, as well as his fear of desertion.

Case 32

Subject 32 was a 55-year-old white male of the Evangelical faith, who had been disabled by emphysema for 18 years and was briefly separated from his wife at the time of his death. He was born and lived his entire life in the St. Louis area. His father, a factory worker, died of a myocardial infarction when the subject was 37 years old. His mother had diabetes but lived to age 86. She had lived with him and his wife until 3 years before his death. He had no known school problems. His only major legal difficulty was a conviction for breaking and entering with several other teenagers at age 17. He served 3 years in a state reformatory, where he completed his secondary education. He was 21 years old when released from the penal institution. According to his wife, he was rejected for military service in World War II due to age (he was born in 1913) and an inguinal hernia. More likely it was because of his felony conviction. He had a tattoo on his arm—a dagger piercing a skull. Despite this unpromising beginning, he read a lot and was "a capable conversationalist" according to his wife. She thought his employment as a beer truck driver was considerably beneath his intellectual level.

An early marriage ended in divorce after about 3 years, due to his drinking. He married his second wife at age 34. He was already a heavy drinker and the relationship was stormy, occasionally punctuated by physical threats. Actual physical violence was not recorded. Medically retired at age 37, he received Social Security benefits and perhaps others as well, but he contributed nothing to the household finances. His wife paid all the household expenses from her salary. He kept his actual income a secret and submitted income tax statements after his wife had signed blank forms. They were separated for a few days before his suicide. His wife told us she was caring for her mother, who was ill. However, she had told the coroner's investigator that they were separated because of her husband's drinking. He had social contacts both in the tavern and with his wife's family, but he would sometimes walk out on the visiting family when he wished to be alone.

He had been a daily heavy drinker as long as his wife had known him, with a capacity for up to a fifth of liquor. He had frequent blackouts, binges, morning drinking, and frequent withdrawal symptoms, with evidence of liver impairment. He once struck a telephone pole while driving under the influence of alcohol. He had outbursts of rage and, from early in the marriage, was physically threatening when drunk. Twice he ran his wife out of the house with a gun, most recently 2 months before his suicide.

Some months earlier he had forced her out of the house at night in midwinter, in her nightgown. Once, 2 years before he took his life, he threatened her with a knife. He had about a year of abstinence early in the marriage but was more belligerent and unpleasant during that time. He had worked for 10 years as a truck driver for a brewery, but he would disappear for days, and even several weeks at a time. He threatened to kill a supervisor who reprimanded him. Owing to a medical disability, he did not work for the last 18 years. His first hospitalization for alcoholism, 20 years before his death, was probably only for detoxification. Another, about 10 years later, was for DTs. Although he admitted he drank too much, he never felt guilty or attempted to control his drinking.

He was described as always moody, chronically irritable, high-strung, sensitive, and given to sudden outbursts of rage. He had frequent anxiety attacks for many years and was uncomfortable in crowds. In the last 2 years he feared the dark and had to have a light on at all times. He was medically disabled for work for the last 18 years of his life, owing to chronic pulmonary emphysema. A spontaneous pneumothorax, treated conservatively with chest tubes, marked his retirement. He reportedly became despondent, saying "I am not a man anymore." He was angry and frustrated over his inability to work, and at his recurrent lung trouble. A recurrence of pneumothorax just a year before his death led to a pulmonary lobectomy.

Two years before his death he underwent fairly extensive right neck and jaw resection for carcinoma of the tongue. Following surgery, while still unable to speak, he wrote to his wife on a slate, "They didn't do me no good by pulling me through this operation. They should have let me go on the table." He became preoccupied with suicide. From that time on, he would point to a prominent vein in his neck and say he could end it all by cutting that vessel. He frequently said to his wife, mother, and other family members that he would be better off dead and would blow the top off his head or cut his throat. He often followed these suicidal comments to his wife with the statement, "But I hate to leave you." His mother feared that might indicate a murder–suicide intention. He felt disfigured, was disgusted with himself and the world, and believed he was a burden. He developed many symptoms of depression, including chronic low mood, anorexia and weight loss, insomnia, anhedonia, loss of energy and interest, social withdrawal, and poor memory. Following his jaw resection and neck dissection, he had to eat soft or pureed foods, which aggravated his malnutrition.

The family history was entirely negative for psychiatric illness, alcoholism, drug abuse or suicide. Family members were described as "very straight."

Circumstances Leading to the Act

Three weeks before his suicide he saw his otolaryngologist, who scheduled him for further surgery for a recurrence of the carcinoma. Removal of his tongue was to be a part of that procedure. He told his wife, "For the first time in my life, I am scared to death." She thought he was overreacting to the impending surgery. He increased his drinking and become even more depressed. His wife had gone to her mother's home a few days before the suicide. She told the coroner's death investigator that she had separated from him because of his drinking. She last saw him drinking at a bar the day after she left him. For 2 days she found his telephone line always busy. On finding his car at home she thought something might be wrong and telephoned the police. They found him in the kitchen with his throat cut, lying dead in a large pool of blood. Reconstruction of the suicide placed the act in the bathroom, where a razor blade was found and the toilet bowl was filled with blood. There were bloody tracks into the kitchen, where the telephone receiver was found off the hook.

A note was found, most of which was illegible due to bloodstains. Addressed to his wife, the note read: "Babe, I am too old to start over again . . ." There may have been more to his wife's leaving than she revealed to us.

Findings and Sources

Clinical Diagnosis: (1) Alcoholism, chronic; (2) major depressive disorder, secondary to the alcoholism; (3) panic disorder; (4) cancer, tongue, recurrent; (5) pulmonary emphysema.
Toxicology: Not performed.
Primary Informant: Wife, married 21 years.
Informant's Opinion of Reason for Suicide: Feared the surgery.

Comment

This man attained both his high school diploma and his majority in a state reformatory. The dates of his first marriage were unknown to the informant, but his drinking caused its dissolution. He could have had a drinking problem for as long as 30 years; 23 years would be a minimum figure. He had an unpleasant disposition—secretive, selfish, verbally abusive, at times physically threatening, but, so far as we learned, never actually assaultive. He had major health problems, of which his pulmonary emphysema was not alcohol related. His retirement after suffering a collapsed lung may or may not have been fully justified on medical grounds alone.

His first oral surgery was disfiguring, and his food had to be pureed. Both added to his already low self-esteem. He had already judged that he would have been better off dying on the operating table than having the tongue-conserving surgery he had undergone. Now he was confronted with losing the free portion of his tongue and thus his speech. He was greatly upset at the prospect. It is remarkable that his wife chose this most unpropitious time to leave him. Although she told our interviewer that she had simply left for a few days to help her mother out, she told the death investigator immediately after his suicide that she had separated from him because of his drinking. His suicide note, saying he was "too old to start over," reinforces that interpretation. The loss of support must have been overwhelming. I included him among the alcoholics with recent loss. Alone, depressed, and facing the unacceptable, he did what he had threatened to do ever since his previous surgery.

Case 48

Subject 48 was a white male, 42 years old, married, and still employed at the time of his death. He was born in the St. Louis area, where he lived all his life. He had one sibling, a sister. His father owned a small business. The family's religious orientation was identified as "Protestant." The parental home was intact but his father drank excessively until 7 years before his son's death. The subject had fights in school as a boy and once was suspended for 3 days because of it. He had graduated from high school and married at age 19. The marriage produced three children, two girls, ages 14 and 17, living at home, and a son aged 19, away at college at the time of their father's death.

He had begun to work in the family business by age 13 and had worked his entire life in it. He had no military service. Two years before the suicide his father announced his plan to retire and commenced the process of turning the business over to him. Building construction was in a decline. The company was losing money and he felt responsible. His sister and her husband had been employees. They had borrowed money from the company on a number of occasions and were asking for more. On the advice of his attorney, he had fired his sister and refused further loans. They were not on speaking terms for the last 6 months.

He was described as always sensitive but generally well adjusted, until the year prior to his suicide. He began heavy drinking about 12 years before his death and within 2 years he was having drinking and driving problems and accidents, as well as arrests for public intoxication and disturbing the peace. He drank daily and sometimes stayed out all night drinking, but he always managed to get to work. He would sometimes sleep on the job or leave work early on these occasions. He did not go on benders. He knew he drank too much and felt guilty about it. His family and friends also thought he drank too much. He had blackouts and withdrawal tremors but no major medical problems related to alcoholism. He had at one time been under the care of a psychiatrist who specialized in the treatment of alcoholism. He did attend Alcoholics Anonymous for an uncertain period up to 1½ years before his suicide. Although no longer attending AA, he was abstinent from alcohol for the last 9 months of his life.

A year before his suicide, he became grandiose and hypertalkative, but for the last 8–9 months of his life he was self-deprecatory. He developed profound symptoms of depression, with constant low mood, joylessness, and feelings of worthlessness and self-disgust. He suffered from hypersomnia, anorexia with a 40-pound weight loss, loss of interest in activities, indecisiveness, poor concentration and memory, low energy, and suicidal thoughts. He was underactive and withdrew socially. He feared he was losing his mind. He was under the care of a psychiatrist and had last seen him less than a month before his death. He had been given an unidentified antidepressant for 15 months prior to his suicide. His wife had thought he was feeling somewhat better in the weeks just before his death. He had almost no social life in the final year of his life.

His physical health was good, although he had complained of occasional sharp chest pain and fatigue for at least a decade. His only hospitalization was for prostate trouble 7 years before his end.

His mother had a depression when he was 29 and was hospitalized for electroconvulsive therapy. His father's alcoholism had been in remission for 7 years. A maternal cousin was also alcoholic. Further family history was not obtained.

For the last 5 years, he occasionally said, when drinking, that the family would be better off without him. On two occasions, a month or so before taking his life, he said to his wife, "I can see why someone would get in a car and turn it on" (referring to suicide by carbon monoxide inhalation). He did not speak directly of wanting to die. However, he often made reference to his sense of worthlessness, guilt, and inadequacy in his business. At some point he had said to his wife, "I can't go on." The future looked bleak to him. Ironically, a month after his death the company began to make money again as a result of his earlier efforts.

Circumstances Leading to the Act

Nothing much changed. He felt overwhelmed with business worries. On the day of his death his wife drove him to work. He held a meeting with his employees at which he told them there would be less overtime pay because business was poor. He went to the post office and returned. Then he said he was going out to make an appraisal. Instead, he returned to his home, went into the garage, closed the door, and started both cars. He was dead by the time he was found. There was no note.

Findings and Sources

Clinical Diagnosis: (1) Alcoholism, chronic; (2) major depressive disorder, probably bipolar, secondary to the alcoholism.

Toxicology: Blood alcohol concentration insignificant (0.01 g%), blood carbon monoxide saturation 63%.

Primary Informant: Wife, married 23 years, had known him 26 years.

Other Sources of Information: Coroner's death investigation report.

Informant's Opinion of Reason for Suicide: (1) Worried about the business; (2) had lost self-confidence; (3) sick.

Comment

This man might have been expected to have started drinking earlier, given his disciplinary problems in school and his father's alcoholism. He didn't, for whatever reason. When he did start, at age 30, it quickly got out of hand, except that it didn't seem to affect his working to a significant extent. He was undeniably an alcoholic, but it wasn't the drinking that got to him in the end. He had a brief hypomanic episode followed by a rather severe depression. This occurred in a context of increasing business responsibilities in an unfavorable business climate. With onset of the depression he stopped drinking altogether. He felt personally responsible for the business and tortured himself for his failure to turn things around. Suicide became a psychologically acceptable solution in the last month of his life. There was no specific precipitating event, just continuing depression and the overwhelming burden of his sense of responsibility. He didn't live to see business improve as a result of his efforts.

Case 50

Subject 50 was a 65-year-old married white male unemployed accountant. He was born in Illinois and lived most of his life in the St. Louis area. He was raised in the Roman Catholic faith. His father, an alcoholic with no steady job, died 7 months before his son's suicide. His mother ran a decorating shop to support the family, which was physically intact, although troubled. If there were siblings, they were not mentioned. He was not known to have had any school problems. He earned a college degree and worked as an accountant. He served in a nonmilitary capacity with the Army Corps of Engineers for a short time early in World War II. He did not marry until he was 35. The couple had two sons. The older one was 29 and living elsewhere; the younger one was 19 and living at home at the time of the subject's death.

His sexual relationship with his wife had been poor for years and that was a source of tension. He blamed her, saying she was a poor sex partner and that they should have had more children. She thought the exclusive use of the "rhythm method" of birth control had been disruptive to their sex life from the beginning of the marriage. She always refused his sexual advances when he was drunk, and since he was that a lot of the time, they didn't get together much. They had not slept together for many years and had not had sexual intercourse for several years. They had had separate bank accounts for 10 years. She didn't trust his judgment in money matters and didn't want him spending her money.

He was described as having been high-strung, sensitive, easily hurt, and readily moved to tears. He was a shy man, not a mixer. When drinking he became moody. His social life was a mystery to his wife. He would often leave home at night, returning the next day, and she had no idea where he went. The fact that she knew nothing of his habits outside of the house is further evidence of estrangement. Apart from the possibility that he spent those nights with a friend, he appears to have had little in the way of social life outside of work.

He began heavy drinking at about the time he married. It was a problem from the beginning. There was a 1-month separation because of it, 10 years before he ended his life. His wife came back to him when he promised to stop drinking, but of course he didn't. He drank daily with progressive loss of control, up to a fifth or more of liquor per day. He realized he drank too much but did not feel guilty about it and did not try to stop. His family and others objected to his drinking. About 3 months before his death, his wife and younger son said they would take him to no more family parties, as he got very drunk, sometimes passed out, and embarrassed them.

He had morning drinking, blackouts, tremulousness, and probably mild hallucinations on withdrawal. He was first fired for problems related to drinking 9 years before his death. He then was able to keep a job for 2 years or less before being fired again. He had lost four jobs in all due to drinking. His last job was in the City Hall and when he was fired, 6 months before his death, he was unable to find any other work.

He had outbursts of verbally expressed rage when drinking, but he did not get into fights when drunk and was never arrested for any reason. His capacity for alcohol had diminished. He had no significant period of abstinence until he was placed in an alcoholism treatment center 4 months before he ended his life. He spent nearly 2 months in treatment but did not respond well. Upon release he drank more heavily than ever, or at least showed it more.

His only contact with a psychiatrist was during his admission for alcoholism treatment. He was not followed subsequently. Loss of interest in activities had been present for 8 months. He had been noticeably sad for 6 months and was diagnosed as depressed at the time of his discharge from the treatment center. For the subsequent 2 months he hadn't eaten regularly and had lost weight. For the last 6 weeks he had constant low mood, suicidal thoughts and a possible suicide attempt, fatigue, inertia, poor concentration, and impaired memory. (He had had insomnia for 30 years.) When his father died, 7 months before he took his life, he was sad about it but said it was a relief. His wife did not connect those feelings to the depression that he developed a short time later.

He appears to have been in fair physical health. His only medical hospitalization was for plastic surgery for rhinophyma 3 years before his suicide. He had intermittent middle ear trouble (Ménière's syndrome) that produced vertigo. He complained of "neuritis" and trouble with his feet the last few years of his life. He had mild liver function impairment when admitted to the alcoholism treatment center and some degree of pulmonary emphysema, but no major medical illness.

His father was alcoholic and all of his uncles and cousins on that side of the family were heavy drinkers or alcoholics. There was no history of mental illness or suicide.

The first indication of suicidal thought was 6 weeks prior to his ending his life, when he sat down in front of a gas stove and turned on the gas. This was only discovered later when his wife found the chair in front of the stove and the gas on. He merely laughed when confronted on the matter. About a month before his suicide he bought a hose, which the family believed was intended for use in a suicide attempt. His son threw it away, but he surreptitiously bought another. About the same time his wife urged him to take better care of himself and to see a physician. He replied, "I'm not worth it. You'll see." His only attempt to put his affairs in order was to tell his wife, a week before his death, to take care of their son and to be honest with herself. He never specifically mentioned suicide, wanting to die, or that the family would be better off without him.

Circumstances Leading to the Act

He had been unable to find work for 6 months. His wife refused to give him money, so his only source of income was his small savings and dividends from stocks. It was probably not much money. In retrospect, his wife thought this affected his self-esteem and wished she had not been so unyielding. Her and their son's decision not to take him to any more family parties pained him. His depressive syndrome increased considerably after his discharge from inpatient alcoholism treatment. The day before his suicide he drank scotch all day, as he had for 2 months. That evening he argued with his wife over a frequent visitor being in their home. She told him the visitor could stay as long as she (the wife) wished. He left home, drove his car to his brother-in-law's house, parked in the driveway, connected the hose he had purchased to the exhaust, and put the other end in the car window. He was found dead in the car the following morning. An empty pint bottle of gin was on the front seat, but no note.

Findings and Sources

Clinical Diagnosis: (1) Alcoholism, chronic; (2) secondary depression.
Toxicology: Blood alcohol concentration 0.41 g%; blood carbon monoxide saturation 66%.

Primary Informant: Wife, married 30 years, had known him 33 years.
Other Sources of Information: Hospital records, son, coroner's death investigation report.
Informant's Opinion of Reason for Suicide: (1) Sad life—didn't get along with his spouse; (2) alcoholic; (3) no job; (4) bad health.

Comment

This man sacrificed his self-esteem to whatever he thought alcohol did for him. Nevertheless, it pained him. He had felt rejected sexually from very early in the marriage, and that may have been a major factor in his drinking. Originally, it may have resulted from his wife's commitment to the rhythm method of birth control. Subsequently, she refused sex if he had been drinking. That was a circular process. They had had separate bedrooms and separate bank accounts for 10 years. When he lost his last job, 6 months before his death, his means were sharply curtailed. She refused to give him any financial assistance. She decided he wouldn't go to any more family parties. On the evening of his suicide, she told him, in effect, that entertaining guests in their home was at her discretion, not his. Intoxicated and depressed, he was moved to carry out what he had been planning for a month. He must have felt a total loss of status in the family. Granted that he brought it on himself, he had lost every shred of dignity.

Case 36

Subject 36 was a 52-year-old married white Protestant male, retired on disability from the insurance business. He was born in the St. Louis area and lived most of his life there except for military service time. His father was a writer in very poor health at the time of the subject's death. He did poorly in school, was truant a great deal, and dropped out after the 10th grade. He served in the military during World War II from age 24 to 29 without problems, receiving an honorable discharge.

He married in the early days of the war but was away during most of the marriage. His wife objected on religious grounds to his drinking, and they were divorced after 4 years of marriage. They had a son, aged 27 at the subject's death. He remarried at age 30 and sired two children, a daughter aged 19 and a son aged 17 at the time of his death. This son was still living at home. He tried to be a good husband and father but neglected the children when he was drinking. He was not close to his mother but was "emotionally dependent on his father," whose health was failing.

He began to drink at age 15, and drank heavily as a young adult. He lost control about 15 years before his suicide but had drinking problems from at least age 31. Following military service, he had a series of jobs as an insurance adjuster. His drinking led repeatedly to job trouble, usually resulting in his quitting before he was fired, and finding another job. He started his own company 11 years before his death and did well at first, but alcohol soon began to interfere again. Nine years before his suicide, he was diagnosed as having multiple myeloma. He did not work at all after that. His alcoholism probably played a part in his retiring at age 43. His employees carried on for him for a few years, but the company folded up 5 years before his death. From that point on, his only income was Social Security disability. After he quit working, he drank up to a fifth of vodka a day, with morning drinking, blackouts, and three seizures, presumably due to alcohol withdrawal. He had had two arrests for DWI and other arrests for public intoxication, none during the last year of his life.

Although generally an honest man, as executor of his uncle's estate, he misappropriated and spent $1,000 from that account about 1½ years before his death. This may not have come to light prior to his demise. He did not abuse drugs of any sort, but took chlordiazepoxide (Librium) in the morning under a doctor's prescription. Three years before his death he attended Alcoholics Anonymous meetings a few times. Two years later, he initiated a 6-month period of sobriety, but he relapsed for the last 6 months of his life. He was described as feeling miserable during periods of abstinence. He drank with his wife and with friends at his and others' homes as well as in lounges. His wife had problems with alcohol after his death, and probably before as well. She claimed he had "20 close male friends."

He was described as high-strung, sensitive, and easily hurt. After the diagnosis of multiple myeloma was made, he drank more than before and began to speak of suicide. His inability to work caused him to feel inadequate. He had seen psychiatrists for treatment of his depression during his last year of life, but he was never hospitalized. Because of his suicidal preoccupation, a psychiatrist was concerned about his lifelong passion for guns. He warned the informant to get rid of the guns but the subject would not allow her to do so. Although she estimated the duration of his depression as 2 years, she dated some of the criterion symptoms as of 2–3 months duration. In either event, he did become gloomy and pessimistic, feeling guilty and worthless. He was concerned that he was not doing anything to support his family and his invalid father. He had trouble sleeping and thinking, and he lost interest in sex. He had frequent anxiety attacks when drunk.

For the last 2 years of his life he was progressively disabled by pain and recurrent infections secondary to his multiple myeloma. This led to frequent admissions to the Veterans Administration Hospital. His last hospitalization was 6 weeks before his death, for pneumonia. Two weeks earlier he had been admitted for a pathologic fracture of the sternum. He was given radioactive cobalt treatment at that time and was being followed in the VA outpatient clinic. His last clinic visit was on the day of his suicide. Some blood tests had been done, and he held high hopes of being admitted for treatment that would arrest his disease. Nothing was offered him but a return visit in 1 month. He appeared to be quite disappointed that nothing further was done.

The only recorded family history of alcoholism was in a maternal great uncle. There was no other mental illness or history of suicide in the family.

He stated explicitly, when he learned his diagnosis, that he would not die in a hospital bed but would shoot himself instead. He expressed that sentiment to almost all family members and friends. All of his friends had heard him say it at least once. He spoke with increasing frequency of suicide toward the end, almost weekly. However, he never made a suicide attempt and did not appear to make any preparations.

Circumstances Leading to the Act

His mother died during his penultimate hospitalization, 2 months before his suicide. His wife did not think that disturbed him much, as they had not been close. The day of his suicide he returned from an outpatient medical visit very disappointed that the doctor didn't mention further treatment of his cancer. He quarreled with his daughter about which TV channel to watch. He and his wife had a dispute about a message he had forgotten to give her. In the course of that argument he took a pistol and walked out of doors, saying "I'll take care of things." He put the pistol barrel in his mouth and shot himself. He was intoxicated at the time. He had not written a note.

Findings and Sources

Clinical Diagnosis: (1) Alcoholism; (2) secondary depression; (3) multiple myeloma.
Toxicology: Blood alcohol concentration 0.21 g%.
Primary Informant: Wife, married 22 years; saw him daily.
Other Sources of Information: Coroner's death investigation report, hospital record (last admission only).
Informant's Opinion of Reason for Suicide: (1) "He was alcoholic and hated himself"; (2) couldn't cope with life.

Comment

The multiple myeloma was apparently quite far advanced. His expectations regarding a cure were seemingly unwarranted. Nevertheless, he had them, along with a depression of at least 2 months duration. This combination of bad news (or absence of hoped-for good news) plus depression might have proved lethal even without the alcoholism. His marriage was not threatened, and he still had friends. A trivial domestic argument was the apparent trigger, but the suicide was just waiting to happen. Rather than being unable to cope with life, I think he didn't care to cope with slowly dying.

Case 45

Subject 45 was a 45-year-old unemployed married Caucasian male who shot himself in the chest with no prior warning. He was born and raised in rural Missouri and lived in the St. Louis metropolitan area for the last 5 years of his life. He had a twin sister and a brother. The family was Baptist. His father, a farmer, died when he was 11 years old. He completed the 11th grade and entered military service at age 16 during World War II. He served again during the Korean conflict for 3½ years and was in combat there. Later in life he was somewhat troubled by having killed men in combat. After his honorable discharge from the military service at age 27 he worked as a carpenter both in St. Louis and in Arizona. He lost a good job in Arizona 6 years before his death, then returned with his family to St. Louis where he worked out of the union hall. He was usually able to hold employment except for seasonal variations.

He was married at age 28 and had two children, a son aged 15 and a daughter aged 16 years at the time of his death. The family lived together in a three-room apartment. He had received unemployment compensation for 3 months, owing to a strike. The unemployment benefits ended, and for the last month he was unable to find work and had no income. He had no social life at all in his last weeks, and perhaps none before that.

He developed a serious drinking problem at age 32, thirteen years before his suicide. That same year he was found to be ill with tuberculosis and was hospitalized for

4½ months. Although he did not drink in the hospital, he resumed this habit after taking his unauthorized departure. It progressed to a daily consumption of up to two fifths of liquor a day. In the last 2 years of his life he "went downhill" and was unable to start the day without a few drinks. He knew he drank too much, felt guilty, and tried unsuccessfully to quit. Frequently, he would say, "When I finish this bottle I'm quitting," but he always got another bottle.

His wife and family were concerned about his drinking. Two years before his death his wife tried to commit him to the Veterans Administration Hospital for alcoholism treatment but alleged she was told "a relative" had to do this. She appears to have been a classic "enabler." He stole money from her for drink. She would give him money to pay rent and utility bills and he would spend it on alcohol. Then she would be furious with him but would do it again. She once told him she would kill him if she found him in a bar again. But she would buy liquor for him to help him deal with the shakes.

He was fired 6 years before his death for missing work. He had gone on four 1-week binges over an 18-month period, each episode being precipitated by his wife's admission to a hospital. (What occasioned these admissions was not learned, but it is unlikely to have been the result of spouse abuse; see below.) During the last year of his life he had three automobile accidents while drunk but was never charged with drunken driving. He did not get into fights outside of the home.

His wife had become very angry about his drinking. Ten months before his death he and she had a physical fight. She beat him severely enough to fracture three ribs and cause a concussion and demanded that he leave. He went to live with his mother in the town where he grew up, receiving outpatient treatment for his injuries there. Four months before his suicide he was jailed for 2 weeks for failure to pay family support. His drinking caused problems at his mother's home and his brother came from out of state to tell him to either stop drinking or move out. He thereupon returned to live with his wife for the last 5 weeks of his life. He stayed at home drinking while she worked. He was trying to cut down on his drinking and was suffering daily mild withdrawal tremors.

He was never seen by a psychiatrist or treated for alcoholism by any physician. He had been complaining of headaches and blurred vision for the last 2 years of his life; he also had diminished appetite and believed he had cancer, but he did not seek medical attention for these complaints. He had never appeared to have any emotional problems apart from alcoholism, nor was his personality unusual in any way. The only symptoms of possible depression were anorexia for 2 years and fatigue and hypersomnolence for the last 6 months of his life. He did not appear depressed and did not speak of low mood, guilt, worthlessness, hopelessness, or suicide at any time.

The only serious illness recorded was "far advanced pulmonary tuberculosis" discovered at age 32 and thought to be of 6-month duration. He was hospitalized and treated in a research protocol with INH (isonicotinic acid hydrazide) and PAS (para-aminosalicylic acid) with shrinking of cavities and conversion of sputum to negative for the acid-fast tubercle bacillus. He was not yet scheduled for discharge but became impatient and eloped from the hospital 4½ months after admission. His only other significant medical contact was hospital outpatient treatment for fractured ribs and concussion resulting from being beaten by his wife.

He had a paternal cousin with alcoholism and cirrhosis. His twin sister was described as "nervous" but there was no other family history of mental illness and none of suicide.

Circumstances Leading to the Act

It appears possible that his wife was preparing to make a major decision about the marriage, as she had said, "We can't go on with you drinking." He was trying, with limited success, to cut down on his drinking but she was increasingly angry about it. They were not communicating at all well at the time of his death. He, she, and their son had returned from a Boy Scout parent–son camping weekend during which he had experienced alcohol withdrawal tremors and had to be driven by his wife to a nearby town to obtain liquor. On Monday morning he was again tremulous, stayed in bed, and began drinking again. He told his wife she should not try to work with an injured leg (no details obtained) and she replied angrily, "Someone has to." She also said, "You'll never stop drinking as long as someone buys liquor for you." He responded, "You'll never know." This vague reply turned out to be his only hint that he was thinking of suicide. His wife left for work and when the children arose at 11:00 a.m. they found their father had shot himself in the chest and expired.

There was a note addressed to the family in general:

> To all. [Son] gets my tools and Van or bus as you may call it. The rest goes to [wife's name and daughter's name]. I have a brain trouble, and a lung trouble, plus stomach. [Son] do not let Miss come were [sic] near me are [sic] our family. [victim's first name]

Findings and Sources

Clinical Diagnosis: (1) Alcoholism, chronic; (2) healed pulmonary tuberculosis.
Toxicology: Not performed.
Primary Informant: Wife, married 17 years, had known him 20 years.
Other Sources of Information: Coroner's death investigation record, hospital record (pulmonary).
Informant's Opinion of Reason for Suicide: He was sick, alcoholic. Other family members doubted that his fatal wound was self-inflicted.

Comment

This man had been thrown out by his wife 10 months before his suicide, thrown out of his mother's home 6 months later, was back with his wife, but had been out of work for 4 months. His wife was thoroughly fed up with his drinking. Although described in the coroner's death investigation report as "in depressed mood," confirmatory symptoms were denied to our interviewer by his wife. He was not being successful in moderating his drinking and his wife's patience had worn very thin. She was continuously angry with him. It is purely speculation that she was planning to leave him. No specific precipitation is identifiable. His note says he saw himself as sick in more than one way. It does not mention a threatened separation. If his wife had killed him, as some family members thought, I doubt that she would have consented to be interviewed. If loss of self-respect is sufficient motive for suicide, it gets my vote. He was also estranged from his mother 5 weeks before his death. I nominated him for recent loss of a close interpersonal relationship on the basis of that estrangement. His wife was fed up with him, too. If your mother can't tolerate you, who will?

Case 20

Subject 20 was a 50-year-old white separated Roman Catholic male, born in St. Louis. He was minimally observant of his religion until the last 2 years, then not at all. His mother, widowed since the subject's father committed suicide when the subject was 6 years old, worked in a laundry for a number of years thereafter. She had a history of alcoholism. More than 3 years before his death, she had lived with him and his second wife for 2 or 3 months. During that time she got drunk nightly, and sometimes was found drunk on the street.

It is thought that he finished the eighth grade. He had 3 years of military service during World War II without going overseas and received an honorable discharge. His age at his first marriage was not learned. He was divorced by his first wife about 15 years before his death, and married his second wife 3 years later. That marriage lasted 12 years, ending when he died. There were no children from either marriage. He had worked for the City of St. Louis as a street maintenance man for 12 years but was fired 2 years before ending his life. He was unable to find work after that. Earlier, he worked in construction and his wife thought he might have made more money then. His total working life was more than 30 years. He had no friends, even at the tavern he frequented.

It is not known when he began drinking, but his second wife believed his first wife divorced him because of it. That would place onset of his problem drinking earlier than age 35, with a minimum duration of 16 years. His second wife objected to his heavy drinking throughout the marriage. She had separated from him, after about 5 years of marriage, because of it. Around that time he lost consciousness in a bar while sober and was hospitalized. His wife took him back upon his release. Records from that admission were unobtainable.

When drunk, he was moody and cried easily. For the 3–4 years before his suicide his behavior when drinking included yelling, screaming, throwing things, and trying to tear up the house. However, he did not physically assault anyone. His behavior worsened 2 years before his death, around the time when he lost his job. During the last 6–8 months of his life he would sit secluded in his room nightly and talk as though someone were there, pause, and talk again. His wife thought he was hallucinating. His memory had become very bad and he was generally confused about things such as the time of day and place, even when not drinking. He often couldn't find his way home without help. People at the bars he frequented wouldn't talk to him because he was irrational. He had a decreased tolerance for alcohol for the last 6–12 months. When drinking, he thought he had money when he really didn't.

He drank before breakfast and had a history of benders. Two years before his death he was fired from his job of 12 years with the City Street Department because of drinking on the job, walking off the job, and failure to report to work. He did not drive a car and had no arrests. He had never had treatment for alcoholism. He had never been concerned about his drinking until near the end of his life, and then not much. Only in the last 2 months of his life did he begin to acknowledge that he drank too much and to feel some guilt about it.

He had lost weight (he was described as "skin and bones") and was chronically tired the last 2 years of his life. He had little interest in anything except drinking and was markedly underactive. He had no sexual relations with his wife in the last 2 years. It was not possible to determine whether his inactivity should be considered psychomotor retardation or simply secondary to his very evident organic brain syndrome.

Five years before his death he had lost consciousness in a bar when he hadn't been drinking and had an electroencephalogram. Two years later he was hospitalized for an inguinal herniorrhaphy. On a hospital admission 2 years before his death, his complaints were of poor appetite, general malaise, and intermittent blood in his stools. He claimed to have had surgery for gastric ulcer 20 years earlier. There was no evidence of abdominal surgery, although the gallbladder was not visualized. Radiographic examination showed duodenal deformity characteristic of inactive duodenal ulcer as well as a rectal polyp. There was also radiologic evidence of an earlier granulomatous pulmonary infection, probably tuberculosis. He last visited a doctor 1½ years before his suicide for "stomach pain and ulcers" caused by excessive drinking. He had that complaint until his death.

His father committed suicide when he was 6 years old. Nothing else was learned of this man. His mother was clearly a habitual drunkard in her later years. He must have had a sister, because he had a brother-in-law. Nothing was reported concerning her.

For 6–12 months before his suicide, when drunk, he would pray that God would let him die in his sleep and would say that he would be better off dead. Three weeks before his death, he told his brother-in-law that he planned to jump out of the window.

Circumstances Leading to the Act

His second wife had filed for divorce 5 weeks before his suicide. She forced him to move out of the house 3 weeks before his death "because he wouldn't work" and because of his persistently unpleasant behavior. She said she hoped it would "pull him to his senses." According to the coroner's death investigation report, he went to his brother-in-law's place and asked for a beer and a place to stay. While there, he walked back and forth constantly. When he was told to leave, he said he planned to jump out of a window. His brother-in-law said, "Why don't you?" Three weeks later he jumped from the window of his third-floor room in a rooming house where he had been living since his wife put him out. The window, which faced a sidewalk, was raised and a small kitchen chair was at the window. Fresh scuff marks were on the window ledge. He was found dead on the sidewalk with a pool of blood at his head. No note was found.

Findings and Sources

Clinical Diagnoses: (1) Alcoholism, chronic; (2) secondary dementia with organic hallucinosis; (3) probable secondary depression (DSM-III-R definite).

Toxicology: Blood alcohol; none detected.
Primary Informant: Wife, married 12 years, had known him 14 years; saw him daily until the last 3 weeks.
Other Sources of Information: Brother-in-law, through coroner's death investigation report, hospital records.
Informant's Opinion of Reason for Suicide: Accidental fall.

Comment

It is difficult to assess the role of depression in this case, as several of the criterion symptoms (weight loss, lack of energy, loss of interest, impaired thinking) are equally likely to be attributable to his dementia. This man's only identifiable interest was in drinking. It cost him two marriages, a steady job, the positive regard of others, and, ultimately, adequate brain function. He became disoriented and irrational, and he hallucinated. He had so alienated his brother-in-law that, after his final separation, when he expressed to him the thought of jumping out of a window, the response was, "Why don't you." He had no social support whatever. He cannot have felt anything but superfluous. He was not drinking just before his suicide. Perhaps he was out of money, too. Expulsion from his home 3 weeks before his suicide puts him in the "recent loss" category.

Case 39

Subject 39, a 54-year-old married white male brewery worker, ended his life unexpectedly by gunshot wound. Born and raised in the St. Louis area, he lived there his entire life. His parents were both born in Ireland and were Roman Catholic. His mother died of "uremic poisoning" when he was 1 month old, presumably the result of toxemia of pregnancy (eclampsia). His father then married her sister. He ran an insurance agency. There was no mention in the record concerning siblings. He had an unremarkable childhood, completed the 10th grade, and went to work. He worked steadily in local breweries for most of his adult life and was considered a good worker. According to the custom of the industry, beer was freely available on the job. He took full advantage of that opportunity. His only job problems were related to his health. His last job consisted of cleaning brewing vats, and he became unable to work a full day due to shortness of breath secondary to chronic pulmonary emphysema. At the end he was subjected to ridicule by fellow workers, but whether this was owing to his dyspnea, his drinking, or something else was not learned. He married at age 30 and had two daughters, who were 23 and 22 at the time of his death. Both were married and out of the home, so just he and his wife were there. He had not been in military service.

He began drinking heavily at age 35 and drank daily, with progressive loss of control. He had two periods of spontaneous abstinence of 6 months each, 2 and 4 years before his death. His typical pattern was five or six shots of liquor in the morning and then continuous beer drinking during the day, from the supply readily available to him on the job. He sometimes had mild alcohol withdrawal tremors but no serious withdrawal symptoms. His drinking was not reported to have resulted in problems at work, nor did he have arrests or driving problems related to drinking. His wife objected to his drinking and they argued over it. Only during the last 3 years of his life did she regard him as alcoholic. During his 20s and 30s he had temper outbursts when intoxicated. When in arguments with his wife, he would fly into a rage. That behavior disappeared later, and he was never physically abusive.

A year before his death his wife attempted suicide with an overdose of medication because she felt she couldn't live with his drinking. Their older daughter had made a suicide attempt 5 years before his death, for unknown reasons. He felt guilty about these attempts, as he was no doubt supposed to do. He felt guilty about drinking and knew he drank too much. However, he did not seek treatment or attend Alcoholics Anonymous. His drinking aggravated medical problems, particularly his emphysema and a hiatus hernia which developed in the last 2-3 years of his life. He had been drinking more heavily for 6 months. He worried a great deal about his failing health and inability to work a full day. He felt guilty about not being a good provider. During the last 1 or 2 months, his drinking increased even more. For the last 3 weeks of his life he was unable to retain solid food, probably as a result of alcoholic gastritis. "Everything he ate would come back up." During that time he "lived on beer." His wife said he had at least 15 close friends, who "would do anything for him." There was thus no evidence of social isolation.

He was always sensitive and easily moved to tears, although he tried to hide this from his wife and others. During the last year of his life he lost interest in activities, including sex, and was impotent for the last 6 weeks. His wife thought it troubled him. He gave up his season football tickets, saying he was getting too old to go out on Sunday and freeze. During the last 6 months he complained of fatigue. "His whole personality changed in the last 3 or 4 months." His appetite became poor and he lost 30 pounds. He spoke of being worthless, blaming himself for the family's troubles and for being a poor provider. He felt no one was with him and there was no hope for him. He said he was not sure whether he was losing his mind, but supporting symptoms are lacking. He became nervous, jittery, and irritable. He never saw a psychiatrist or any other physician for treatment of either depression or alcoholism, and he took no psychotropic medications. His wife didn't think he looked depressed, but his symptoms and behavior are highly characteristic.

He was hospitalized twice at age 30 with kidney trouble, twice for back surgery at age 49, and once at age 53 for a hernia repair. It is not clear if the latter was for his diaphragmatic hiatus hernia or for an inguinal hernia. He was under the care of a physician for chronic pulmonary emphysema as well as the hiatus hernia, both of which became much worse in the last 3 months of his life. His dyspnea limited his ability to work and thereby reduced his income. He slept poorly, frequently being awake much of the night coughing.

There was no family history of alcoholism, mental illness, or suicide. Hs daughter had made a suicide attempt.

For 3 months he said there was no hope for him and his wife didn't need him. He never directly spoke of suicide or of dying. He did refer to his wife's and daughter's suicide attempts, for which he felt ashamed and responsible. His last words—"I'll show you how to do it"—were his only direct reference to suicide. The act was a great surprise to everyone who knew him. He was regarded as "the last person to commit suicide."

Circumstances Leading to the Act

He had considered his fellow workers at his last place of employment "unfriendly." During the last month of his life, they ridiculed him. On the day of his death he left work early, went to a bar, and drank for several hours. He returned home about 9:30 p.m. When he entered the house, intoxicated, his wife started to remonstrate with him. He stared at her for a few moments and said, "Well, [their daughter] tried it and you tried it, and I'll show you how to do it," referring to their suicide attempts. He then walked into the bathroom, lay down in the empty bathtub, and shot himself in the head with a .38-caliber revolver. He died in the hospital several hours later.

Findings and Sources

Clinical Diagnosis: (1) Alcoholism, chronic; (2) pulmonary emphysema ; (3) hiatus hernia. Diagnosis of major depression is withheld.
Toxicology: Blood alcohol concentration 0.21 g%.
Primary Informant: Wife, married 24 years; saw him daily.
Other Sources of Information: Coroner's death investigation report.
Informant's Opinion of Reason for Suicide: Guilt about being less than the best provider.

Comment

A diagnosis of depression is withheld here. Advanced pulmonary emphysema is characteristically attended by weight loss, interrupted sleep, fatigue, and, ultimately, inability to work. Although it is possible for such symptoms to have more than one source, the informant's statement that he never looked depressed negates an essential criterion for the research diagnosis. Loss of interest can substitute for depressed mood under DSM-III-R, and he does meet those criteria. It is relevant that he was said to have exhibited a major personality change in the last 3–4 months of his life, and with it, hopelessness, concern about losing his mind, an increase in drinking, and rapid decline in both physical health and capacity for work.

Alcohol thickens bronchial secretions and thus worsens the symptoms of pulmonary emphysema, so increased drinking and worsening of physical state go hand in hand. The supervention of a major depression would account best for his personality change, his increased drinking, and his feelings of guilt and hopelessness. However, there is a legitimate alternative explanation for a number of his depressive symptoms. The precipitants of this suicide are, then, somewhat circular: a progressively incapacitating medical illness complicated by and complicating alcohol abuse; guilt about impairment of his provider role, contributed to both by his emphysema and his alcohol abuse; and being ridiculed at work. In the end, impairment of his provider role damaged his self-esteem. His progressive pulmonary disease and his out-of-control drinking were additive factors.

Case 5

Subject 5 was a 57-year-old white divorced Protestant male, born and raised in St. Louis. His father was a tavern owner. Our informant did not know whether he did or did not have an alcohol problem. His mother died when he was 16, and his father when he was 18. In neither case was the cause of death known to the informant. He lived with his sister from age 18 to 20 and completed schooling on his own, graduating from college with a degree in electrical engineering. He married at the age of 31 and had four sons, aged 24, 20, 18, and 13 at the time of his death. He was divorced at the age of 44, thirteen years before his suicide. Although he had little social life while married, he later became active in the Masonic Lodge and in his last 5 years was additionally active in his church, both regularly attending Sunday services and participating in other social activities. He had additional social life in taverns.

After his graduation from college, he worked for the federal government as a hydraulic engineer until he entered military service as an officer in the Army. He served overseas, was decorated, and was honorably discharged when he was 35 years old. He worked again, briefly, in his previous capacity, then took similar employment with a private concern. He held that job for 19 years until 9 months before his death. He gradually developed persecutory and grandiose delusions and was forced to take "early retirement" 9 months before he took his life. With the end of his employment, his monthly income dropped to 20% of its previous level. He was unable to find work for many months, meanwhile remaining grandiose and delusional and harassing his former employer. He secured employment as a security guard 2½ weeks before his death. It was the only work he could find.

He had his first drink in his late teens and drank occasionally in college and in the military service. Following his military discharge, he was described as a social drinker, but by age 39, some 18 years before his suicide, he was drinking each evening and "heavy" on the weekends. (In response to a different question about when he became a heavy drinker, his ex-wife said he was a heavy drinker by age 25.) He usually drank beer, and occasionally whiskey. His weekend binge drinking became heavier, and with it he exhibited increasing hostility toward his wife. Gradually, he became more verbally aggressive and on two occasions assaulted her physically. That led to their divorce 13 years before his death. He was unable to understand why such behavior should result in divorce. His heavy weekend drinking continued until the time of his death. He frequently had morning "shakes" but no other reported physical effects of his drinking. He had one arrest, for peace disturbance, in the last year of his life.

There are hints of persecutory thinking as early as the time of his military service. He blamed the influence of another officer for his failure to be promoted from first lieutenant to captain. Later in the marriage he blamed his wife for a good deal of what occurred and some things that did not. He spoke also of suspicions concerning attitudes and behavior of some co-workers. This gradually became more open. His job performance declined, he refused to follow orders, and he expressed persecutory delusions about other workers. Eighteen months before his death, he was forced by his employer to accept hospitalization for "complete evaluation." To quote from the discharge summary of this admission:

> The complaints on the part of the Company were that he was developing certain theories involving the use of hydropower for production of electrical current; these theories were extremely bizarre and grandiose. The patient also felt he was being assigned menial tasks and was refusing to accept assignments from his supervisor of personnel. He began to be suspicious that those that worked with him were singling him out to ridicule and depreciate, and at times he became rather angry.

His physical status was unremarkable. Oddly, the workup did not include a psychiatric consultation.

He seemed somewhat better for 3–4 months, but then his earlier behavior returned. Nine months before his suicide he was forced to accept "early retirement." Thereafter, he hounded his former employer almost daily with accusations and delusional schemes of a grandiose character, and he demanded to be given work to do. Four months before his death, he had a 2½ week psychiatric hospitalization on the advice of his minister when his former employer was about to take legal action to stop his harassment. At that time, he was described as appearing chronically ill, somewhat depressed, and withdrawn. At the same time, his behavior was sometimes overactive and inappropriate. His speech was described as circumstantial and tangential. He was clearly delusional. He improved somewhat with phenothiazine medication and was discharged with diagnoses of chronic alcoholism and paranoid reaction. Apparently after that hospitalization, he no longer harassed his former employer. Although he was described as appearing depressed at times, his ex-wife was unable to report any actual depressive symptoms.

Five years before his death, he was hospitalized for a herniorrhaphy. He had no known chronic medical disease.

His oldest son, age 24, had had two psychiatric hospitalizations and had been unable to work for the previous 4 years. He was being treated with phenothiazines and his illness appeared to have a chronic, deteriorating course, like schizophrenia. The informant knew nothing of his parents. A paternal uncle had been quiet, withdrawn, and unable to work for several years.

Thirteen years before his death, when his wife left him, he told her, "I'm going to kill myself." However, he took no action at that time. For about the last 2 years of his life, he said occasionally to his ex-wife, "I don't know why I go on." He never made a suicide attempt and made no other communications of suicidal intent.

Circumstances Leading to the Act

Nine months before his death, because of chronic persecutory and grandiose delusions, he lost a job he had held for the previous 19 years. He was unable to find suitable work and was in financial distress. He had bought an apartment building 5 years before his death. Since losing his job, he was unable to make payments on it or to keep it up, but he hadn't lost it. He finally accepted employment far below his level of education and experience, as a security guard. Two and a half weeks later, while on the job, he shot himself in the head with a .38-caliber revolver. It was the day before his 57th birthday. He did not leave a note.

Findings and Sources

Clinical Diagnosis: (1) Alcoholism, chronic; (2) delusional disorder (possible paranoid schizophrenia).
Toxicology: Not performed.
Primary Informant: Ex-wife, who knew him for about 27 years; saw him two to three times a week since the divorce.
Other Sources of Information: Hospital records, coroner's death investigation report.
Informant's Opinion of Reason for Suicide: (1) Lost a good job; (2) financial obligations; (3) let everyone down.

Comment

Symptoms of a depressive syndrome had not been noted by this subject's ex-wife, who saw him two to five times a week throughout the 13 years since their divorce. A delusional syndrome, both grandiose and persecutory, had developed gradually over a period of years. He had shown a strong tendency to project blame as long as 25 years before his death. The expression of delusional material seems to have come under a fair degree of control with medication in the last 3–4 months of his life. Despite that disorder, he was reported to have had quite a substantial social support system. It was most probably his delusional disorder, rather than his drinking, that cost him his good job, although he did experience a number of serious consequences of his drinking. The only recent loss that can be identified was a major one. He was in financial straits as a result of losing a good job, and he was reduced to accepting night work as a security guard. The loss of status was extreme. He was not reported to have commented upon it to his ex-wife, but with the whole night to contemplate the course of his life, it seems to me this must have been sufficient occasion for his suicide. Whether he was drinking at the time he shot himself was not determined.

Case 22

Subject 22 was a married white male of no known religious persuasion. He was 62 years old at the time of his death. He was born in Texas, the second of two boys. His father, occupation unknown, had been alcoholic in his younger years. His mother was so opposed to liquor that she kept a liquor bottle in the house marked with a "skull and crossbones." He was described as "uncontrollable" as a child, and punishment was ineffective in keeping him at home and abiding by family rules. He would fight with anyone, regardless of size. However, he did complete high school satisfactorily and was good at football. He had no military service, having just missed military draft at the end of World War I. He had had many jobs in Texas until his move to St. Louis nearly 9 months before his suicide. During the last 20 years of his life he worked mostly as a salesman. He had also briefly worked in aircraft maintenance and as a resort and apartment manager. At the time of his death, he was a hardware store manager.

He was married at age 20 and had sired five children, two girls and three boys. They ranged in age from 40 to 23 at the time of his death. The second youngest boy was killed in military combat 2 years before the subject's suicide. His wife left him first in February of the year of his death to come to St. Louis. He followed her in April. She left him again on the day of his suicide, in late December. She described him as well liked by others, but unaware of it. He would pick up the tab for the group when he went out. "He had to be top dog." Throughout their relationship, he was jealous of any attention paid to his wife by other men. They could not go dancing because he would accuse her of flirting. She had to stay right by him, could not even visit the children by herself. Despite his faults his wife and children loved him. He was generous, usually kind, and helped with raising the children.

He is described as drinking little at the time of his marriage at age 20, but he was a regular weekend drinker by age 30. He was having problems from drinking by age 39 and was out of control by age 44, with increased fighting with his wife and sons, gradual social withdrawal, expressions of disgust with the world, spitefulness, and anger when he was intoxicated. His pattern was a weekend binge about every 3–4 weeks, beginning Friday evening and continuing until late Sunday. He consumed about a fifth of wiskey a day and required 2 days to sober up.

When he was 45, his wife had surgery for pelvic cancer and was told she had 6 months to live. He sold the family farm for $7,000 to use for his wife's care. Instead, he quit traveling as a salesman and spent the money on women and liquor. The next year his wife had exploratory surgery and was found to be free of cancer. He accused her of squandering the money. Between ages 47 and 50 he had frequent anxiety or panic attacks while sobering up. He drank before breakfast at times. He had varying periods of abstinence. The longest was about 5 months, ending in a binge just a few days before his death.

He had been arrested twice, with overnight incarceration for public intoxication, at about age 46. On the first of these occasions, as a result of his physical abuse, his wife telephoned their son, who was in the military service. He came home and together they had him arrested and tried to get him admitted to an alcoholism treatment program. He was held in jail for 2 days, but the effort at hospitalization was unsuccessful. He failed to return to his then current job following the attempt to force him into treatment. He was jailed for indecent exposure in February of the year of his suicide. That occurred in the same month his wife left him and moved to St. Louis, but the temporal sequence was not clear.

He had at least eight different jobs in the last 10 years of his life, was fired from two of them, and quit at least two others. He was physically abusive and dangerous to his wife when drunk, and had had one fight while at work. His wife was afraid of him. On at least one occasion he threatened her with a shotgun, and he voiced suspicions that she was unfaithful to him. He beat her severely enough to require hospitalization on two occasions, 4 and 1 year prior to his suicide. On the day before his death he attempted to choke her, and she left him. He did acknowledge that he drank too much, and family and friends held that opinion. However, he did not lose friends. He had progressive loss of control and failed attempts at abstinence. No serious medical problems resulted from his drinking.

His only contact with a psychiatrist was one office visit at age 35, for undetermined reasons. He was described as always having been moody, with rapid mood changes and occasional periods of elation, but "no happy medium" according to his wife. He never had periods of depression lasting longer than a week until the last year or two of his life. At age 57, he suffered a head injury in an automobile accident. He was reportedly not intoxicated at the time. He was unconscious for 2 hours and hospitalized for 3 weeks. He received a $4,000 settlement, which he quickly used up. Following the head injury he was more vindictive, more critical of others, and more violent when drinking. He developed panic attacks characterized by dyspnea, palpitation, and chest pain, which his wife stated were worse when he was recovering from a binge. He also became agoraphobic at that time and remained so to the end of his life.

In the last 5 years he seemed to have less energy. He gave up golf and wouldn't drive on trips anymore. The last 3 years he was slow and had trouble calculating, but he was not disoriented. During the year prior to his death he had a weight loss of 15–20 pounds, decreased interest in activities, indecision, a persistently sad expression, interval insomnia, and an increased sex drive. He manifested no psychotic symptoms (unless his pathological suspiciousness is so regarded) and did not seek psychiatric treatment, but heavily used chlordiazepoxide, (Librium), propoxyphene hydrochloride, (Darvon) and meprobamate, (Equanil), which he obtained from physicians. He occasionally mentioned casually that he thought he was losing his mind.

Had two hospitalizations at age 60, one for a "checkup" to investigate nervousness and a question of a "heart attack." The other was for surgery for a ruptured cervical disc, which continued to cause neck and back pain and was the justification for large amounts of analgesics and tranquilizers, which he took in combination with alcohol for at least a decade. The ruptured disc antedated his auto accident by about 3 years, occurring just after his son's death. He was under treatment with an osteopathic physician for his back and neck pain and was seen about 1 month prior to his death. Requests for medical and hospitalization records were not responded to.

His father was an alcoholic as a young man, but nothing is known about his later years. A paternal uncle was also alcoholic. There is no known history of mental illness or suicide in the family.

Earlier in his life he had repeatedly predicted he would "never reach 50," but he did. For the last 4 to 5 years he had occasionally said, while drinking, that he would be better off dead, but he wouldn't talk about a burial policy or a plot in a cemetery. In his last 2 years he occasionally said he wished he could drink enough to go to sleep and not wake up, but he made no specific mention of suicide or of method of suicide. His comment "I'll make it legal" (see below) probably referred to suicide.

Circumstances Leading to the Act

His wife had left him in February and moved to St. Louis because of his violent behavior toward her. She allowed him to join her in April, with the understanding that she would leave him permanently if he drank again. He may have done so within about 3 months, as they had been back together for 8 months and she reported that he had 5 months of abstinence from alcohol prior to his death. He began drinking again after an interpersonal dispute just before Christmas. ("A 'punk' had 'cussed him out' while he was looking for a car.") Three weeks before his death, his wife had to call the police because he had locked their granddaughter in the bedroom. Drinking was not mentioned in connection with that event. During the holidays, his wife reiterated her warning that she would leave him if he continued to drink. He was too intoxicated to return to work after the holiday.

A day or two before his death he told his wife, "I know what you're doing [with the apartment maintenance man]. I'll make it legal" (a reference to his pathological jealousy). At the time, she thought he was threatening her. After the fact she believed it was a suicide threat. He also said he would kill the police if they came after him. On December 28, he became enraged at his wife over food she was preparing for him, and he began choking her. A telephone call from their daughter interrupted the fracas and his wife told the daughter she "had better get over here." She believed he was going to get his shotgun, with which he had threatened her in the past. In fear for her life, she left home and spent the night with her daughter. Early the next morning she returned home together with her daughter and son-in-law, to find the subject dead, lying on his bed with an abdominal wound and the shotgun lying nearby. He took his life the day after the eighth anniversary of his son's death in Korea. There was no note.

Findings and Sources

Clinic Diagnosis: (1) Alcoholism, chronic; (2) major depressive disorder; (3) history of head injury with some personality change.
Toxicology: Blood alcohol concentration 0.30 g%.
Primary Informant: Wife, married 42 years; saw him daily.
Informant's Opinion of Reason for Suicide: "He was tired of trying to stop drinking, tired of living and trying to cope."

Comment

This man was rebellious as a child and erratic in his work history. His alcoholism had a long incubation period, during which he was able to establish a loving relationship with his wife and children. He became physically abusive toward his wife in the last 20 years of their marriage when drinking. Following a head injury 5 years before his death this abusiveness worsened, and his wife finally fled from him to St. Louis 10 months before he took his life. She agreed to let him back into her life 2 months later, with the understanding that if he drank and became abusive again, that would be the end of the marriage.

It is possible that she had tolerated one further bout. He certainly fell off the wagon shortly before Christmas and couldn't reestablish sobriety. During that episode she reiterated her intention to leave him if he did not straighten up. When he attacked her physically on seemingly trivial grounds (he objected to what she was preparing for dinner), she escaped and spent the night with her daughter. He shot and killed himself shortly after she left. She said she left in fear for her life and did not mention an intention to separate permanently at that moment. It might be argued that her leaving was temporary, not a true separation. My interpretation is that he knew he had exceeded her tolerance with little or no justification and that he was incapable of doing better. He did not wait for her return. I think the separation, however informal, was the final straw, although I did not include this subject in the tabulations of recent loss. At a minimum, loss was threatened.

Case 35

Subject 35 was a 50-year-old married white male investment broker and land developer at the time of his death by gunshot wound. He was born in the St. Louis area and lived there most of his life. He had two older sisters and a younger brother. His professed religious affiliation was Congregational. Observance was not learned. His father was a pharmacist who, late in life, worked as a stockbroker. There were no known childhood problems and the home was conventionally middle class. He graduated from high school and had one semester at a local university. He entered the Army at age 19, two years before World War II, and served until the end of the war. He saw combat but escaped injury and disciplinary or drinking problems. After his honorable discharge at the end of the war, he joined a firm of investment brokers and continued with them until his death.

He married at age 27 and the couple had two daughters who were 17 and 22 at the time of his death. Eleven years before his suicide he started a contracting firm but had little business success and many conflicts with his employees. He didn't seem to know how to manage people. At the end, he was getting deeper in debt, while expressing unrealistic optimism about being on the verge of making large amounts of money. During the last 5 years, his brokerage clients increasingly left him for other brokers.

He had his first drink at age 15, but his wife did not think his drinking was a problem until about 10 years before his death. During the next 4 years it became a serious problem. Drinking heavily, he abused his wife. She left him and filed for divorce 5 years before his death, then returned to him 2 days later when he agreed to stop drinking beer and to stop hitting her. He substituted vodka for beer, but he did cease his physical abuse of her. He drank daily, except on Sundays. The amounts of alcohol he drank are not known, but he often drank in the morning and continued to drink during his long working day. He lost business clients as a result. He lost friends also, for this reason, and his secretary of many years quit her job 5 years before his suicide because of it. He received several tickets for driving while intoxicated and had several accidents, but no serious legal consequences. His wife had called the police to their home several times during the period when he was physically abusing her. No arrest or other intervention occurred as a result.

He felt guilty about his drinking but was unable or unwilling to try to stop. He had visible tremulousness during the last 2 years. Alcoholic gastritis led to several hospitalizations but he was never treated for alcoholism as such. He used a combination of alcohol and an over-the-counter sedative to deal with insomnia but did not abuse stronger drugs. He had not seen friends at home in 4 years. He had little meaningful contact with his wife and daughter, not even taking meals with them except on the weekend. His only social life appears to have been at bars. How much time he spent there, as opposed to drinking alone in his office, was unknown.

He was described as always high-strung, sensitive, and easily moved to tears. He became more moody and sensitive when his drinking increased. When intoxicated, he had outbursts of rage. His preoccupation with job and financial worries increased. Although he almost continuously expressed unrealistic optimism about his business prospects, he had constant low mood, fatigue, general loss of interest, and insomnia for about the last 2 years of his life. His appetite became poor just in the week prior to his suicide. He saw a family physician at infrequent intervals, but he never saw a psychiatrist.

He received cortisone injections regularly from a dermatologist, for psoriasis as well as treatment for "jungle rot" (fungal infection), but he had not seen his internist for over a year. He was hospitalized for cellulitis of his right leg 2 years before his death, and twice for abdominal pain diagnosed as chronic cholecystitis 3½ years before his death. Six months earlier, a hospital admission for acute abdominal pain with suspected bowel obstruction culminated in a diagnosis of gastroenteritis. The informant thought that all three admissions for abdominal pain resulted from alcoholic gastritis. His only other known hospitalization was about 10 years earlier, for stripping of varicose veins of the left lower leg.

The only family member thought to have had mental illness was his father, who had a period of heavy drinking just after World War II. He had changed jobs from his lifelong career as a pharmacist to work as a stockbroker in the same firm that employed his son. He was doing poorly and stated at a business meeting, "I'm going to give myself two more months." Two months later he was found dead in his room. The death was signed out without autopsy as a heart attack. The informant suspected it was a suicide, since the man was not known to have had heart trouble.

Throughout their marriage this subject had regularly "kidded" his wife about dying before she did. This increased in the last 10 years. A few months before his death he began to say to his wife that he would be better off dead, and that he wanted to die. There was no specific mention of suicide.

Circumstances Leading to the Act

The older daughter was away at college. His younger daughter would leave for college in a few months. His wife thought he believed she would leave him when both girls were gone. He believed he was once more in serious financial trouble in his contracting firm. He had taken a second mortgage on his home for $15,000 and two business loans amounting to another $12,000. He feared repossession of the two family automobiles. Whether these fears were realistic was uncertain.

He seemed much more calm during the week before his suicide. He did not drink for the last 2 days. Sunday morning, his wife went to church, leaving him and their 17-year-old daughter at home. He tried several times to get his daughter to leave, saying, "There will be a disturbance." She interpreted this to mean a fight between him and her mother and finally left the house. Just as his wife was driving up to the house she heard what sounded like a gunshot. She ran into the house, calling her husband's name. Getting no response, she went to a neighbor's house for help. The neighbor investigated and found him in the basement, dead of a gunshot wound of the head, with a .30-06 military rifle clutched in his left hand and lying across his body. A gun cleaning kit was open on the workbench. He had borrowed the rifle from his father-in-law the day before.

A note written on brown paper reportedly found on the kitchen counter is purported to have said: "Dear [wife's first name], I love you." The police never saw the note, as the widow said she was unable to find it again.

Findings and Sources

Clinical Diagnosis: (1) Alcoholism, chronic; (2) secondary affective disorder.
Toxicology: Blood alcohol concentration 0.003 g%.
Primary Informant: Wife, married 23 years; saw him daily.
Other Sources of Information: Coroner's death investigation report, police investigation report, hospital records, dermatologist's office record.
Informant's Opinion of Reason for Suicide: (1) "His drinking finally got through to him. He was always sorry for himself"; (2) "Anxious and depressed a good deal of the time."

Comment

The timing of this suicide is not as easily understood as many of the others. Several commonly encountered factors were present, but why did the act occur just when it did? He was remarkably isolated, not even taking meals with his wife and daughter except on weekends. He had been recognizably depressed for 2 years, and perhaps the depression had worsened in the last week, as his appetite had become poor just then. The extent of his financial problems was unreported but must have been known to the informant, as the interview took place 10 months after his death. The fact that she said he *believed* he was in serious financial difficulty, rather than that he *was,* I take to be significant. She was still living at the same good address as when he died. We are left with the probability that his concerns were, at least to some degree, delusional and consistent with his mood. If he was gravely concerned about the consequences to the marriage of their second daughter leaving for college, the event was 5 or 6 months in the future.

The suicide was not impulsive. "In the last week, there was a calmness in his personality not seen earlier." In the last 2 days he did not drink. He borrowed the rifle from his father-in-law the day before he took his life. The police report is, in part, illegible, but it *appears* to say that her father would not tell the subject's wife the reason he gave for borrowing the gun. I conclude that in the absence of evidence of a current threat to domestic stability, worsening depression was the key to this suicide. The gun cleaning kit on the workbench must have been an attempt by the subject to make the death look like an accident, perhaps related to life insurance. The note, reported by the wife but never seen by the police, undercuts the accident scenario and perhaps that is why she "couldn't find it." There is nothing here to suggest foul play.

Case 41

Subject 41 was a 35-year-old white male used car lot operator. Little of his history was learned, since the informant knew him only for the last 2 years of his life. He was born in Detroit, and was nominally Roman Catholic. His alcoholic father committed suicide when he was a young child. He dropped out of school after eighth grade at the age of 13 and went to work. He had spoken of having been in the Navy, but not in detail. He had been an automobile salesman most of his adult life, working in Michigan and California before moving to St. Louis 5 years before his death. He was reported to have been successful and had no job problems. For the last 3 years he worked at the same used car lot.

There is a notable lack of reliable information about his marital history. According to his secretary/bookkeeper, the primary informant, he had been trying unsuccessfully for the entire 2 years she had worked for him to bed, or, if necessary, wed her. He may thus have been less than forthright about his past life. He had told her he was single but had had two long-term common-law relationships. His first "wife" (or wife) was unfaithful. He claimed to have shot her lover (with unspecified result) and they were divorced. His second marriage (or relationship) was allegedly from age 30 to 32. From that relationship he claimed two daughters, one aged 3 years, the other 3 months at the time of his death. At least one and perhaps both children were thus born after the alleged end of the relationship.

His death certificate showed that he went by a last name different from his father's. It listed him as married. The surname typed in under "surviving spouse" was different from either of these but the same as the name of the automobile lot where he worked. The space on the death certificate designated for "informant" was signed with the first name of the "surviving spouse" and the last name used by the subject. Two brief suicide notes were addressed to her—first name only. One was addressed to another woman not otherwise identified in the investigation but evidently married to a different person. None was addressed to the informant. Was he married or wasn't he? Legally or common-law? His secretary/bookkeeper said he was successful in his business and had $250,000 in the bank. As his bookkeeper, she would have known. They apparently spent a good deal of time together after business hours.

Neither the duration of his abusive drinking nor earlier problems with it were known to the informant. In the last 2 years he was a daily drinker with a reported capacity of up to four cases of beer or three fifths of liquor a day. He also had binges and drank in the morning. Daily drinking had begun to have an impact on his effectiveness. He sometimes stopped drinking for a week at a time, but never longer, and had tremulousness on withdrawal. He did not think he drank too much but those who knew him did. He seems to have had no legal problems with drinking (unless he did shoot his "wife's" lover). One month before his suicide he had a single-vehicle automobile accident while drunk. After that, he began sleeping in his office, and occasionally at a motel, rather than drive home drunk again, since he was regularly drunk by the end of the day. His health seems to have been good and his drinking had not led to hospitalization or psychiatric treatment. He often called his secretary/bookkeeper, intoxicated, late at night, with pleas for a more intimate relationship.

For the last 2 years of his life, he had outbursts of rage when drunk. He would then argue with dissatisfied customers instead of being conciliatory. He had friends or acquaintances at bars and played cards with his friends, but sexual conquest seems to have been most important to him. Given his intense preoccupation with alcohol in the final month, it seems unlikely that he could have had much of a social life during that time.

He was unhappy about his failure to entice his secretary/bookkeeper to either marry or go to bed with him. He was openly jealous of her and accused her of sleeping with other men. Nine months before his suicide she quit the job and left town. She was gone for 7 weeks. During that time he shot a hole in the ceiling of her house. After she returned to St. Louis and to work for him, he told her it had been a suicide attempt.

Other than insomnia and anorexia, which he had had for 2 years, his history is largely lacking in symptoms of major depression or other psychiatric problems. Low self-esteem and feelings of worthlessness and anger reportedly appeared only when he was drunk. He was described as sensitive and, for the last 2 years of his life, high-strung, crying easily.

He complained of daily headaches and frequently took over-the-counter analgesics. He was not under the care of a physician and is not known to have been hospitalized at any time.

His father was reportedly alcoholic and committed suicide. There are no other details known of alcoholism, mental illness, or suicide in family members.

His shooting a hole in the ceiling of his secretary's home, which he claimed was a suicide attempt, she regarded as having been a manipulative act to try to influence her to capitulate. He was not known to have made any other reference to suicide until the evening of his death (see below).

Circumstances Leading to the Act

An employee had fallen from a ladder 3 months before the subject's suicide and was "trying to sue." A customer was bitten by a dog (whose?) at the car lot a month before the suicide and was suing him. He claimed he could "take care of" both suits and seemed unconcerned. An aunt in Detroit had died the week before he did. He did not seem upset about it, saying she had been in pain and was better off dead. None of these events was thought to have played a significant role in his suicide.

For the last month of his life, he had been drunk every night. Early on the evening of his death he was quite drunk and began making phone calls every 15 minutes to his secretary. In those calls he said he would be better off dead, that he had nothing to live for and wanted to die. "It takes a man with a lot of guts to shoot himself." He repeatedly asked her to move in with him, which she refused to do. She also refused to say she loved him. During his last telephone call, near 11:00 p.m., he actually shot himself in the head with a .32-caliber pistol. She called the police, who found him dead when they arrived.

There were several rather incoherent suicide notes. The first:

> This is addressed to [woman's first and last name] of St. Charles, Mo.   Please see that she get this message.
>
> Thank you,
> [his nickname].
>
> [first name of above addressee]!
> You all right be good to your husband and don't never let anything interfere.
> This is
> [his nickname].
> Goodbye your
> Sweet

The second note:

> [wife's first name]:
> I'm sorry, Things just didn't work out.
>
> [printed] [his nickname]

Table 5.1 Background Characteristics: Men with Onset Age 25–44 Years, by Age of Onset

Patient Number	Age at Suicide	Parental Home[a]	Family History[a]	Education (yr)	Civil State
1	50	div (<1 yo), grandmother raised	mother: deserted (6 mo)	10	m
17	30	father: died (16 yo)	father: depressed probable suicide; mother: depressed	20	m
38	42	intact to age 15	negative	8	m
40	56	father: died (5 yo) sister raised	NI	NI	s
6	49	div (8 yo), grandparents raised	father: alcoholic	18 (MS)	sep 30 days
8	57	intact	brother: alcoholic; uncle, niece: suicides	12	m
32	55	intact	negative	12	sep
48	42	intact	father: alcoholic mother: depressed, ECT; maternal 2nd cousin: alcoholic	12	m
50	65	intact	father: alcoholic; uncles, cousins: "drank"	16	m
36	52	intact	maternal great uncle: alcoholic	10	m
45	45	Father died (11 yo)	paternal cousin: alcoholic	11	m
20	50	father: suicide (6 yo)	father: suicide; mother: alcoholic	8	sep 3 wk
39	54	mother: died (1 mo); father married her sister	daughter: A/S	10	m
5	57	mother: died (16 yo); father: died (18 yo)	oldest son: probable schizophrenic	16 (BA)	div
22	62	intact	father: alcoholic; paternal uncle: alcoholic	12	m
35	50	intact	father: brief alcohol problem, probably suicide	12-1/2	m
41	35	father: suicide (few yo)	father: alcoholic, suicide	8	NI

Key: 0 = none; A/S = attempted suicide; apt = apartment; div = divorced; DK = don't know; ECT = electroconvulsive therapy; m = married; NI = no information; sep = separated; wk = week(s); yo = years old; yr = year(s).
[a]Age given in parenthesis is that of the subject at the time of the occurrence.
[b]Deceased.

MEN WITH ONSET OF ALCOHOLISM FROM AGE 25 TO 44

Number of Marriages/ Duration (yr)	Age and Sex of Progeny	Living Circumstances	Drinking Locale	Social Support
1/25	16♂	wife, son	tavern, home	tavern wife ±
1/7	5♂, 3♀, 2♀	wife, children	taverns	2 friends
1/22	21♀, 20♂, 17♂, 14♂, 11♂, 10♀, 3♀	wife, 7 children	home, elsewhere	0
0	0	alone	bar, rooming house	bar/tavern
1/24	23♂	alone house 1 mo	secretly	0
1/36	31♀, 30♂	wife	alone	home poor, 2 close friends
2/3, 21	0	alone 2–3 days	home, tavern	little (wife left him)
1/23	19♂, 17♀, 14♀	wife, 2 daughters	bars	almost 0
1/30	29♂, 19♂	wife, son	home, out (DK where)	wife, distant
2/4, 22	27♂, 19♀, 17♂	wife, son	friends' homes, home	good
1/17	16♀, 15♂	wife	home	angry spouse only
2/?, 12	0	alone	tavern	0
1/24	23♀, 22♀	wife	work, home, bar	reported good
1/13	24♂, 20♂, 18♀, 13♀	alone apt (owned)	tavern	reported good
1/42	40♀, 39♀, 37♂, 20♂,[b] 23♂	alone overnight	home	wife, children change <1 day
1/23	22♀, 17♀	wife, daughter	tavern	bar/tavern, avoided family
2 (?)/?, ?	3♀, 3 mo♀	alone office × 1 mo	place of business, bars	bar/tavern

Table 5.2 Alcohol-Related History: Men with Onset Age 25–44, by Age of Onset

Patient Number	Age at Suicide	Drink Onset/ Duration (yr)	Fights[a]	Arrests[b]	Abusive[c]	Serious Health Problems[d]
1	50	25/25	0	0	0	0 [gout]
17	30	25/5	+	0	P	0
38	42	25/17	A	F	P	0
40	56	25/31	A	F	assaultive	brain damage, cirrhosis, HT
6	49	27/22	0	0	V	CP, HT, ASCVD
8	57	30/27	0	V	V	cirrhosis, DU
32	55	30/25	V	0	threats with gun	cancer tongue, emphysema, cirrhosis
48	42	30/12	0	P	0	0
50	65	30/20	0	0	V	0
36	52	31/21	0	P, V	P	multiple myeloma
45	45	32/13	+	0	abused	[TB, thought he had cancer]
20	50	<35/15+	0	0	V	dementia [DU history]
39	54	35/19	0	0	0	pulmonary emphysema
5	57	39/18	A	F, P	P	0
22	62	39/23	A	F, P	P	[cerv disc]
35	50	40/10	+	0	P+	0
41	35	?/?	0	0	V	0

[a] A = arrest; + indicates fights without arrests.
[b] P = peace disturbance; V = vehicular offense; F = fighting.
[c] P = physical; V = verbal.
[d] 0 = none; ASCVD = arteriosclerotic cardiovascular disease; cerv = cervical; CP = chronic pyelonephritis; DU = duodenal ulcer; HT = hypertension; TB = pulmonary tuberculosis.
[e] 0 = none; cerv = cervical.
[f] 0 = none; 2° = secondary; AD = affective disorder; BAD = bipolar affective disorder.

The third note, which was not addressed:

>Thank you very much.
>   I tried.

And the fourth note:

>[wife's first name]
>   I asked you to come, so I hope you happy now.
>
>   [his nickname].

Last Hospital Treatment	Employment	Other Diagnoses	Other Substance Abuse	Suicide Attempts
4 mo alcoholism	unemployed 2 mo	2° AD	0	0
0	employed (self)	2° AD	chlordiazepoxide 12/day	0
10 days detox	part time (self)	0	0	0
4 mo detox	unemployed (med) 5 yr	2° AD	0	0
21 mo seizure	employed, 0 × 3 wk	0	hypnotics, many	0
3 wk detox	lost or about to lose	2° AD	pep pills	0
1 yr pulmonary lobectomy	unemployed 18 yr	2° AD	0	0
7 yr prostate	employed	BAD 2° Alcoholism	0	0
2 mo alcoholism	unemployed 6 mo	2° AD	pep pills	+
6 wk pneumonia	retired 9 yr	2° AD	0	0
13 yr TB	unemployed 4 mo	0	0	0
2 yr "malaise," melena	unemployed 2 yr	0	0	0
1 yr hernia	employed part time	0	0	0
4 mo psychiatric evaluation	employed	delusional disorder	0	0
2 yr cerv disc	employed 1 wk	2° AD	propoxyphene, chlordiazepoxide	0
2 yr cellulitis	employed	2° AD	0	0
0	employed	0	0	claimed

Findings and Sources

Clinical Diagnosis: (1) Alcoholism, chronic; (2) possible personality disorder, unspecified.
Toxicology: Blood alcohol concentration 0.19 g%.
Primary Informant: Secretary/bookkeeper, had known him 2 years.
Other Sources of Information: Coroner's death investigation report, ex-wife.
Informant's Opinion of Reason for Suicide: Drunk enough and depressed enough to do it.

Comment

The informant's knowledge concerning this subject's marital status was sparse and unreliable. Indeed, the death certificate contains conflicting information in that regard. There seem to have been two preoccupations in this man's life, at least as the informant presented it. One of them was alcohol; the other was getting her into bed with him. There is the flavor of a monomania with increasing frustration, an effort to damp it down with greater quantities of alcohol, and a culminating effort to wring from her even an admission of feelings of love for him. He failed.

There were additional problems in the last 3 months—a threatened lawsuit by a former employee, his automobile accident, an actual lawsuit over a dogbite, plus deteriorating automobile sales as he spent increasing amounts of time in an intoxicated state. These all seem pale by comparison to his major preoccupation. Reading the record, I do not get the impression that this woman was on an ego trip in picturing herself as the object of the subject's ardent desire. Her relationship with him was certainly ambivalent. His behavior distressed her, but so did his distress. Alcoholism and rejection were possibly exacerbated by depression, although that diagnosis can't be supported with confidence.

I counted this as acute loss of a close interpersonal relationship. She heard the shot that ended his life, so the suicide notes had already been written. His last telephone call was his final, desperate attempt to win concessions. Her refusal precipitated his suicide.

DISCUSSION

There were 16 men with age of onset reported to have been between 25 and 44 years and 1 for whom no information could be discovered as to when he began to have trouble with alcohol. As he died at 35, I thought it was conservative to put him in this group.

All but 1 subject in this group had married, 12 (75%) of them only once (Table 5.1). Ten of those first marriages (83%) were intact, 5 of them remaining supportive. In all but 2 cases of intact first marriages, the onset of alcohol problems had followed the marriage. In contrast, 18 (82%) of those with early onset had ever married, but only 11 (61%) of them just once. Five (28%) had intact first marriages, only 2 of them (Numbers 34 and 37) seeming to have remained supportive.

Type 1 versus Type 2 Alcoholics

Onset of alcoholism later than age 25 is a defining characteristic of Cloninger's (Cloninger et al., 1981) Type 1 alcoholic. They are said to experience more guilt, to be unable to abstain from drinking, to go on binges, and to develop cirrhosis. Thirteen (76%) reportedly felt guilty about their drinking, but a quantitative measure of "more" guilt is beyond the scope of the data. Three (18%) had hepatic cirrhosis (Table 5.2), a rate half as high as in the early onset group. Two had a diagnosis of duodenal ulcer and 2 of pulmonary emphysema. In all, 7 (41%) were reported to have had serious health problems, about two-thirds as high a frequency as in the first group. Of the 3 men with cirrhosis, 2 had daily drinking; 1 had an alcoholic father. These 3 and 6 others had both guilt and benders. Benders, implying loss of control of drinking, was not more commonly reported in this group—11 of 17 (65%). Of 12 with relevant information, 11 had been unable to stop drinking. In all, 16 of 17 (94%) reportedly had evidence of loss of control, not different from the men with early onset alcoholism (95%).

Although minor trends were observed, none was in the predicted direction. Sample sizes are small, and no comparison approached statistical significance. The range of duration of alcoholism is not as great in this group—5 to 25 years—but it is proportionately not much different. The mean age of onset of alcohol problems was 31.1 years, tending to be early in the age range 25 to 44 years, compared to a mean of 20 years in the earlier onset group. It is not obvious why the careers of this later onset group should have been 5 years shorter, 19.4 years versus 24.8 years. The possibility of a ceiling effect has to be considered, and will be seen to be further supported by the oldest group of male alcoholics. Eleven (65%) had an affective disorder diagnosis.

Comparison of early with later onset alcoholics provides little clarity regarding Type 1 versus Type 2 alcoholism.[1] It is altogether possible that we didn't ask the right questions. It is generally the case that histories given *about* someone will be less detailed and less comprehensive than those obtained directly from the subjects. Perhaps it is a mistake to expect much from these comparisons. Since we had systematic data on most of the issues, including estimates of age of onset, it seemed worth a try. As it is, nothing can be said about the participation of Type 1 versus Type 2 alcoholics in suicide. The longer duration of drinking in the earlier onset group is associated with greater loss of social support and more instances of serious illness, but not to a statistically significant degree. Overall, the lives of those with early onset were more chaotic, including fighting, arrests, divorces, and suicide attempts, as might be expected of the less socially mature. There are enough negative consequences of alcoholism in all of the groups to suggest that these may more strongly characterize alcoholic suicides than living alcoholics. That matter is taken up in detail in Chapters 8 and 9.

6

Men with Onset of Alcoholism at Age 45 Years or Later

Onset of alcoholism as late as the mid-fifth decade is unusual but does occur. In this series we found four such cases.

CASE HISTORIES

Case 43

Subject 43 was a 46-year-old separated unemployed white male who ended the life of his girlfriend and then his own in a murder–suicide. He was born and raised in the St. Louis area and lived there most of his life. His religious preference, if any, was not reported. His father was a construction materials contractor, and both parents were still living at the time of his death. He dropped out of school after the 11th grade for unknown reasons. He entered military service at age 18, during World War II, was honorably discharged at age 21, and joined his father and brother in the materials contracting business. After suffering a foot injury 5 years before his death, he was no longer able to pursue that work. He went to California and tried to run a restaurant, which failed after a year. Returning to St. Louis, he worked for 3 years as manager of a school of broadcasting. Either that business failed or he failed at it. He obtained a job with another broadcasting school but quit after a few months because of nonpayment of his salary. That was about 4 months before his suicide, when he was spending and drinking excessively. Unemployed until 2 weeks before his suicide, he got a job as an automobile salesman. He had trouble getting along with the manager and either quit or was fired after 2 days.

He had married at age 29 and had one daughter who was 18 at the time of his death. There were no serious marital problems until the last year of his life, when he became restless, excited, and grandiose, and he started drinking heavily. Ten months before his suicide he left his wife "to start anew." He got an apartment and started to date the ex-wife of an old friend. He spent lavishly, using credit cards beyond his means, and began to experience job problems. He and his girlfriend drank and used tranquilizers together. He wanted her to marry him but she was reluctant, and her refusal seems to have precipitated the dire outcome. Divorce from his first wife was in process, but on whose initiative was not learned. He was reported to have had two good friends. Considering how insensitively he behaved toward the man who had taken him in, I think it more likely that he was on the edge of no support at all.

He had been a heavy social drinker for years and occasionally got very drunk at parties, but had no associated problems. After a myocardial infarction about 3 years before his death he quit drinking alcohol. Around the time he separated from his wife he commenced heavy daily drinking starting in the morning. He had concern and guilt about his drinking, and he and his girlfriend had tried unsuccessfully to stop. He was not reported to have had any significant withdrawal symptoms or medical problems caused by drinking. During the last few months of his life he had job problems aggravated by heavy drinking. Lacking both money and employment, he moved in with an old friend, the ex-husband of his girlfriend, a month before his death.

He appears to have had onset of a hypomanic episode about a year before his suicide, characterized by grandiosity, spending sprees, excitability, and circumstantiality. In that frame of mind he left his wife 10 months before his suicide, bought new clothes, and began playing the role of a "gay blade." His work performance became erratic and he began to have interpersonal difficulties with supervisors and management. He was unable to work at all during the last few weeks of his life. For the last 2 months he was depressed and had anorexia, weight loss, fatigue, and suicidal thoughts. The informant didn't know if he had insomnia. Indeed, it is unlikely that he would have known much at all about the subject's late-developing symptoms, as he saw him about once every 3 months. The subject was not known to have sought psychiatric care, his only treatment consisting of an unknown tranquilizer, which, according to his apartment mate's report to the coroner's team, he used in excess.

His personality was described as high-strung, sensitive, and moody. However, until the last year of his life he seems to have been reasonably well adjusted and was not perceived to have had emotional problems. At the end, some who knew him thought him "crazy." Information was inadequate for diagnosis, but his marked behavior change in the last year of his life strongly suggests a late onset bipolar illness. He was seen regularly by the physician who treated his myocardial infarction. Last medical contact was less than a month before his death.

He had a brother who suffered from alcoholism. The family history is otherwise negative for alcohol or drug problems, mental illness, or suicide.

He was known to have mentioned suicide only once, about 4 to 6 weeks prior to his suicide. In trying to persuade his girlfriend to marry him, he stated that if she did not, he would kill himself. He had not discussed wanting to die, being hopeless, or thinking that others would be better off with him gone. Family and friends were entirely surprised at news of his death.

Circumstances Leading to the Act

Following a hypomanic spell, he became depressed. Out of money, out of work, and in debt, he had been living for about 4 weeks with the ex-husband of the woman he was dating. That person was unhappy with their dating and had told him to stay away from her, because he still loved her. Nevertheless, the subject persisted in trying to persuade her to marry him. Some 4–6 weeks before his suicide he told her he would kill himself if she didn't. She said she did not love him that way, but only thought of him as a friend. He was reportedly despondent about his very large debts and inability to get a job, and he was drinking heavily every day. He had worked only 2 days in the last 4 months, but he was to have returned to work on the day following his suicide, at the school of broadcasting where he had first worked. On that final night he took his girlfriend out to dinner and was drinking with her. She was last seen by her daughter in his company that evening as they left the restaurant. She was crying. He drove to a secluded spot and shot her with a .22-caliber pistol, after which he shot himself.

A note was left which purported to be written and signed jointly by the subject and his victim:

> To those we love and there are many but few who think much of us. We're sorry this is the way it must be. We hope we can be forgiven.
> Love, [subject's first and last name].
> Call [telephone number of his apartment mate, ex-husband of the other victim].
> Call [telephone number and brother's name].
> Love, [girlfriend's first and last name].
> P.S. Everything goes to my children [girlfriend's first name].

The other victim's ex-husband stated that her "signature" was not in her handwriting. He believed that this was a murder–suicide rather than the suicide pact it was intended to resemble.

Findings and Sources

Clinical Diagnosis: (1) Alcoholism, chronic; (2) undiagnosed, possible primary bipolar affective disorder, depressed.
Toxicology: Not performed.
Primary Informant: Subject's brother; saw him once every 3 months.
Other Sources of Information: Coroner's death investigation report, friend with whom he had been living.
Informant's Opinion of Reason for Suicide: Despondent because he had no job.

Comment

Our informant had very little contact with the subject. He saw him about every 3 months. Recency of last contact was not recorded. He was able to sketch the broad outlines of the problem, but he was not in a good position to know about the less obvious symptoms of depression. His negative responses to questions regarding sleep, interest, guilt feelings, and impaired concentration reflect, I take it, his lack of awareness of their presence, not knowledge of their absence. The subject's roommate described the subject to the death investigator as "despondent." Unfortunately, we did not resort to that individual for additional information regarding depressive symptoms. It was he who had given the clearest description of the alcohol abuse to the coroner's death investigator. In light of the rather clear evidence of hypomanic behavior directly preceding the despondency, I think we are on safe ground in *supposing* a depression, but information is insufficient to support a diagnosis of bipolar affective disorder.

His excessive drinking was of uncertain duration, reportedly only 1 year, but was serious enough to meet our strict criteria for alcoholism. The final impetus to suicide was his girlfriend's refusal to marry him or even to say that she loved him. He had said he would kill himself in that event, and he did. How he enticed her to the remote spot where he shot her and himself is a mystery. Her daughter's report of seeing her mother in tears as she and the subject left the restaurant, presumably on their way to their deaths, conjures up a picture of a confused, distraught, and possibly intoxicated woman going along because she couldn't sort it all out. It is unfortunate that toxicologic studies were forgone.

The girlfriend's rejection of his proposal of marriage some 4–6 weeks before his suicide would have qualified him for the "recent loss" category, had he not taken matters into his own hands. As it was, she died before he did, and that settles it. If he couldn't have her, no one could.

Case 7

Subject 7 was a white married Protestant male, who was born and lived all 55 years of his life in St. Louis. His father was a policeman and his mother a cook. He had one sibling, a sister. His father committed suicide when he was 13 years old. He completed the eighth grade and was rejected for military service because of a longstanding history of bronchial asthma. He married for the first and only time at the age of 36, some 19 years before his suicide. Four children were born of that union, ages 16, 12, 11, and 9 at the time of his death, all living with the subject and his wife. He had worked in the printing trade continuously from the time of his marriage. No information was obtained as to previous employment; however, it was stated that he had never been fired, quit without having another job to go to, or had periods of unemployment. He is not known to have had any trouble on the job as a consequence of either his drinking or his health problems. He had five close friends and socialized with them in his home and others' homes until the last month of his life. He did not frequent taverns.

His wife said that he did not abuse alcohol before the age of 49, although it cannot be said with certainty that he did not drink at all prior to that time. In the same year that he had a subtotal gastrectomy for a bleeding gastric ulcer he reportedly became depressed and began to drink beer on a regular basis. His upper gastrointestinal pathology antedated his drinking by at least a year. A quiet drinker, he did not abuse his wife, and there was no report of the marital relationship being threatened. His marital and family relationships were affected, however. His wife thought that he drank too much. He had one period of abstinence lasting 3–4 months following a hemorrhoidectomy 2 years before his death. He then resumed drinking as usual. He drank only beer, more heavily on Saturdays (up to 10–12 bottles) and did not drink at all on Sundays. He did almost all of his drinking at home, thereby avoiding vehicular or other arrests.

Three weeks before his suicide his wife was released from a hospital. The reason for and duration of that admission were not recorded. On her return home, he admitted for the first time that drinking was a problem for him and talked of getting help. He felt guilty about it. His wife suggested AA but "a friend" talked him out of it. A fractured rib that may have been incurred while he was drinking caused his hospitalization 10 days before his death. Four days before he took his life he was discharged from the hospital and did not return to work, but he resumed drinking at the rate of 10–12 bottles of beer a day. On a daily basis, as opposed to Saturday peaks, that represents an increase in intake.

For 3–4 years before his death he had had occasional spells during which he would "just sit and cry." He had decreased sexual interest for about the same length of time. During a hospitalization 2 years before he died he was noted to have a "reactive depression." For about the last month he looked constantly depressed, lost interest in both social contacts and other activities, was less active physically, expressed ideas of guilt, and talked of suicide. He complained of "tiredness" to his physician a week before his death. He had had sexual intercourse only one time in the last 3–4 months of his life. He was more severely depressed and irritable the last 2 days. On the day before his suicide he accused his wife of having an affair with a friend.

He had had bronchial asthma since childhood and in late years had chronic bronchitis and chronic pulmonary emphysema as well. At age 49, six years before his death, he had an episode of tarry black stools (melena) followed by abdominal pain, for which he was hospitalized. A laparotomy revealed a sealed-off perforated gastric ulcer and a pelvic abscess which was secondary to the perforated gastric ulcer. The abscess was drained and an incidental appendectomy was performed. The duodenum was also noted to be scarred, as from an old, healed duodenal ulcer. Sixteen months later he had another episode of gastrointestinal bleeding and a subtotal gastrectomy was performed, revealing a large, benign (i.e., noncancerous) gastric ulcer. The scarred section of duodenum was resected as well. Large, inflamed hemorrhoids were noted, but no mention was made of alcohol consumption on either admission.

Two years before his death he experienced gradual onset of fatigue; when hospitalized he was found to be markedly anemic. His extensive bleeding hemorrhoids were resected. A history of drinking "considerable beer" was recorded and his liver was noted to be enlarged and tender. Ten days before his suicide he was hospitalized with pleuritic chest pain and a fractured sixth rib was found. Only late in the hospitalization did he recall that he had injured the rib "on a pantry door." In addition to the fractured rib, chronic pulmonary emphysema, asthmatic bronchitis, and pulmonary fibrosis were diagnosed. His liver was again noted to be enlarged and slightly tender. Liver function tests were never performed and a diagnosis of hepatic cirrhosis was never made. However, two widely separated observations of an enlarged, tender liver and hemorrhoids severe enough to require surgery strongly suggest liver disease.

His father had had two admissions to the St. Louis State Psychiatric Hospital in the 1920s for unknown reasons. He committed suicide when the subject was 13 years old. He is not known to have been alcoholic. A maternal aunt had committed suicide. His sister became alcoholic at the age of 50 and had made a suicide attempt.

Six or seven years before ending his life, he had said to his wife and to some others, "I wish I was dead." One day before his suicide he said to his son, "I'm not going to be here after this weekend." He said to his wife, "I just want out." His wife asked, "Do you want a divorce?" and he answered, "No, I just want out." He had never made an attempt prior to his successful suicide.

Circumstances Leading to the Act

He had been more depressed for about a month before he took his life. During that period he admitted for the first time that he had a problem with drinking. However, he did nothing about it. Ten days before his death he resumed daily drinking. For the last 3 days of his life he voiced suspicions of his wife's fidelity. On the day before his suicide, he accused her of having an affair with a friend. On his last day alive he refused to go to church with his wife and children, and they went without him. They returned to find him comatose in the kitchen. On the table were empty amobarbital (Tuinal) bottles and empty beer bottles. He was dead on arrival at the hospital. No note was found.

Findings and Sources

Clinical Diagnosis: (1) Alcoholism, chronic; (2) secondary affective disorder (meets criteria for *probable* depression, DSM-III-R definite).
Toxicology: Blood alcohol concentration 0.22 g%; blood barbiturate concentration 4.3 mg%.
Primary Informant: Wife, who lived with him continuously for 19 years and knew him for a total of 20 years.
Other Sources of Information: Hospital records, coroner's death investigation record.
Informant's Opinion of Reason for Suicide: No opinion.

Comment

The first link in this chain of events seems to have been the development of peptic ulcer disease, coming to light by way of surgical exploration following an episode of melena at age 49, six years before death. He reportedly became depressed at that time. Following a subtotal gastric resection 16 months later he began to drink beer regularly, especially heavily on Saturdays. (It is of interest that his sister had onset of alcoholism at age 50, about the same age as the beginning of his own drinking problems.) There was a rapid progression of problems, including liver enlargement and severely bleeding hemorrhoids. A 6-day hospitalization seems unusual for treatment of a fractured rib. He had not been at work for an undetermined time before that and did not return to work on discharge but drank continuously until his suicide. This was a rather superficial interview, with ample medical records. Depression is not as well documented as we might wish. Symptoms not listed as present were not clearly known to have been absent. There was documentation for probable, but not definite (Feighner criteria) major depression by history. A depressive episode of about 1 month's duration is identifiable, and this alone appears to account for his suicide. In his depression, he drank more, which cannot have improved the situation.

Case 14

Subject 14 was a 54-year-old white widowed male, born in the eastern United States. His parental home was intact and he had no siblings. Both parents were killed in an automobile accident at time unknown to the informant. He was a college graduate, had 3 years military service during World War II, and received an honorable discharge. He married at age 30 and settled in St. Louis, where he sired three children, two boys and a girl, ages 22, 20, and 14 at his death. At age 51 he was transferred by the government agency for which he worked to Chicago, where he lived with his wife and three children for about 2 ½ years. His wife died from breast cancer 23 months before his suicide. After her death, he started to drink heavily, usually at home. He occasionally went to a tavern to play cards with friends. He retired or was fired 15 months after his wife's death and sold his home. In the next 2 months, he spent about $14,000, thought to be the proceeds of the sale. He then moved back to St. Louis, where he lived in a rented apartment with his mother-in-law and his 14-year-old son. The informant says the subject became "shy" after his wife's death. He did not go out with women. He sat at home and watched TV most of the time. He slept late, getting out of bed at around noon most days. He had virtually no social contact except with those he lived with. At the time of his death, he had been back in St. Louis for 6 months.

He reportedly started drinking heavily at the age of 52, six months after his wife died. If so, he got into it very rapidly. During that same year he was hospitalized for 5 days after he fell out of bed and struck his head. This was believed to have resulted from his being drunk. His physician, who had known him for 8 years, said he had "a severe problem with alcohol" but did not state the duration. Hospital admission records of 5 and 7 years before his death do not mention alcohol use or abuse.

His drinking was sporadic but progressive, and his job attendance deteriorated. He sometimes drank for 2 days, missing work, then stopped for several days at a time. His supervisor talked with him repeatedly, sometimes for as long as 4 hours, about his absenteeism. It is not clear whether he was finally fired from his job or retired voluntarily. He told his mother-in-law that he would quit drinking, but he never did. She inferred from this that he felt guilty about his drinking.

He was brought home by friends 3 months before his suicide after having fallen, either while drinking or from an episode of vertigo or weakness secondary to emphysema. His physician said he had hepatic cirrhosis and hemorrhoids. While he was known to drink a case of beer a week, empty wine and liquor bottles found after his death suggested that he augmented his overt alcohol intake. He took "capsules" for sleeping. The informant did not know whether he took them daily or occasionally, but the prescription was renewed every month.

The informant seemed to know little about his symptoms, despite having shared an apartment with him for several years. She described him as "depressed" after his wife's death and said he never worked regularly again, despite his supervisor's entreaties. She could not identify weight loss or anorexia, but she was aware that he got up several times a night. He was markedly inactive, possibly with psychomotor retardation. He complained of fatigue and exhibited loss of interest both in work and in socializing. If he experienced self-reproach or guilt of a depressive nature, the informant didn't know of it, nor was she able to report on whether his thinking or concentration was affected. She did not think he was *more* depressed shortly before his suicide. He had no previous psychiatric disorder and had had a good work record. His physician told me he did not think he was depressed, but he had given him amitriptyline-perphenazine (Triavil) 10–25 mg three times daily for 2 months, about 6 months before his death, as well as amobarbital (Tuinal) for insomnia. He had been prescribed a major tranquilizer at some time in the past. He meets Feighner's criteria for "probable" major depressive disorder and DSM-III-R criteria for major depressive disorder.

Five years before his death he was hospitalized in Chicago for bronchitis, and a diagnosis of pulmonary emphysema was made. Bilateral cataract extractions were noted in the records. About 2 years before his death he was hospitalized after he fell out of bed striking his head. Four months before his death, on hospital admission for hemorrhoidectomy, the diagnosis of pulmonary emphysema was upgraded to "severe." About 2 months before his death he complained to his doctor of dyspnea on exertion. His physician reminded him of his diagnosis of emphysema and told him to stop smoking. He interpreted this advice as a warning that he would die in a year if he didn't stop smoking. (The doctor denied giving him any such dire prediction.)

Family history was unknown.

He spoke of thinking that he would die soon if he did not stop smoking. He asked his mother-in-law to take care of his 14-year-old son should he die. He told his older son in a letter that he would die in 6 months. Specific suicidal ideation was denied.

Circumstances Leading to the Act

He retired early (or was fired) 15 months after the death of his wife. He sat at home and drank most of the day. The informant thought he worried unduly about financial matters. The day before his death, he talked about getting a job at his former occupation. At the same time, he had been planning a vacation with the family. The informant did not think he had seemed more depressed in the last month. The day before his suicide he had gone to bed at the usual hour and the following morning at 11:30 a.m. was found in a crouched position on his bed by his 14-year-old son. Since he was in the habit of sleeping until noon, the informant did not disturb him. About 5:30 p.m., the informant sent his son to wake him. He found his father in the same position, dead, holding an empty pill bottle in his hand. Missing were amobarbital (Tuinal), 8 capsules; ephedrine and phenobarbital (Quadrinal), 68 capsules; and promazine (Sparine) 50 mg, 84 tablets. The informant did not think he committed suicide, but rather that he accidentally took too much sleeping medication. He did not leave a note.

Findings and Sources

Clinical Diagnosis: (1) Alcoholism, chronic; (2) probable major depressive disorder (DSM-III-R definite).
Toxicology: Blood alcohol concentration, 0.02 g%; blood barbiturate concentration, 1.6 mg%; urine grossly positive for phenothiazine derivatives.
Primary Informant: Mother-in-law.
Other Sources of Information: Coroner's death investigation report, hospital records, family physician.
Informant's Opinion of Reason for Suicide: Accident, not suicide.

Comment

The diagnosis of alcoholism is unquestionable. Its duration is uncertain. Our primary informant said he started drinking heavily only after his wife's death. If that were true, one would expect to find a major depressive episode behind the drinking. Onset of primary alcoholism at this age is very infrequent. On the other hand, his physician, a general practitioner who had known him for 8 years—antedating both his wife's death and his moving to Chicago—told me simply that he had a severe problem with alcohol. I didn't pin him down on duration, because that conversation preceded the primary interview, so drinking may have been of longer duration. His hepatic cirrhosis would make one think so. The doctor said he "never saw him looking depressed. Alcohol was his problem." However, he had prescribed an antidepressant. In spite of conflicting information, a diagnosis of "probable" major depressive disorder is the least we can say.

The mother-in-law's seemingly superficial knowledge concerning the man with whom she had shared living quarters for at least 3 years raises a question as to just how isolated this man may have been. He had cut off contact with all but those he lived with, in any event. The informant's opinion that the death was an accident suggests that she wasn't tracking fully. I think a major depression, probably reactive to bereavement, is the major culprit. Alcohol and social isolation played significant roles. Concern about his health may have been of delusional proportions.

The subject was reportedly planning a family vacation for the near future. Planning pleasant events for the future while planning suicide is not rare.

Case 42

Subject 42 was a 63-year-old married unemployed black male of Methodist affiliation. He was born and raised in metropolitan St. Louis. The informant, his third wife, knew little of his family and childhood, although she had known him for the last 27 years of his life. A hospital record made 2 years before his death included the information that he had eight siblings, three of them deceased, that his father had died at age 52 of unknown causes, and that his mother was living and 102 years old. After completing the eighth grade he had no further schooling. He worked in a packing house, as a chauffeur, and in an ammunition plant. At age 35 he joined a local police department and had a successful career for 21 years without job problems. His reasons for quitting or retiring are obscure and he appears to have regretted the decision. Immediately upon leaving the force he became a partner in a tavern. Following a fall with head injury 3 years before his death, he did not return to the tavern. After a while he worked sporadically for private security firms until about 6–8 months before his suicide. At that point, saying he just didn't feel like working, he worked no more.

He was married three times, for 5, 9 and 25 years. The first two marriages ended in divorce for what was described as his unreasonable jealousy. He accused his third wife of infidelity also, but the marriage endured. The couple had no children of their own but had adopted a girl, who was 13 at the time of the subject's death.

Although he was probably a moderate to heavy social drinker most of his life, he was not thought to have had a drinking problem until the last 7 years. It began when he became a partner in a tavern. His wife thought he felt disgusted with himself for having left the police force. He drank gin and vodka heavily on a daily basis, often beginning in the morning, without binges. He had had tremulousness. His wife and friends thought he drank too much. It caused him to lose friends. He never had job problems, fights, or vehicular or other arrests in connection with drinking. His wife found it difficult to tell how much he drank and he probably developed significant tolerance. There is no suggestion that he thought he drank too much, ever sought treatment for his drinking, or tried to control or stop it.

A little over 4 years before his death he was hospitalized for gastritis with singultus (hiccups) and vomiting. His liver was noted to be enlarged and one liver function test was abnormal at that time. Two years later he was found unconscious after closing time in his tavern. He was hospitalized, semicomatose, with a probable concussion. It was thought that he had fallen while drunk, as he had a cut over his left eye. There were no focal neurologic signs, but he was disoriented throughout the 9-day admission, with residual confusion on discharge. He did not return to the tavern but did resume daily drinking. He was again described as confused when admitted to another hospital 2 months later with an alleged 70-pound weight loss but denial of any complaint by the patient. (Information given the death investigator was that this hospitalization was for alcoholism.) A psychiatric consultation did not include a mental status examination. His inability to give a coherent history was interpreted as "massive denial."

Depression was not noted on any of the three hospital admissions described. (Given the era, the early 1970s, this is not unusual.) Nevertheless, he told his wife that he was depressed during his last year and he looked it. He had anorexia and profound weight loss, beginning more than 2 years before his death. (At 6 feet, 2 inches tall, he weighed 139 pounds at his death.) He was reported to have exhibited irritability and low mood, social withdrawal, low energy, and fatigue for at least a year. He had a poor memory, probably secondary to head injury. During the last 3–4 months of his life he frequently asked the date and neglected his personal hygiene (he was previously immaculate in his grooming). He had had little interest in sex for the last 5–6 years of his life, but he often accused his wife of being interested in other men.

Most of his medical problems appear to have been consequences of heavy drinking: head injury, gastritis, mild liver impairment, and dizzy spells unexplained by any medical tests. He had early bilateral cataracts and generalized arteriosclerosis but had not seen a physician in the last 2 years.

There was no information available on alcoholism, mental illness, or suicide in his family.

About 6 months before his death, he began to speak occasionally of having nothing to live for, of being sick and tired, and thinking that he would be better off dead. He said to his wife, "I have enough nerve to kill you or [their daughter] but I couldn't kill myself." He had never actually threatened either family member or to kill himself, but he was clearly preoccupied with dying. His wife was uncertain whether he was intoxicated when making these statements. About a month before his suicide he abruptly asked her if his insurance was paid up. He also said, "When I die don't spend money on me." He never made a suicide attempt.

Circumstances Leading to the Act

On the day of his suicide he awakened looking pale and tremulous and complained to his wife of being sick. She was not sympathetic. He went back to bed. On her way out to work, she said she would bring him a bottle when she returned. He replied, "You won't need to." When she came home that evening she found him dead, having shot himself in the chest. He did not leave a note.

Table 6.1 Background Characteristics: Men with Onset Age 45 and Older, by Age of Onset

Patient Number	Age at Suicide	Parental Home[a]	Family History	Education (yr)	Civil State
43	46	intact	brother: alcoholic	11	sep 10 mo
7	55	father: suicide (13 yr)	sister: alcoholic, A/S; father: PH (2x), suicide; maternal aunt: suicide	8	m
14	54	intact, DK how long	NI	16	w 23 mo
42(B)	63	NI	NI	8	m

Key: apt = apartment; (B) = black; barb = barbiturate; DK = don't know; m = married; mo = month(s); NI = no information; PH = psychiatric hospital; sep = separated; tav = tavern; wk = week(s); w = widowed; yo = years old; yr = year(s). yrs = years.
[a]Age given in parentheses is that of the subject at the time of the occurrence.

Findings and Sources

Clinical Diagnosis: (1) Alcoholism, chronic; (2) moderate dementia, alcoholic versus traumatic; (3) probable secondary depression (DSM-III-R; organic mood syndrome versus major depressive disorder).
Toxicology: Blood alcohol concentration 0.09 g%.
Primary Informant: Third wife, married 25 years, had known him for 27 years.
Other Sources of Information: Coroner's death investigation report, hospital records.
Informant's Opinion of Reason for Suicide: (1) Alcohol; (2) depressed.

Comment

A user of alcohol all of his adult life, this man appears to have had a late onset of problem drinking, with a rather fulminating course. The head injury he sustained 2 years before his death seems to have left him with a postconcussion deficit. That could

Table 6.2 Alcohol-Related History: Men with Onset Age 45 and Older, by Age of Onset

Patient Number	Age at Suicide	Drink Onset/ Duration (yr)	Fights	Arrests	Abusive	Serious Health Problems
43	46	45/1	0	0	0	ASHD, MI
7	55	49/6	0	0	0	emphysema
14	54	52/2	0	0	0	cirrhosis, emphysema
42(B)	63	56/7	0	0	0	brain injury

Key: 0 = none; 1° = primary; 2° = secondary; AD = affective disorder; ASHD = arteriosclerotic heart disease; (B) = black; fx = fracture; MI = myocardial infarction; prob = probable.

7

Alcoholic Women

Women comprised 14% of the suicides in this study—a not-unexpected proportion.

CASE HISTORIES

Case 47

Subject 47 was a 32-year-old single unemployed black woman born in Arkansas and living in St. Louis for the last 20 years of her life. Her mother died when she was about 3 years old. She lived with her father, a retired laborer, two sisters, and her 2-year-old son in a four-room rented house. All of them were on some form of public assistance. She had a brother as well, living in St. Louis until the day of his death and hers. The family's religion was Baptist. She had gone as far as the sixth grade in school, presumably in Arkansas, but had been "put out of school" at that point, according to hospital records. She could neither read nor write and was considered to be mentally retarded. She had worked only 2 or 3 days of her life, as a domestic at age 28, but found the work too taxing for her. She received around $100 a month in AFDC (Aid for Dependent Children) and Social Security Disability payments.

She had had an ongoing relationship with a married judge (probably a local magistrate) for a number of years and it was believed that it was he who had sired her 2-year-old son. She was much troubled with having a child, complaining that he tied her down. She had a lot of trouble finding baby sitters while she went out to bars or with the judge. The child was "getting on her nerves." The Child Welfare worker periodically asked her if she wished to give the child up. She always declined. Her sister-in-law thought she had appeared depressed for about a year over this burden. Her relationship with the judge had been deteriorating for about the same length of time, owing to her increasing drinking and her tendency to fight with him (and others) when drunk. He had told her on a number of occasions to leave him alone and not come to his office anymore.

She began drinking at age 16 and quickly developed a drinking problem. She had had multiple arrests for drunkenness and for disturbing the peace over the last 10 years of her life. The police would often take her home or to the county hospital. She would drink whenever she could get it or whenever she could get out of the house. Men would buy her drinks at the bars. She would sometimes go off for 2–3 days at a time and drink continuously. She knew she drank too much but did not express guilt or try to stop. Her family and others objected to the amount she drank. In the last year of her life she drank more than ever, became abusive, and would fight with her family, her lover, or others. As a result, she had alienated her lover and perhaps others. The informant was uncertain whether she ever had shakes or any other physical consequences of her alcohol abuse.

Her sister dated onset of the subject's psychiatric illness to her teens. However, the subject herself had told the admitting physician during one hospitalization that she had been "hearing voices" since she was little. She was said to have had a 1½-year stay in the St. Louis State Hospital for this condition. Hospital records were obtainable for only the last 5 years of her life. At age 26 she was admitted to the psychiatric service of the St. Louis County Hospital because of bizarre behavior. She was noted to be hallucinating. She received a course of seven ECT treatments and was discharged with diagnoses of mental retardation and catatonic schizophrenia. She was readmitted 3 weeks later, mute, with catatonic posturing. She was "hearing voices." When responsive, she gave incoherent answers and exhibited thought blocking. Chlorpromazine (Thorazine) brought only modest improvement.

On several subsequent admissions the diagnosis made was chronic undifferentiated schizophrenia. For the last year or two of her life she was receiving biweekly injections of fluphenazine (Prolixin Decanoate) as well as daily chlorpromazine by mouth. A diagnosis of chronic alcoholism was entered for the first time on her last psychiatric admission, 2 weeks before her death. She had allegedly taken an overdose of unknown medication. She did not appear to have endangered herself and was discharged 2 days later to follow up in the outpatient department. There was no record of her attendance there.

On hospital admission at age 26 she had a marked iron deficiency anemia. It was attributed to excessive menstrual bleeding and she underwent a D&C. She adamantly refused to take iron tablets. Extensive public hospital records contain no evidence of other surgical or medical illness. She was described as emaciated on the last two hospital admissions.

No history was obtained of alcoholism, mental illness, or suicide in the family. If the brother's death was related to any of these or to drugs, we did not learn of it.

Apart from the hospital admission for a medically inconsequential overdose 2 weeks before her death, she was not known to have made any reference to suicide. She had a sort of tantrum behavior, lying on the ground kicking and crying for as much as 30 minutes at a time, saying that nobody liked her. She would do this when she wanted someone to look after her child.

Circumstances Leading to the Act

On the morning of her death, her brother became involved in an argument and was shot to death. When she heard of it, she became agitated and tearful and began walking up and down the street in front of their house. She refused to come in and continued walking for several hours. When she finally entered the house, she said that she wanted to "join" her brother. Her family said she had not been drinking at that time. That evening she drank, then went to the judge's office in his home. The judge let her in and she reportedly went to his desk where he kept a .38-caliber pistol. She shot herself in the head.

Findings and Sources

Clinical Diagnosis: (1) Mental retardation; (2) schizophrenia, chronic undifferentiated; (3) alcoholism, chronic.
Toxicology: Blood alcohol concentration 0.12 g%.
Primary Informant: Sister, lived with subject for 28 years.
Other Sources of Information: Coroner's death investigation report, hospital records.
Informant's Opinion of Reason for Suicide: Doesn't think she did it. She and others suspect the judge or his wife shot her.

Comment

This unfortunate woman was born into a family whose every member received some sort of public assistance. Mentally retarded and probably hallucinating since childhood, she could hardly be expected to rise above that level. She spent her days—when she could escape from her family's supervision—hanging out in bars, where men would buy her drinks. A 2-year relationship with a married public official was deteriorating rapidly, because of her increasingly erratic and abusive behavior. She killed herself in his office, within hours of hearing that her brother had been shot and killed. She was intoxicated at the time. How close she was to her brother was not learned, but that "recent loss" was clearly precipitating. He was the only sibling not still living at home.

Schizophrenia is a diagnosis not often encountered in community studies of suicide (Table 2.1) but amply represented in studies of deaths among psychiatric hospital inpatients where schizophrenics comprise 30%–60% of the population compared to 1% in the general population (Roy, 1982; Allebeck & Wistedt, 1986). Suicides of schizophrenics often appear impulsive. In this case, mental retardation complicated the schizophrenia. Alcohol intoxication was facilitative. She gave notice of her intent only some hours before the act.

Case 49

Subject 49 was a 40-year-old unemployed married Caucasian woman, born into an old southern family and spoiled as a child. She had a younger brother. Her father was an attorney, an alcoholic for 20 years. Her mother was a homemaker. Religious affiliation was "Christian." The family was intact until both of her parents died when she was 22. How they died was not recorded, but they reportedly died together. She is said to have had suicidal thoughts as early as the age of 5 years. She completed college and graduate school, earning a master's degree. She was married for the first time at age 19 and had two daughters, who were 16 and 18 at the time of her death. That marriage lasted 8 years and ended, according to the account in one hospital record, with her husband's death in an airplane crash. The informant said it was ended by divorce.

She married a second time at age 29 and had another daughter, who was now 8 years old. She fought with this husband and the marriage ended in divorce after 7 years, 4 years before her death. Her third marriage, when she was 38, was even more stormy. Her husband left her a number of times but always returned, and they were living together at the time of her death. They had moved to a nicer home 3 months earlier. The last few years of her life were chaotic, with multiple suicide attempts, multiple hospitalizations, and loss of jobs. She was a compulsive shoplifter, but was never arrested.

She married professional men of adequate means and did not need to work. Her first employment that we learned of began after her second marriage ended. In the last 4 years of her life she had four jobs. After working in a governmental agency for 1½ years she was fired for reasons thought to have been related to a lesbian affair with a friend's wife. She quit another job after 2 weeks. She worked at a public hospital for 3 months and was fired. Her last job, with a city department, was terminated 9 months before her death because she refused to sign a release of information that would have revealed her history of alcoholism. She was described as always having been high-strung, moody, sensitive, and given to sudden outbursts of rage. She had almost no social life in her last 9 months.

She began drinking at age 17 with 6 weeks of almost constant alcohol intoxication in Paris. Drinking and its attendant behavior probably caused the dissolution of her first marriage. It certainly ended her second marriage and troubled the third one. It was during the second marriage that her drinking problem became more severe and she began a series of suicide attempts. She did a poor job as a mother since her alcoholism and suicide attempts rendered her incapable of parenting much of the time.

She became physically violent and sometimes dangerous when drunk. Most of her suicide attempts were made while markedly intoxicated. On several occasions she threatened or assaulted her third husband. Just a year before her suicide she pointed a gun at him and said she wanted to kill him. He left her and they were divorced but then remarried within a month. Nine months before her suicide she beat her youngest daughter and drove her out of the home. (She returned later.) Around the same time she killed several puppies that were whining because she didn't like the noise. About 8 months before her demise she stabbed her husband with a knife. He left her again, but he returned in about 2 weeks.

She customarily drank liquor daily. At times she would quit drinking for up to 2 weeks, but she always went back to it. She went on binges, indulged in occasional morning drinking ("only on Sundays"), and experienced withdrawal tremulousness and DTs leading to several hospital admissions. She once took disulfiram (Antabuse), but for what duration or with what effect was not learned. She had automobile accidents while drunk and was arrested twice for traffic violations during the year prior to her suicide. She thought she drank too much and felt guilty about it but was unable to maintain sobriety. Family and friends objected to her drinking. She had profound interpersonal and psychiatric problems but no medical problems related to her alcoholism.

She had been under the care of a succession of psychiatrists over the years, receiving a variety of diagnoses on different occasions. Alcoholism was always one of them. In addition, cyclothymic personality, personality trait disorder, and reactive depression were invoked by different psychiatrists. For the last year of her life she was described as having a constant low mood and frequently voiced feelings of guilt and worthlessness. She lost interest in social contact and had almost none in the last 9 months. She became much less active, talked of suicide, and made a number of attempts. The informant linked her insomnia to her drinking. She was anorexic and disinterested in sex in the last 2 weeks. She had not been noted to complain of fatigue or impaired concentration, and she was neither agitated nor retarded. During the last 2 weeks she hid under the bed much of the day, drinking heavily, and was totally withdrawn. She seemed confused and disoriented.

Her father had had a 20-year history of alcoholism when he died of unknown cause. A paternal uncle, also alcoholic, committed suicide. Her brother was thought to have a problem with alcohol.

She first had thoughts of suicide at age 5 years. Her first suicide attempt was at age 34, some 15 years before her death. She had many hospitalizations during the last 7 years of her life for suicide attempts, eight in the last 2½ years. Seven of these attempts were by overdosing with chlordiazepoxide (Librium) or other medication plus alcohol and one was by slashing her wrists. One overdose episode occurred just 2 weeks into her third marriage. She once lay on the railroad tracks as a suicide threat. Once she impulsively crashed an automobile. She had threatened to shoot herself with a shotgun. A year before her death she threatened to jump from a 10th-floor window of a hotel. Often—usually when intoxicated—she said she would be better off dead. Persons who knew her were convinced that she would eventually commit suicide.

Circumstances Leading to the Act

She had been drinking a fifth of liquor a day for 2 weeks, often hiding under her bed during the day. She was uncommunicative, confused, and seemed to be disoriented. This was new behavior for her. On the day before her death she climbed onto the third-floor balcony and threatened: "Don't come near the door or I'll jump. I've got the nerve to do it and I'll do it." The police were called and she was persuaded to come back into the house. The following night, when others were asleep, she again went out onto the balcony, grossly intoxicated, and leaped to her death. Nine notes were found, all reading simply "To whom it may concern."

Findings and Sources

Clinical Diagnosis: (1) Alcoholism, chronic; (2) probable secondary depression (DSM-III-R; major depressive disorder); (3) probable acute delirium.
Toxicology: Blood alcohol concentration 0.324 g%
Primary Informant: Husband, married 2 years.
Other Sources of Information: Hospital records, coroner's death investigation report.
Informant's Opinion of Reason for Suicide: "Tired of life. She set her aspirations high and failed to attain them."

Comment

This woman's whole life seems to have been stormy. Her father was alcoholic. She had thoughts of suicide from childhood on. Her marriages were filled with strife, mostly of her own creation, owing to her excessive drinking. She was physically assaultive and violent, driving her husbands and her daughter away. Strangely, they always returned. It was not—so far as we learned—a separation or threat of separation that led to her demise. She was depressed (diagnosis of *probable* depression based on the husband's report) for the last year, probably worse for 2 weeks. During that time she drank especially heavily and behaved in a manner suggesting delirium. She was disoriented, fearful, and hid under the bed, but she was lucid enough to threaten suicide without appearing to be responding to frightening hallucinations. She was at least drunk out of her mind (BAC 0.324 g%) as well as depressed. That was enough.

Case 16

Subject 16 was a 44-year-old married white woman of no identified religion. She was born in New Jersey, had three sisters, and lived most of her life in the Northeast. Her father was a banker, her mother a homemaker, and the family was intact. She had graduated from high school and married at about age 24. They had one daughter, who was 19 years old at the time of the subject's death. Her husband had become an executive in a national corporation during the course of their 21-year marriage and was transferred by his firm to St. Louis 10 months prior to her suicide. He seemed to have remarkably little exact knowledge about his wife's problems, symptoms, and behavior.

She had been employed as a salesperson in a department store for about a year when she was 37 years old. She quit either because she found the work too hard or because she became ill. She had held no other employment outside the home. She had never been a tidy housekeeper, but in the last 3–5 years she neglected the house considerably. She had taken very good care of her daughter until the last 4 months, when she began attacking her daughter verbally for no evident reason.

She had used alcohol throughout the marriage. Use before that time is unreported. She started drinking daily at about age 26, 3 years into the marriage. This antedates by 3 years her hospitalization for pulmonary tuberculosis. She drank vodka with fruit juice and in late years consumed about half a fifth of vodka a day. Her family objected to her drinking. She had had no friends for 10 years. During the brief time that she worked she was warned of tardiness that was related to her drinking. In the last 5 years she expressed a desire to stop drinking, but her efforts in that direction were unsuccessful.

She had no arrests for drinking problems, as she went out of the house only rarely. "She just sat at home and drank." Her drinking increased somewhat in the last year of her life. Her behavior toward the family deteriorated badly in the last 4 months. The verbal attacks on her daughter were "irrational." Her daughter was described as previously "the apple of her mother's eye." Her husband could not say whether there was morning drinking, tremulousness, or blackouts. They didn't speak much, except to argue. It is uncertain what role her alcoholism played in marital conflict or in her several psychiatric hospital admissions, but they cannot have been totally unrelated.

She had been in psychotherapy intermittently from about age 24. Her family physician described her as "always in a 'slow burn' frame of mind." She was described as very sensitive to criticism, and although self-deprecatory, she became enraged at any criticism of her actions. At times she verbally attacked her husband without apparent cause. A scalp laceration noted on one admission for "chronic fatigue and insomnia" may have resulted from a fall or an altercation. The record does not state.

She was described as having a very negative view of life. "Everything was bad or no good." She realized that she was difficult to get along with but said "that's just tough" for her husband. She complained of fatigue for nearly all of the marriage and had even less energy for at least 10 years. She stayed up late drinking for the last 15 years and slept poorly. She disliked crowds and left the house only rarely in the last 5 years (it was unclear whether she was agoraphobic). She had isolated herself socially long before the move to St. Louis. She was clinically depressed for the last 2–5 years of her life, with low mood, decreased sex drive, and decreased interest and activities. She neglected the house and the care of her family, cooking very little during that time. Self-deprecation, fatigue, poor appetite, and insomnia were of longer duration.

In addition to alcohol, she took barbiturates daily. On hospital admission about 1 year before her death she was noted to be taking 100 mg. pentobarbital (Nembutal) two times a day as well as tranquilizers. During the last 2 years of her life she frequently accused her husband of having a girlfriend. That led to heated arguments. He contended the accusation was unfounded. She denied him sex for the last year. On several occasions she became so irrational, aggressive, and hard to handle that her husband put her in a "rehabilitation center" (actually, a private psychiatric hospital in another state) for 1–2 weeks until she calmed down (or dried out?). The last such admission occurred 5 months before her suicide. Very sketchy hospital records do not identify alcohol abuse symptoms, although "moderate to heavy" alcohol use is noted. She last saw a psychiatrist about 6 weeks before ending her life.

She had been hospitalized for pulmonary tuberculosis at age 27–28 and had a left upper lobectomy. She also had an appendectomy and unilateral oophorectomy. She had had pneumonia at age 37 and had various other minor complaints.

According to the informant, her mother and all three of her sisters "drank too much." One sister had a "nervous breakdown" a year before the subject's death, treated by her family physician. Another was psychiatrically hospitalized for an unknown time about 5 years before the subject's suicide.

She had talked intermittently of committing suicide for 8–10 years and had made suicide attempts at ages 35 and 43, by overdose of medication. During the last year of her life she told her husband and daughter on several occasions that she would be better off dead and talked of being "a bother" to them. She had stated after the last previous suicide attempt that next time she wouldn't "botch it up." A close friend, a nun, had died 4 months before she did and she was very upset about it. She asked, "Why should I be alive if my good, kind friend is dead?" There had been increasing suicidal communication the last 4 months, beginning when her husband mentioned chronic hospitalization. The timing of her last communication was not learned. She owned several books pertaining to suicide and homicide and had talked about these on several occasions in the 2 years before ending her life.

Circumstances Leading to the Act

She had been depressed for at least the last 5 years, increasingly in the last 2 years. The relationship with her husband was extremely strained. He knew so little about potentially observable aspects of her behavior that it seems a fair assumption that he came to ignore her. Toward the end, she hardly spoke except to argue. Four months before her suicide he broached the possibility of long-term hospital commitment, owing to her increasing irritability, unhappiness, constant drinking, and perhaps her general unpleasantness, irrationality, and aimlessness. She said she would kill herself instead. About that time she began attacking her daughter verbally without provocation. Because of this, the daughter was looking for an apartment in order to get out of the house. She was unable to control her behavior, feared hospitalization, and perhaps perceived that it would not be long before she was involuntarily committed. However, none of the feared events had yet occurred. On the day of her suicide, she wrote a note to her husband, drank an excess of alcohol and took an overdose of barbiturates. Empty pill bottles included Tuinal, Valium, and Triavil.

> [daughter]–[daughter],–Mother and whoever else might care—please forgive and try to understand—I just cannot fight to operate any more. I realize that I am doing damage to put it mildly—but [daughter]—remember what Dr. L_____ said—you are basically strong and I am counting on that. You can be stronger and I'm counting on that too. For the rest—I am not strong. I am tired & weak & stupid & worn out—and there is no future for me. I love but I'm being sloppy, and horribly selfish. Obviously there is a great deal of hate in me or I wouldn't repeat what I'm doing. It isn't directed at any one of you—I just feel used up and useless. For what it's worth and despite Missouri's dubious laws—[daughter] owns my three drawered bed table & the glass table in the living room plus contents—They were only given to me in keeping for her. Also what "family jewelry" as there is—and most of all the sampler & "primitive" hanging in the living room, & the [family name] silver, plus bill of sale which will be found in the ammo box in my closet. Needless to say the "hers to his to hers" M.J. will is my desire & I know [husband] loves [daughter] as I do— more, since he has the courage to live. If there is any question of ownership as stated, refer to [name of person] of Las Vegas, and [name of person] of [town], N.Y.—but gently, please. There are other things—the dining room chairs, the mantel clock, the blue and silver tea pot—the Delft vases! Other things—help is needed. Most of "mine" is hers, just waiting for the right age & time.
>
> Please, [husband]—you know most—when Sis or B_____ are able, they can identify more—don't let them take them away from [daughter]—they are a heritage which I hope she can see and understand beyond my illness.
>
> I hope you can too. I love you & have loved you, but too destructively for either of us. Please don't take your anger at me out on anyone else. No one caused my action but my own inability to cope. You'll be better off in the long run—& so will [daughter]—I feel worst about mother who won't understand—please be kind—lie if need be.
>
> Good night— + I hope this won't mean another hospitalization & more expense— I don't think so. I do think [daughter] will make it with your help—just don't be bitter please—it won't help either of you and wasn't caused by either of you—lord knows I had all the help you could have provided.
>
> [first name]

Findings and Sources

Clinical Diagnoses: (1) Personality disorder, mixed; (2) alcoholism, chronic; (3) major depressive disorder, secondary.
Toxicology: Blood alcohol concentration 0.18 g%; barbiturate concentration 2.3 mg%; salicylates 3.7 mg%.
Primary Informant: Husband, married 25 years; saw her daily, in some sense.

Other Sources of Information: Coroner's death investigation report, hospital records (incomplete).
Informant's Opinion of Reason for Suicide: Fear of institutionalization.

Comment

Because of her housebound housewife lifestyle, this subject did not expose herself to arrests. The paucity of other symptoms of alcoholism seems to be owed to the husband-informant's lack of observation rather than to a possibly mild degree of alcohol abuse. Drinking had been her vocation for years. The marital relationship was severely strained. It appears that her husband ignored her existence to the extent possible. With her daughter planning to move and her husband threatening psychiatric commitment, she was facing further isolation. Only a thin barrier seems to have separated her from this act for quite a long while. I think these recent threats of loss, added to her depression, breached the barrier. The suicide note does not suggest an acute precipitating event.

Case 10

Subject 10 was a 46-year-old white thrice-married Protestant secretary, born in Georgia, the only child of U.S.-born parents. Her father was a dentist and an alcoholic. He died of unknown cause when she was 7 or 8. Her mother was a homemaker. She completed 14 years of schooling without difficulty. She was first married at the age of 18 and divorced 2 years later on grounds of physical cruelty. She was next married at 23 and divorced at 29 for unknown reasons. She was married for the third time at age 30 and remained in this marriage to the time of her death. She had one child, a daughter, from the second marriage. The daughter was aged 17½ at the time of the subject's death.

Twelve years prior to her suicide, her mother came to live with her, her husband, and her daughter. She was described by the subject's husband as "a dissatisfied and domineering person, wanting to know everything she was doing, and who tried to make all decisions for her." The subject felt quite hostile toward her mother but permitted her to continue to live with them. Two years before her suicide, her mother died.

She worked only sporadically, having a total of five jobs in her whole life, mostly as a secretary. She had done well in her jobs and had never been fired or been in trouble at work. In the last year of her life she was performing her household work so poorly that her husband threatened to "take over" in that department. As a secretary, she had apparently worked right up to the time of her death. Her drinking did not seem to affect her employment. She was reported to have had five friends and no change in her relationship with them.

According to the informants, the subject started heavy drinking at the age of 35, in her third marriage, in order to relieve anxiety symptoms. She was a "spree" drinker who drank irregularly, drank before breakfast, thought she drank too much, and felt guilty about her drinking. Her husband objected, as did others, and she lost friends on account of drinking. She was unable to control it and during the last 6 months of her life contacted AA for help. Rather than becoming abstinent, she drank more than usual, up to a fifth of hard liquor a day. She had shakes and blackouts but no arrests. When drinking, she sometimes became morose.

She was described as always sensitive, with easily hurt feelings. In her 20s, she began having mild anxiety symptoms. At about age 35 these became severe, and she consulted a psychiatrist in California. The anxiety symptoms improved after a year's treatment but were exacerbated with the mother's death 2 years before her own. Following that event, she expressed feelings of guilt that she had not done right by her. She seemed to go downhill from that point, with more anxiety symptoms. A suicide attempt led to a brief hospitalization. For the last year of her life, she was more indecisive than previously. For the last 6 months, she looked sad, lost interest in things, complained of fatigue, performed her housework poorly, lost appetite and 10 pounds of weight, and looked depressed. Slightly over a month before her death, she was hospitalized for depression and given a low dose of antidepressant medication. Her psychiatrist described her as "depressed, lonely, agitated, with insomnia and anorexia." She was released from the hospital 3½ weeks before she ended her life. She saw her psychiatrist 2 days before her death. He said he had wanted her back in the hospital because of the severity of her depression. He also noted that she suspected her husband of having affairs with other women. "He travels a *lot*!" Her internist thought her suspicions might have been justified.

There was no evidence that her general health was impaired in any way. She had last seen her family physician almost a year before her death, for a complaint of vaginitis. Her only hospitalizations were for suicide attempt and depression.

Her father was alcoholic and may have died of that disease. Her mother was hospitalized for an unspecified psychiatric illness 6 years before the subject's death, received ECT, and recovered. Presumably she suffered from depression. There was no information concerning collateral relatives.

Her psychiatrist understood her to have made a suicide attempt by overdose at age 40. Her family physician said she had made two suicide attempts, one by overdose and one by cutting. Her husband reported that she had made a suicide attempt by overdose at age 44, for which she was briefly hospitalized. In the last 2 years of her life, and only when drinking, she spoke of committing suicide, said she would be better off dead, spoke of wanting to die, spoke of killing herself by taking "dope," said the family would be better off if she were dead, spoke of wanting to give her body to science, and had spoken recently of changing the insurance benefits to her daughter. She also said she had nothing to live for.

Circumstances Leading to the Act

She had been upset since the death of her mother 2 years before her own. She had been increasingly depressed for the last 6 months of her life and drinking more. She had become suspicious that her husband had other interests and was going to leave her. When she was drinking, he sometimes did threaten to do so. When she was sober, he assured her that he would not. She was also concerned that her daughter would be leaving her in a few months (probably about 6 months) to go to college. Her sister-in-law died 3 months before she did, and she was quite upset about it. For 3 days before her death, she was upset over a number of things: (1) friction with her husband because of her drinking; (2) an unsuccessful attempt to effect a reconciliation between a friend and her husband (She was accused of being a "meddler."); (3) on the day before she died, she was upset when she learned that her daughter had received a traffic ticket. On the evening of the suicide, her husband and daughter went to bed around 11:00 or 11:30 p.m. She stayed up, drank, and then went to the car in the garage and asphyxiated herself with carbon monoxide. Her husband saw her put a piece of paper in a notebook beside her bed when he came home from work. It proved to be a suicide note.

> I will kill myself—why not? All my life I have had to fight—and by the same token understand and look after other people—They could care less as long as I'm of use—FINE—But when I'm not—well—that's why—I believe we are a long way from solving problems as I have no matter what one does. The doctors can't make the people who surround me different—I am glad to go to sleep—

Findings and Sources

Clinical Diagnoses: (1) Alcoholism, chronic; (2) generalized anxiety disorder; (3) secondary depression.
Toxicology: Blood alcohol concentration 0.23 g%; blood CO saturation 80%.
Primary Informants: Spouse and daughter, who knew subject for 16 and 18 years, respectively, and saw her almost daily.
Other Sources of Information: Psychiatrist, general practitioner, coroner's death investigation report.
Informant's Opinion of Reason for Suicide: (1) Felt cheated of happiness life should provide; (2) guilt that she hadn't done right by her mother.

Comment

No obvious external precipitant is found here. A chronically insecure alcoholic, she was anxious about the stability of her marriage as she became progressively more depressed, and, as her suicide note suggests, angry. She seems to have been brooding about unfairness, but why did the suicide occur just when it did? Did her husband, our primary informant, neglect to mention something? Absent this, her depression and alcoholism together are sufficient to account for her suicide.

Case 25

Subject 25 was a married homemaker, 53 years old at the time of her suicide. She was born in Louisville, Kentucky. Her father was a professional gambler, a ne'er-do-well, and an abuser of alcohol. He was absent for long periods while she was growing up ("away for a year, then back for a week") and at one time spent 5 years in prison. Her parents were divorced sometime after the subject's marriage. Her mother was a deeply religious woman, an adherent of a fundamentalist protestant sect. That brand of religion had been the subject's major preoccupation as well, until about the age of 30. She had four siblings (two brothers), but age relationships were not learned. She had no school performance or conduct problems, and no record of inappropriate behavior until, in the 10th grade, she and a friend decided to leave Joplin and visit Kansas City for several weeks. She never returned to school.

She was married at 19 to a man she had known for 5 years. He progressed to the position of a sales executive in the building materials field. They had three children, two boys and a girl, who were 32, 24, and 22 and all out of the home at the time of her death. She was never employed regularly outside the home. A major problem in the marriage involved her fundamentalist religious beliefs or practices. This led to a separation after they had been married for 5 years. She took her 3-year-old son and moved to Los Angeles, while her husband worked near Las Vegas and supported them. They were reconciled after a year, at the cost of her breaking with her church. Her husband entered military service at about that time.

She was described as having few interests ever, but being a meticulous housekeeper. After suppressing her religious interests she became preoccupied with her own mental health. She blamed her mental state on her husband's lack of attention. She became increasingly introverted, shy, easily hurt, and moody. In the last 6–7 years of her life, she avoided friends and relatives. She was fearful of being alone and also of driving an automobile.

Her excessive drinking began at about age 41, in the course of a major depressive episode, possibly her first, 12 years before her suicide. From age 46 to 49, she drank up to a quart of liquor a day. During that period and prior to their moving to St. Louis, she ended all of her friendships and established no new ones after the move. She even ran her sister away. Thus for the last 6 years of her life her husband was her sole social contact. She was fearful when he traveled and left her alone, as happened with some frequency. She drank before breakfast, thought she drank too much, felt guilty about drinking, and tried to stop. She eventually was successfully abstinent for a period of 4 years. Just a month before her suicide she resumed drinking for unknown reasons. When intoxicated she fought with her husband, who also thought she drank too much. She once picked up a knife and threatened him. The husband's response was to lock up the firearms and rid the house of ammunition.

She became neglectful of household responsibilities in the last 2–3 years of her life, during her period of abstinence. She experienced no problems in legal or economic areas, as she was little exposed to those risks, and was not known to have medical problems secondary to drinking. She rarely left the house except to purchase liquor. Owing to a rather poorly informative interview, she meets strict criteria for probable alcoholism. She was verbally combative and once threatened her husband with a knife, so probable versus definite alcoholism depends on one's definition of "fighting."

She was always sensitive to criticism and easily angered. At about age 39, fourteen years before her death, she suffered onset of a recurring major depressive disorder. She was hospitalized for it six times over a period of 5 years, receiving ECT, insulin coma, and symptomatic treatment with sedatives and tranquilizers, which she eventually abused and was unable to stop. She stopped driving after her depression began, because she was fearful in traffic. She felt anxious, worthless, guilty about her abuse of medication, she cried easily, found life sad and joyless, suffered from insomnia, poor memory, loss of interest, and low energy, and had persistent suicidal thoughts. She sometimes gained as much as 20–30 pounds during depressed periods, attributing it to the medication she took (amitriptyline).

Her excessive drinking began in the context of a major depression. During the last few years of her life, she continued to see a psychiatrist but was hospitalized only once more, 4 years before her death. Her St. Louis psychiatrist diagnosed her as having a schizoaffective disorder and treated her with thioridazine (Mellaril) (an antipsychotic medication), in addition to the antidepressant. Apart from her self-imposed social isolation, a schizophrenic flavor did not come through in the husband's description. Hallucinations and delusions were specifically denied.

She was generally in good health but was often concerned about headaches, palpitation, chest pain, backache, severe premenstrual tension, and other somatic complaints for which she took "up to a bottle" of aspirin a week. She had a hysterectomy at age 36 and a hemorrhoidectomy at 40.

Her father was described as a ne'er-do-well, an alcoholic, and professional gambler. One sister was emotionally unstable, married four or five times, and abandoned her child to her parents. No other family history was known to the informant.

At age 40 she took an overdose of medication after her husband had gone to work and the daughter to school. She was found unconscious and hospitalized. The following year she cut her wrists, one of them badly. In neither case was the husband able to cite a precipitant for the act. During the last 8 years of her life, she frequently said she had little to live for, was a burden to her family, and wanted to die. She had stopped speaking of suicide several months before her death.

Circumstances Leading to the Act

She had resumed heavy daily drinking a month before her death, after 4 years of abstinence. Her husband last saw her in bed, before he left town to attend his cousin's funeral. She had been expected to accompany him but declined that morning, saying she didn't feel like it. On his return the next day, he found her dead. A whiskey glass and empty medicine bottles, which had contained ethchlorvynol (Placidyl), chlordiazepoxide (Librium), thioridazine (Mellaril), and amitriptyline (Elavil), were in the room, together with a suicide note.

> Of course notify police, abulance [*sic*] & a doc immediately.

> Now I don't want a funeral, just a brief legal burial, cheap as possible. And don't be stupid enough to notify the 3 kids or mom. It'd only disrupt their lives. If you do— it will only be because you have self pity! Mail them these cards after one week. Bury me in this old black dress. I want C _____ to have fur, pearls & my rings. She'll want to go through everything, trunks, etc. And keep pictures etc. Send _____ & _____ their old things if they want them. After you & C _____ have gone through everything & you are ready to move, have _____come in & take all you don't want.
>
> [first and last name]

Findings and Sources

Clinical Diagnosis: (1) Primary affective disorder, recurrent depression; (2) secondary alcoholism; (3) sedative tranquilizer abuse.
Toxicology: Blood alcohol concentration 0.14 g%. Blood drug levels: chlordiazepox-

ide 0.1 mg%; ethchlorvynol, "small amount"; negative for thioridazine, barbiturates, and salicylates; analysis not reported for amitriptyline (the most likely intoxicant).
Primary Informant: Husband, married 34 years; saw her about daily.
Other Sources of Information: Coroner's death investigation records, attending psychiatrist and internist.
Informant's Opinion of Reason for Suicide: "She got depressed . . . her early life had a lot to do with it."

Comment

This woman had a chaotic childhood, with a sociopathic father who was gone much more than he was home. Her mother found refuge in a fundamentalist religion, and so did she. When she married, some unspecified aspects of her religion came between her and her husband, leading to a separation. She made a forced choice between her religion and the marriage after a year, and her life was apparently uneventful then, for a number of years. Her depressive disorder began 9 years later and in turn gave rise to alcohol abuse within 2 years. She stopped entertaining about 6 years before her death and cut herself off from all of her friends and her family for undisclosed reasons. The timing does not coincide with her hospitalizations, but she was drinking a fifth of liquor a day by then. Her last psychiatric hospitalization occurred 4 years before her suicide. The reason for it was unstated, but she became abstinent from alcohol at that time and remained so until a month before her suicide. Then she resumed daily drinking. She was clinically depressed. The combination appears to have been lethal, as in so many other cases. No added stress was reported. For a woman of a previously strong religious bent, her expressed wish for "a brief legal burial, cheap as possible," speaks of a high degree of self-rejection. Low self-esteem characterized her.

This was a peculiarly arid history, considering the customary thoroughness of the interviewer who recorded it. The personality of the woman just doesn't come through. It is possible that she had little personality. It is also possible that her husband was unable to relate to it. The children are reported to have complained that he neglected them. Her abruptly leaving school in the 10th grade to go to Joplin with a friend seems out of character for her. It seems to have been an isolated incident with the outside possibility of an early hypomanic episode without recurrence.

Case 44

Subject 44 was a 55-year-old divorced unemployed white female who ended her life by overdose of propoxyphene (Darvon) and alcohol. She was born and raised in the St. Louis area where she lived all her life. She had three sisters. Her father was a hod carrier and her mother a homemaker. The family, of Roman Catholic faith, was intact. She had no known major childhood problems and completed eighth grade. She married for the first time at age 25 and her husband died 18 years later. She remarried 2 years after his death, this time to an alcoholic who beat her. She divorced him after 6 years of marriage, when she was 51. She never had children. She bought and operated a tavern for about 3 years, then sold it to her sister. She continued to work there as a barmaid for 4 years. A little over a year before her death she began working as a cook in her niece's restaurant. That business was sold 6 months later and she was either unable or unwilling to look for other work. She had worked only for herself or members of her family.

She was described as having always been a sensitive and moody person. Prior to the death of her first husband she seemed to have been well adjusted and free of major emotional problems. For the last 4 years she lived alone, maintaining infrequent contact with two sisters in the city. The informant, one of her sisters, saw her about three times a month. She had at least one friend outside of her family, a woman who reportedly was not told about the suicide. For the last 8 months of her life, she was unemployed and was living on savings, which were almost totally exhausted. Her social contact was minimal during the last 6 months of her life.

She began drinking heavily at about the time of the death of her first husband, 12 years before her suicide, and developed a daily drinking pattern. She drank beer, both during work at the tavern, and often continuing to drink into the early morning hours. Although she frequently had the withdrawal symptom of tremulousness and drank before breakfast to steady her shaking, she never missed work or was obviously impaired on the job. She knew she drank too much and felt guilty about it. Her family also told her she drank too much. She never received any treatment for alcoholism and never tried to stop drinking. Some 7 or 8 years before her suicide she fell at home while intoxicated and was hospitalized with an ankle injury. She had rectal bleeding during the last year of her life but refused medical attention despite her family's urging. Two weeks before her demise she fell three times in one day, and thereafter complained of pleuritic pain. Although she was said not to have seen a physician, she must have, as she had obtained propoxyphene (Darvon), which she used in a suicide attempt and subsequently in her suicide.

She was never seen by a psychiatrist or treated for any mental condition. She had a poor appetite for the last 5 years of her life. During the last 6 months she had persistent low mood with feelings of guilt and worthlessness and neglected her personal hygiene, a behavior characteristic of psychomotor retardation. When in her cups she frequently became tearful and often verbalized feelings of worthlessness and sadness. She stopped going to movies, ostensibly to conserve what little money she had. She lost interest in socializing and stopped playing cards with relatives during the last 6 months. The informant had no knowledge of her sleep pattern, energy, or thought processes.

She appears to have been in good health during most of her life and had little reason to seek medical care. Her only known hospitalization was for an injured ankle. During the year preceding her death, her sister noted blood on her dresses and learned she had rectal bleeding. She rejected her sister's urging to see a physician, using the excuse that she could not afford a doctor, despite the family offering to pay for her care. She believed the bleeding was due to a cancer.

There was no known family history of alcohol or drug abuse, mental illness, or suicide.

During the last 6 months of her life, she had intermittently spoken of suicide to her sister when drunk. She remarked that she had no children and was not needed. A week before her suicide she told her sister, "If pills would kill you, I took enough this week that I should be dead." She had taken an unknown amount of propoxyphene.

On the evening of her suicide she told her sister of her suicidal thoughts and advised her on disposition of some of her belongings.

Circumstances Leading to the Act

She had no income and only $30 in the bank. She had long been worried about impoverishment but would not accept proffered financial help from her family. She had fallen three times in one day and was having chest pain, as well as worries of possible cancer causing her rectal bleeding. A week after her suicide attempt she called her sister at her tavern around 8:00 p.m. and told her that she felt like committing suicide. She asked her sister to come to her apartment, three blocks away. The sister agreed to do so in an hour. She asked if her sister had a key, and when told she did not, said she would leave the door open. During the conversation she said, "let [a nephew] have the furniture." Apparently not taking this suicidal talk seriously, her sister did not visit that evening as she had promised. The following morning the other sister (the informant) and her daughter went to the subject's apartment and found her dead.

Findings and Sources

Clinical Diagnosis: (1) Alcoholism, chronic; (2) probable secondary affective disorder (DSM-III-R; major depressive disorder).
Toxicology: Blood alcohol concentration 0.23 g%; blood propoxyphene in trace amounts; bile propoxyphene 54.5 mg%.
Primary Informant: Sister, known all her life; saw her about three times a month.
Other Sources of Information: Coroner's death investigation report.
Informant's Opinion of Reason for Suicide: To get attention. Others: "She didn't really mean to do it."

Comment

The informant's lack of knowledge of whether this subject experienced insomnia, fatigue, or impaired thinking or concentration deprives us of a confident diagnosis of major depressive disorder. Criteria are sufficient for a *probable* diagnosis (DSM-III-R, definite). Her belief that she had cancer and her refusal to seek treatment for it, as well as her feelings of redundancy, are best understood in association with that diagnosis.

She may have been a rather timid person, never working for anyone but herself or family members. Yet, how does a timid person run a tavern? She did not actively try to find work after the restaurant was sold. Her financial plight was extreme at the end, but she would not accept proffered help from her family. She apparently didn't apply for unemployment compensation either. She seems to have tired of her rather empty existence. Depression, lack of money, and belief that she had cancer were enough. Falling and hurting herself probably hastened her decision. There was more "cry for help" in her communications than in most suicides. Had her sisters responded more vigorously, she might have lived.

Case 23

Subject 23 was a 57-year-old white married woman, born in a small town in Illinois. Her father was a machinist and her mother a homemaker. She had one brother, about whom no details are known. The parental home was not unusual. She progressed uneventfully through high school and was married at 19 to a man about her own age whom she had known for 2 years. She worked as a clerk in variety stores from age 18 to 27, while her husband completed his education. After that she was a homemaker. She had one stillbirth and three spontaneous abortions before she bore a daughter when she was 30. She and her husband adopted two girls when she was 37. He was a very busy executive at the time of her death.

The family moved to the St. Louis area 12 years prior to her death. Of a liberal Christian denomination, she attended church regularly and taught Sunday school. Five years later, her mother, who lived with them, became senile. She died after a stormy 3 years in which she repeatedly accused others of stealing from her, soiled herself, and generally showed her senility. Her mother's senile behavior and her death were very troubling to the subject, who was described as high-strung, moody, sensitive, and given to crying easily.

Since about the age of 39, she had taken an occasional social drink of beer. That pattern changed at about age 50, when her mother became senile. For a time she began to believe that she, too, was losing her mind. She began drinking hard liquor surreptitiously. Five years before her death her husband was hospitalized with his second myocardial infarction. Their daughter confronted him with evidence of her drinking, which he seemed not to have noticed. After he returned home she did not moderate her drinking. Indeed, she no longer prepared meals on time and stopped attending church. Her mother died the next year. Her drinking pattern had rapidly evolved into daily drinking (up to two fifths of bourbon per 3 days) with additional 3- to 4-day binges.

She and her husband had occupied separate bedrooms for years, at first ostensibly because of differing preferences regarding air conditioning, subsequently because she was usually drunk and asleep when he came home. She arose daily at 6:00 a.m., drank to relieve her tremulousness, and returned to bed before the informant arose. She had granted him her sexual favors only one time in the last year, protesting fatigue, or "not in the mood" on other occasions. She had used sedatives regularly for about 4 years, and nightly for the last 2 years. During the last few months of her life she used prescribed sedatives during the day as well as at bedtime. She had frequent falls, after which she would be found unresponsive. On one such occasion she sustained a fractured clavicle.

She seems to have been agoraphobic, leaving the house only rarely since her heavy drinking began. As a consequence, she had no driving trouble or contact with police. Whether she had her liquor delivered or her husband purchased it is unknown. She went to the store for liquor on the day of her death. Her husband remarked that that was uncharacteristic of her.

In addition to abandonment of all household duties, she withdrew from social contact with friends. She had frequent quarrels with one adopted daughter concerning her drinking. In the fall of the year before her suicide her husband confronted her about her drinking. He told her that if she did not seek help for the problem, he would have her institutionalized. She threatened suicide but did nothing. She managed to remain abstinent for 3 months, after which she relapsed with a progression of symptoms.

In her last 3 years she was noted to exhibit anorexia with weight loss and insomnia. Loss of interest was of longer duration—not less than 5 years. She exhibited psychomotor retardation in the last 3 days. These symptoms, plus recurrent thoughts of suicide, are sufficient to establish a diagnosis of major depressive disorder, secondary to her alcoholism.

Her first contact with a psychiatrist was about 5½ months before taking her life. At that time she had had a severe drinking problem for over 6 years. Relatives from out of town were passing through and telephoned her. She said she was not feeling well and suggested they not visit. They decided to stop by and see if they could be of assistance, knowing that her husband was out of town. (He returned the next day.) They found her unconscious in her bedroom from an overdose of medication, probably amobarbital (Tuinal) and alcohol. They called her daughter, who had her hospitalized at a local psychiatric hospital where she remained for 15 days under the care of a psychiatrist whose name had been picked out of the telephone book. The diagnosis made was acute alcoholic psychosis.

After discharge from the hospital, she continued to see the psychiatrist every 3 or 4 weeks, receiving chlordiazepoxide (Librium) 10 mg four times daily and amobarbital (Tuinal) 200 mg at bedtime. She was described as making very little therapeutic progress and professed not to know why she was seeing him. He, in turn, had complained to her husband that she wouldn't "open up" with him, so his efforts to help her were frustrated. Her last office visit was just over 3 weeks before her death. No other diagnosis was made. The psychiatrist did not think she was depressed, just alcoholic. He last refilled her prescriptions 3 days before her suicide.

She had been hospitalized at age 43 for a generalized allergic skin rash with chronic secondary excoriations, and for a hemorrhoidectomy at age 48. She had a surgical procedure for occluded tear ducts at age 56. The last year of her life she was hospitalized because of hypertension, weight loss, and anemia, all attributed to her alcoholism. That same year, she had a second hospitalization for tear duct surgery. It was noted on that admission that she suffered from chronic bronchitis with emphysema. A diagnosis of duodenal ulcer was made by her internist as well, but not as a part of the hospital workup. Her fractured clavicle has been mentioned.

A maternal aunt, an almost lifelong alcoholic, died in a nursing home about 4 months before her suicide. A maternal uncle was hospitalized as a young man and was reported to have died in the hospital (i.e., presumably did not recover). There was no other history of alcoholism or mental illness in the family, and no suicides. Her father died of gastric cancer at age 68, her mother of "senility" at 78.

One and one-half years before her suicide, she had told her youngest daughter she would kill herself. About a year before her death she again spoke of suicide in the context of her husband's threat to institutionalize her. She is reported to have said that if the car keys had been available she would have taken the car out and put an end to herself in a high-speed accident. Her overdose, a serious attempt at suicide while her husband was out of town, was discovered by accident, as described.

Circumstances Leading to the Act

One week before her suicide, her adopted daughter left for a vacation in Honolulu with a boyfriend of high school days and his parents. She and her husband were planning to leave soon on a vacation and she was thought to have been looking forward to it. She was abstinent from alcohol for 3–4 days, but she made no other preparations for the trip. She appeared to her husband to be depressed. The day of her death she knew he did not plan to be home until late evening, because of a dinner engagement with a business associate. She began drinking in the afternoon. He believes she also took a sedative, probably amobarbital (Tuinal), as her medicine bottle could not be found. At 10:45 p.m. he returned home to find the garage door locked, which was unusual. He entered the garage to find the car not running but the engine still warm. His wife was sitting in the front seat of the car, unresponsive. Resuscitation was attempted by a police officer and a passer-by. She was dead on arrival at St. Louis County Hospital at 11:08 p.m. If there was any acute precipitant of the suicidal act, it was not reported.

A note by the subject was found in the house: "Creamation [sic] please; don't tell [an adopted daughter], no memorial; thanks for being good to me."

Findings and Sources

Clinical Diagnosis: (1) Alcoholism, chronic; (2) major depressive disorder, secondary.
Toxicology: Blood alcohol concentration 0.08 g%; CO hemoglobin saturation 70%. No other toxicologic results reported.
Primary Informant: Husband, married 38 years; saw her about daily, in passing or passed out.
Other Sources of Information: Internist, psychiatrist, coroner's death investigation record.
Informant's Opinion of Reason for Suicide: "No reason. Just alcohol."

Comment

There was a substantial educational and vocational discrepancy between this subject and her husband. She had worked as a variety store clerk while he completed his master's degree. She sought no education beyond high school. He was very intense about his work and always "on the go." He probably spent few evenings at home or with his wife. They occupied separate bedrooms—at least in part because of her drinking. She had given up her domestic interests and volunteer activities over the last several years, and except for contact with her husband and her adopted daughter, had entirely isolated herself socially. It appeared that he had isolated himself from her as well.

Nevertheless, she and her husband were planning a vacation in a few days. She was thought to be looking forward to it. She had obtained a 2-week supply of amobarbital from her doctor, in order to have an adequate supply for the trip. She stopped drinking for 3–4 days, but she did nothing else in preparation for it. She went out for

Table 7.1 Suicide Mortality as a Proportion of Overall Mortality of Alcoholics by Sex

Reference	N		n	%	Dead N	%	Suicides N	%	Combined Rate (%)
Fremming (1951), Denmark	61	M	59	97	14	23	2	14	14
		F	2	3	0		0		
Selzer & Holloway (1957), United States	86[a]	M	62	72	12	19	1	6	6
		F	24	28	6	25	0	0	
Kessel & Grossman (1961), Scotland	218	M	172	79	20	12	11	65	52
		F	46	21	3	7	0	0	
Tashiro & Lipscomb (1963), United States	1,692	M	1,431	85	107	7	6	6	2
		F	261	15	17	7	0	0	
Helgason (1964), Iceland	241[a]	M	229	95	77	34	12	16	15
		F	12	5	3	25	0	0	
Wieser & Kunad (1965), Federal Republic of Germany	153[a]	M	140	92	54	39	12	22	22
		F	13	8	6	46	1	17	
Ciompi & Eisert (1969), Switzerland	1,386[a]	M	1,232	89	976	79	94	10	10
		F	154	11	102	66	4	4	
Gillis (1969), South Africa	802	M	690	86	86	12	10	12	12
		F	112	14	9	8	1	13	

Study	N	Sex							
Schmidt & DeLint (1972), Canada	6,478	M	5,359	83	639	12	47	7	7
		F	1,119	17	99	9	4	4	
Lindelius et al. (1974), Sweden	257	M	139	54	25	18	3	12	23
		F	118	46	19	16	7	37	
Choi (1975), United States	863	M	714	83	38	5	2	5	4
		F	149	17	7	5	0		
Combs-Orme, Taylor, Scott, & Holmes (1983), United States	1,289	M	1,005	78	182	16	7	4	4
		F	284	22	64	22	3	5	
Berglund (1984), Sweden	1,312	M	1,192	91	495	42	85	17	16
		F	120	9	42	35	3	7	
Nielsen et al. (1987), Denmark	408	M	324	79	36	11	15	42	40
		F	84	21	9	11	3	33	
Lindberg & Ågren (1988), Sweden	4,872	M	3,910	80	1,141	29	98	9	9
		F	962	20	191	20	21	11	
Wells & Walker (1990), New Zealand	616	M	524	85	66	13	1	2	4
		F	92	15	17	18	2	12	
Totals	20,734	M	17,182	83	4,562	26	456		9.1
		F	3,552	17	3,968	23	406	10	
					594	17	50	8	

[a] N recalculated to reflect number of probands successfully followed up, not original N.

Table 7.2 Background Characteristics: Women by Age of Onset

Patient Number	Age at Suicide	Parental Home[a]	Family History	Education yr	Civil State
47(B)	32	mother: died (2–3 yo)	NI	6	s
49	40	intact	father: alcoholic; paternal uncle: alcoholic, suicide; brother: ? alcoholic	18	m
16	44	intact	mother, 3 sisters: abused alcohol; sister: NBD, PH	12	m
10	46	father: died (7 yo)	father: alcoholic; mother: hospitalized, ECT	14	m
25	53	father: mostly absent	father: alcoholic sociopath	10	m
44	55	intact	negative	8	div
23	57	intact	maternal aunt: alcoholic; maternal uncle: depressed	12	m

Key: 0 = none; (B) = black; div = divorced; ECT = electroconvulsive therapy; m = married; mo = month(s); NBD = nervous breakdown; NI = no information; PH = psychiatric hospital; s = single; yr = year(s).
[a]Age given in parenthesis is that of the subject at the time of the occurrence.

Table 7.3 Alcohol-Related History: Women by Age of Onset

Patient Number[a]	Age at Suicide	Drink Onset/ Duration (yr)	Fights[b]	Arrests[c]	Abusive[d]	Serious Health Problems[e]
47(B)	32	16/16	+	P	P	0
49	40	17/23	0	V	P	0
16	44	26/18	V	0	V	[TB history]
10	46	35/11	0	0	0	0
25	53	41/12	V	0	0	0
44	55	43/12	0	0	abused	[rectal bleeding, thought rectal cancer]
23	57	50/7	0	0	0	HT, DU emphysema

[a](B) = black
[b]V = verbal; + indicates fights without arrests.
[c]p = peace disturbance; V = vehicular.
[d]p = physical; V = verbal.
[e]0 = none; DU = duodenal ulcer; HT = hypertension; TB = pulmonary tuberculosis.
[f]S/A = suicide attempt.
[g]1° = primary; 2° = secondary; AD = affective disorder; MR = mental retardation; prob = probable; SCU = schizophrenia, chronic, undifferentiated.

Number of Marriages/ Duration (yr)	Age and Sex of Progeny	Living Circumstances	Drinking Locale	Social Support	Last Hospital Treatment[f]	Employment	Other Diagnoses[g]	Other Substance Abuse	Suicide Attempts
0	2	father, sister, 2 yo son	home, bar	adequate	2 wk OD	unemployed life	SCU MR	0	+
3/8, 7, 2	18♀, 16♀, 8♀	husband, 8 yo daughter	not stated, probably home	almost 0	3 mo S/A 2 ×	unemployed 9 mo	prob 2° AD	chlordiazepoxide	+ many
1/26	19♀	husband, daughter	home	husband distant, angry with daughter	5 mo psychiatric (fighting)	unemployed 7 yr	2° AD	barbiturates daily	+(2)
3/2, 6, 16	17♀	husband, daughter	home	five friends?	4 wk depression	employed	2° AD	0	+(2)
1/34	32♂, 24♂, 22♀	husband	home	0, husband avoided	4 yr depression	never	1° AD	sedatives, tranquilizers, prescription only	+(2)
2/18, 6	0	alone	job (tavern) relatives' homes	minimal	7 yr, injury secondary to alcoholism	unemployed 8 mo	prob 2° AD	propoxyphene	+
1/38	28♀	husband, adopted daughter	home	0, husband ignored	5½ mo OD	housewife 30+ yr	2° AD	"sedatives"	+

liquor, knowing he would be home late, drank some, probably took all of her medication (the bottle was not found) and asphyxiated herself in the closed garage.

No acute precipitant was identified in the interview. Five and one-half months earlier she had made a similarly unheralded serious suicide attempt, surviving only by the chance visit of relatives from out of town. Although a full depressive syndrome was not identified at that time, it was not necessarily absent. Psychomotor retardation in the last 3 days, during which she was not drinking, completes the diagnosis. The husband, our informant, had little contact with his wife, although perhaps more than he cared to. She had ceased to function as a homemaker, a companion, or a sex partner. Her life seemed altogether empty and pointless. Drinking, considered alone, would not seem to account for such marked withdrawal. Depression, beginning with her mother's senility and death, and deepening abruptly at the end, joined to her husband's active avoidance of her, was sufficient reason for her suicide.

DISCUSSION

Women comprise 14% of the suicides in this study. A tabulation of all of the follow-up studies of alcoholics I could find in the world literature that include women as well as men in a seemingly unbiased sampling (Table 7.1) shows that women make up about 17% of the total. They contribute 13% of the mortality, and 11% of that by suicide. Thus they have a relatively small impact on the overall statistics regarding suicide in alcoholics. The present sample does differ from that of the men in several respects.

The women who took their lives had almost as wide a range of ages of onset of abusive drinking—16 to 50—as men, but a narrower range of durations of their drinking careers, 7 to 23 years with a mean of 14.1 years. Medical problems were not prominent and none of the women had a history of arrests for fighting, although 3 of them abused their partners, 2 physically, and 1 verbally (Table 7.2). One was herself physically abused. One, a mentally retarded schizophrenic, had multiple arrests for peace disturbance. Another had arrests for vehicular infractions. All had a history of suicide attempt, 6 of them with verbal communication of suicidal thoughts as well. Addictive drinking, as evidenced by benders, was found in 4 of 5 where inquiry was recorded. At least 4 had a family history of alcoholism, with 1 lacking information (Table 7.3). All 7 of the women had psychiatric comorbidity; 6 of them were affectively disordered, 1 had chronic, undifferentiated schizophrenia. What was most striking to me about these women was the profound lack of support and interest on the part of the husbands of those 5 who were married. Lacking careers of their own, they seemed to live in almost total isolation, to a considerable extent self-imposed. The pointed disregard by their husbands might well have felt worse than living alone.

IV

FINDINGS AND IMPLICATIONS

8

Why They Do It

Suicide doesn't just happen. It has a history.
Jan Beskow, M.D. (1979)

INTERPERSONAL LOSS

Original Findings and Pertinent Literature

It was the finding of a large number of loss events and their statistically significant clumping in the last weeks of the self-terminated lives of alcoholics that led to the investigation that provides the data base for this book. Neither frequent loss events nor their recency characterized the largest diagnostic group, suicides with a primary diagnosis of major depressive disorder (Table 1.1). The difference is consistent with the clinical impression that the suicidal concerns of depressives are oriented largely around how they feel about themselves and that they tend to take their lives for internal reasons. Alcoholics, on the other hand, react more to crises and interpersonal issues. We published the finding (Murphy & Robins, 1967), aware that it was discovered, not predicted.

It had long been clear to me that strict replication of our finding was needed. My undertaking of that task was discussed in Chapter 3. The result is displayed in Table 3.3. The single hypothesis being tested was confirmed. Just over one-quarter (26%) of the 50 alcoholic suicides were, indeed, found to have experienced disruption of a major interpersonal relationship within 6 weeks of their suicide ($P < 0.01$), replicating the original finding (Murphy et al., 1979).

Further strong support for this nexus has come from the work of Rich, Fowler, Fogarty, and Young (1988), not only for alcoholics, but for abusers of other substances as well. Those authors found one or more interpersonal losses to have antedated the suicide by 6 weeks or less in 41% of their alcoholics and in the same proportion of drug abusers. In contrast, only 18% of those with pure depressive disorder ($P < 0.02$) and 20% of those with other diagnoses had had a recent interpersonal loss. The specificity of such loss for abusers of psychoactive substances has thus been found three times in similarly conducted studies (Murphy & Robins, 1967; Murphy et al., 1979;

Rich et al., 1988). After psychiatric diagnosis, it is our strongest indicator of heightened risk of suicide (Mitterauer, 1981).

The association between disruptive life events and suicide has been commented upon frequently in the suicide literature (Breed, 1967; Humphrey, French, Niswander, & Casey, 1974; Humphrey, 1977; Ripley & Dorpat, 1981). Loss, actual or subjective, is readily found and anecdotally reported. Two things are missing from these investigations, cumulatively covering hundreds of cases, that limit their clinical usefulness. One is their relationship to specific psychiatric diagnoses. The other is enumeration of these events within a narrow time frame. With timing unrestricted, there may well be no difference. Dorpat and Ripley (1960) did consider psychiatric diagnoses and reported finding no difference across diagnoses in loss of a love object (27% overall) within the last year of the suicides' lives. The frequency and distribution of very *recent* losses was not addressed, and that is where the difference is found.

Scandinavian Studies

A Finnish study of alcoholic suicides, based solely on official records, failed to find evidence of the association we reported (Virkkunen, 1971). Had we restricted our investigation to official records, we would not have found the association either. Death certificates provide no space for sociopsychological data, and there is no tradition for systematically obtaining such information in coroners' or medical examiners' investigations.

A second study, incorporating personal inquiry, reported failure to confirm the relationship between interpersonal loss and suicide in alcoholics. Lönnqvist and Achté (1971) investigated a 7% sample of the adjudicated suicides occurring over a 10-year period in Helsinki. In addition to official records, information "was secured through interview with . . . relatives." Published details of this inquiry are lacking, but it was conducted after the end of the 10-year period (J. Lönnqvist, personal communication, September 27, 1990). Even without knowing exactly what was asked, or of whom, one must be cautious in relying heavily on recall of specific details of timing of events after a lapse of several years. Whether the population studied was comparable is also open to question. Only 60% of the putative alcoholics had abused drink in the last year of their lives and only one in four suicides occurred during or just after a drinking bout. In our (1967) study, all but two subjects were drinking right up to the time of their death. Lönnqvist and Achté may or may not have failed to replicate our work.

Despite the robustness of the finding of recent loss as a predictor of suicide in alcoholics, it nevertheless can be held accountable in no more than 25% to 40% of cases. Since the behavior of alcoholics tends to provoke repeated disruptions in their lives and the lives of those around them, I wondered why the suicide had occurred at this particular time and not another. It would be naive to expect suicide to result always, or even often, from a single, uncomplicated stimulus. The great majority of individuals who contemplate the act never undertake it. The case histories show that each individual reached his or her terminus by a distinctive route having some features in common with others. Interpersonal loss is but one predictor of a suicidal outcome. A major goal of this book is to ferret out those commonalities that occur in the midst of individual differences, in the hope that additional factors predicting increased risk will be uncovered.

In my comment on each case history I have recorded my opinion of the most important *immediate* reasons for the suicide. A condensed version is included in Table 8.5. I have not always judged recent loss of a close interpersonal relationship to be the most important reason for the suicide. Why does interpersonal loss not figure more prominently in my estimation of "most important reason" for suicide?

Disruptions of interpersonal relationships are rather frequent complications of the lives of alcoholics. Even such major losses as marital separation or divorce do not always lead to suicide. Twenty-six subjects (52%) had 38 divorces in their earlier history. Previous marital separations were known to have occurred, even in those still married. Thirteen subjects had experienced such an event recently (6 weeks). Only 6 of them were not known to have had a prior similar loss event. Might other factors be found that heighten the likelihood of a suicidal response to loss? Might they even be suicidogenic in their own right? An accumulation of factors, rather than one alone, characterizes these deaths.

Anticipated Losses

In our original report (Murphy & Robins, 1967) we defined interpersonal losses as those interruptions of relationships that had actually occurred and persisted to the time of suicide. Recent separations followed by reconciliation, for example, were not counted as losses. The focus was on the social system of the alcoholic as of the date of the suicide. By the same token, threatened, impending, or anticipated disruptions were not counted, as their inevitability could not be assessed. Their impact, in the strictest sense, had not been realized. That was not to discount the motivational impact of threats or fears, but only to recognize both their different quality and the uncertainty of their realizability.

Although threatened losses were meticulously excluded from the count of recent losses, they did appear to have played an equally critical role in some instances. Subject 26 had already been told by his wife that she would leave him forever if he drank and abused her again. He did, and she ordered him to leave. He shot himself while packing, as she telephoned her attorney. Subject 22 had a similar marital history, except that his wife left him overnight after he choked her. She returned home the next day to find him dead. Subject 10 feared her husband would leave her, but there was no direct confirmation that separation was pending. Subject 45 feared his wife would eject him, as she had in the past. Subject 8 feared rehospitalization, which his wife was arranging at the moment when he shot himself. In all, six subjects (6, 8, 15, 16, 28, 29) reportedly dreaded rehospitalization and had reason to think it was imminent. The loss anticipated was of their personal autonomy, as well as their self-esteem.

Subject 4 faced a court appearance following a hit-and-run vehicular accident for which he was responsible. There is every likelihood that this accident reactivated painful memories of his daughter's death 11 years earlier in a collision in which he was driving while drinking. He might have anticipated a jail term as well.

Subject 21 was on the run from bill collectors. Subject 32 was facing a second, and more mutilating resection of his tongue for a recurrent cancer. He had expressed a wish not to have survived the first operation and was profoundly pessimistic about the prospect for the second one. Subject 30 was scheduled for amputation of his left forearm, which, to him, meant the end of his working life. He regarded that as unacceptable. Subject 36, suffering from multiple myeloma, had hoped for news of a promising treatment from his doctor on the day of his death. He received no such encouragement. The numbers and proportion of subjects anticipating loss (17; 34%) are greater than for actual loss. At least some of these expectations appear to have played a crucial role in the suicide. Although statistical use of this category is subject to abuse, clinically I would not neglect it.

Other Losses

There were losses of a more symbolic nature that, in my opinion, at times weighed heavily in the decision to end life. Circumstances provocative of shame were evident in this regard: a hydraulic engineer with a long history of steady employment who could, at last, obtain no better job than that of night security guard (Subject 5); a man who found he could no longer command his son's obedience in maintaining his lawn care business (Subject 38); a man bereft of employment and adequate financial support, whose wife told him bluntly, in response to his complaint, that she would entertain whomever she chose in the home (Subject 50); loss of the provider role through inability to control drinking (Subjects 39 and 45). In these cases, self-destruction followed rather swiftly on the confrontation. In other cases, the humiliation was more chronic. A depressive syndrome developed, and, in the absence of evidence of another precipitant, I thought it was this that tipped the balance. Distress over inability to secure further employment figured prominently in the suicides of four alcoholics (Subjects 1, 18, 45, 46). Even more than threatened losses, symbolic ones are highly subjective and not a fit category for statistical treatment. They may, nevertheless, be of substantial *clinical* importance to suicide.

DRINKING

Not every alcoholic who took his or her life had been drinking just before the act. But it is striking that only 2 subjects were in a prolonged state of abstinence. Beskow reported this in only 1 of the 83 alcoholics in his study: "One alcoholic addict, somatically ill and under strong influence from his family members, stopped using alcohol during his last months, but instead developed depressive symptoms." (1979, p. 84). *Continued drinking is an important risk factor for suicide in alcoholics.*

PSYCHIATRIC COMORBIDITY

Fewer than one-quarter (22%) of the subjects of this study were without another psychiatric diagnosis in addition to alcoholism. Altogether, nearly three-fourths (72%) were found to meet criteria for definite or probable major affective disorder by strict (i.e., Feighner et al., 1972) diagnostic criteria (Table 8.1). All of those with the diagnosis of probable major affective disorder by these criteria had a definite major depression according to DSM-III-R.

We are not alone in this comorbidity finding. Barraclough, Bunch, Nelson, and Sainsbury (1974) made a second diagnosis of "depressive illness" in 9 of their 15

Table 8.1 Psychiatric Diagnoses in Addition to Alcoholism

Diagnosis	N	%
Major depression complicating alcoholism	23	
Major depression primary, alcoholism secondary	1	
Major depression primary vs. secondary to alcoholism	1	56
Bipolar affective disorder primary, alcoholism secondary	1	
Bipolar affective disorder secondary, alcoholism primary	1	
Probable depression primary,[a] alcoholism secondary	1	
Probable depression[a] complicating alcoholism	8	16
Undiagnosed, possible secondary bipolar affective disorder	1	
Chronic undifferentiated schizophrenia with mental retardation	1	6
Delusional disorder	1	
Alcoholism only	11	22

[a] By DSM-III-R criteria, all are definite major depressive disorder

alcoholic suicides (60%). Mitterauer (1981) noted a "depressive condition" in 28 of 30 suicides identified as alcoholics in his Salzburg (Austria) study. Kapamadžija, Biro, and Till (1981) found definite depression in 46% and probable depression in an additional 24% of their alcoholic suicides. Rich et al. (1988) found 75% of their substance-abusing suicides to have a major depressive disorder as well. On the other hand, Beskow (1979, Table 16.2, p. 122) diagnosed a depressive syndrome in only 45% of 100 Swedish male substance-abusing male suicides, but the *symptom* of depression in 89%.

In the earlier report of our replication study (Murphy et al., 1979), we mentioned the frequent co-occurrence of major depression almost in passing. It is not to be ignored. A number of subjects were reported to be depressed only when drinking or when sobering up. I did not consider that phenomenon to be of clinical importance. Lacking continuity, it would not merit a separate diagnosis, even though it was an established recurrent pattern. A major depression had to meet our research criteria for that diagnosis, including a duration of a month or longer. It was generally a late complication of a longstanding pattern of alcohol abuse and hence was, by definition, secondary. In some cases, a similar episode had occurred previously.

One woman (Subject 25) had a major depressive disorder and a man (Subject 24) had a bipolar affective illness that antedated their alcohol abuse problems. In two (Subjects 4 and 7), a depressive syndrome was reported to have emerged in the same year as the onset of alcoholism. A strict accounting would put the first two of these cases—one unipolar, the other bipolar depression—in the major depressive disorder group for outcome purposes. They are retained here because accession was by way of identifying the stigmata of alcoholism, which dominated the clinical picture.[1] Deletion of these cases would affect the results only minimally (71% versus 72% DSM-III-R major depressive disorder; 25% versus 26% with a recent interpersonal loss).

Like the alcoholism that is central to this report, the precise duration of the terminal depression was not easy to learn from secondary sources. From our best evidence, its mean duration was 1.5 years, with a range of 2 months to 5 years and a median of 12 months. In only 10 cases was the approximate duration 6 months or less. In no case had it been continuous throughout the duration of the alcohol abuse history.

The findings do not suggest that the *onset* of a complicating depression signals a period of increased risk of suicide, but the *presence* of depression is an important risk factor. It was not more common in those experiencing loss of a close interpersonal relationship within 6 weeks of their suicide (8 of 13 = 62%), nor did the depression appear to have been precipitated by that loss except in one instance. Subject 14, depressed at the time of his suicide, reportedly became so after his wife died, but that was 23 months earlier.

Depression in Living Alcoholics

Depression is not the constant companion of alcoholism. In Ciompi's (Ciompi & Eisert, 1969) long follow-up of Swiss alcoholics, only 1.1% had been given a supplementary diagnosis of depressive syndrome on their first admission. Gillis and Keet (1969) noted "marked depressive reaction" in 13% of nearly 800 white South African alcoholics on hospital admission. Berglund (1984), in a 10- to 31-year follow-up, found 34% of 1,312 first-admission Swedish alcoholics "slightly depressed" on hospital admission and severe depression in only 2%. "Slight" depression referred to nonendogenomorphic depressive mood states with varying degrees of approximation to a depressive syndrome. About half of them (i.e., 15%, or 16%) would be diagnosable as major depressive disorder by DSM-III-R (Berglund, personal communication, February 15, 1991). Among 339 alcoholics referred to an inpatient research facility of the National Institute on Alcohol Abuse and Alcoholism, Roy et al (1991) found that 17% had a current—and 33% a lifetime history of—major depressive disorder. These prevalences are strikingly different from what we found at death, 72% with DSM-III-R major depression.[2]

The Epidemiologic Catchment Area (ECA) Study (Regier et al., 1984) was conducted in six sites across the United States to assess the prevalence of various psychiatric disorders *in the community*. A *lifetime* history of alcoholism was diagnosed in 13.5% of respondents, with 6% recently abusing alcohol. On a lifetime basis, 8% of men and 23.4% of women diagnosed as alcoholic had also experienced major depression and/or dysthymia. Among respondents with recently symptomatic alcoholism the corresponding figures for *recent* depression were 2% and 13% (Robins et al., 1988). Thus the comorbidity of major depression in alcoholics in the community is fairly low.

A comparison of life events in suicides with a primary diagnosis of major depression versus those diagnosed alcoholic (Table 1.1) showed that the kinds of disruptive life events that characterized the alcoholics were, in the pure depressives, rather infrequent and randomly distributed in relation to suicide (Murphy & Robins, 1967). Thus depression itself may be a sufficient occasion for suicide. Uncomplicated by other psychiatric disorders, it accounts for nearly half of all suicides. Added to alcoholism, it continues to exert its lethal effect. *The presence of a major depressive episode in the course of alcoholism is a powerful vulnerability factor for suicide that is substantially independent of acute interpersonal loss.*

LACK OF SOCIAL SUPPORT

Much more common than acute loss of a close interpersonal relationship was a dwindling or near absence of social support. There were frequent reports that the subject had alienated or withdrawn from his or her friends or "had no friends." Relationships with spouses and children were strained, and a number of marriages that had not eventuated in separation were on very shaky ground. Threats or plans to leave had been made. For 35 of the suicides, their only reported social contact, outside of a tenuous, distant, or hostile marital relationship, was with tavern associates or with co-workers on the job—a very thin support system indeed (Table 8.2). It was most strikingly seen in the men with onset of alcoholism before the age of 25. They had the longest drinking careers and were the most often abusive of others. Their social world had been reduced to only bar/tavern companionship or none at all in 18 of 22 cases (82%).

Living Alone

Of the 7 women in this study, 5 were married. All lacked the emotional support of their husbands. Subject 10 feared desertion by her husband, but she had friends. The others didn't have any friends. Subject 47, unmarried, was living with her father and sisters when her brother was killed. She had alienated her lover. Subject 44, divorced and living alone, failed to get the emotional support from her sisters that she needed.

The proportion of subjects living alone was higher than expected among suicides in our original study, both among those suffering from affective disorder ($P < 0.05$ versus the adult population of the United States) and even more so among the alcoholics ($P < 0.001$) (Murphy & Robins, 1967). It was again higher than expected in the present sample ($P < 0.01$), with 19 subjects (38%) living alone, compared to 10% of the U.S. adult population age 25 and older in 1970 (United States Department of Commerce Bureau of the Census, 1985). Living alone was most often a consequence of marital disruption, although the breakup was not always very recent. Nevertheless, more than half of those living alone had been in that status for less than 6 weeks, usually as a consequence of a marital rift. The change was never an improvement in the subject's circumstances. In terms of social integration, it would appear to be a major loss.

Subjects 12 and 45, although still living with their wives, had very little support from that quarter. The wife of Subject 12 had unilaterally separated her husband from both his sole companion and his beloved garden. Subject 45 was living with his angry and abusive wife only because his mother would no longer tolerate him. Although an enabler, his wife had little use for him. In all, 23 of 27 married subjects (Numbers 1, 2, 4, 8, 9, 10, 12, 15, 16, 17, 22, 23, 25, 26, 28, 29, 35, 38, 42, 45, 48, 49, 50) living with their respective spouses had a markedly strained or distant relationship with

Table 8.2 Social Contact/Support of 50 Alcoholic Suicides

	N	%
None at all	14	28
Recent change	3	6
Long duration	11	22
Tavern or work only	15	30
Recent change	5	10
Long duration	10	20
Minimal, other	6	12
Better social support	15	30

their mate, and 19 of them had little or no outside support. Better social support was reported to be present in 4 of the married.

The social support of many of these men and women had dwindled severely. It was common among those who had sustained a recent loss, but it was distributed more broadly as well. It appears that the interpersonal loss we identified in the original study and replicated in this one was most fully capable of precipitating a suicide when it was the last meaningful link to others. Overall, social isolation emerges as a factor of great importance in risk assessment. At a minimum, *relative social isolation appears likely to be a vulnerability factor ranking with depression in frequency and perhaps in its significance for suicide in alcoholism.* It may, of course, be important to suicide in nonalcoholics as well, but that is beyond the scope of our data.

UNEMPLOYMENT/UNDEREMPLOYMENT

Exactly half of the alcoholic suicides in this series were unemployed at the time of their death (Table 8.3). Only 1 (Subject 12) had reached common retirement age. He was 69 years old and had been retired for 6 years because of failing eyesight. In all, 6 men (14%) were medically retired: Subject 12 (noted previously), Subjects 31 and 42 owing to dementia, Subject 32 for emphysema and subsequently cancer of the tongue, and Subject 36 as a consequence of multiple myeloma. Subject 30 had been off work with a shattered forearm for 10 months. It is uncertain whether Subject 14 was retired or fired at age 53, but he was out of the work force.

The remainder of the unemployed men were recently unable to find work or had stopped looking. The duration of their unemployment ranged from 1 month to 5 years, with a mean of 9 months. Just over half (13 subjects) had been out of work for less than a year. Inability to work, or to work steadily, was clearly frustrating for a number of the men. It may have been simply one less source of self-esteem or structure for others. Both the medically retired and the otherwise unemployed were cut off from the approval and self-respect our culture links to gainful employment. They also lacked the social contact that the workplace commonly affords. Two women had never held employment (Subjects 25 and 47) and 1 (Subject 23) had not worked outside of the home in 30 years. Only 1 of the 7 was currently employed.

Of that half of the sample thought to be employed, only 10 may have attended work on the last working day of their lives (Subjects 4, 5, 9, 10, 17, 34, 35, 39, 41,

Table 8.3 Employment Status of 50 Alcoholic Suicides

Employment Status	N	%
Unemployed	25	50
Retired by age	1	2
Medical reasons	4	8
Unemployed < 1 year	13	26
Unemployed > 1 year	7[a]	14
Regularly employed	25	50
Not at work last day	13	26

[a]Two women never worked.

and 48). Of these, 5 were self-employed (Subjects 17, 34, 35, 41, and 48), and 2 of these had nothing to do at the office. Five of the employed had not worked for a week or longer. Alcoholism, and in many cases depression as well, had made substantial inroads into the vocational functioning of this group. *Unemployment or failure or inability to attend work characterized three-quarters of the suicides and appears to be an additive risk factor for suicide,* as will be shown.

HEALTH PROBLEMS

Only 18 of the 50 suicides were without known medical or surgical disease, and 21 without significant or serious health problems. Liver disease was reported to have been present in 11 cases (22%). Duodenal ulcer existed in 5 (10%).[3] Pulmonary emphysema was as frequent (Table 8.4). Four subjects had a history of one or more seizures.

The records do not reveal either the immediacy of the physical threat or the subjective concern occasioned by the various somatic diseases identified. I have somewhat arbitrarily nominated as serious those medically identified conditions with the most serious potential consequences. These include hepatic cirrhosis, duodenal ulcer, pulmonary emphysema, diabetes mellitus, major malignancy, seizure disorder, renal disease, arteriosclerotic heart disease with a history of myocardial infarction, pneumoconiosis, and dementia of more than mild severity. Nine probands had more than one of these serious disorders.

Four additional subjects reportedly believed they had a malignancy without supporting medical evidence. I thought the medically unconfirmed belief in the presence

Table 8.4 Associated Medical/Surgical Disease in 50 Alcoholic Suicides

Disease or Condition	N
Hepatic cirrhosis/liver disease	11
Dementia	9
Moderate–severe	4
Mild	5[a]
Duodenal ulcer	5
Pulmonary emphysema	5
Seizure history	4[b]
Diabetes mellitus	3
Pulmonary tuberculosis (history)	3[a]
Hypertension	3[a]
Malignancy	2
Arteriosclerotic heart disease	2
Gout	2[a]
Chronic pyelonephritis	1
Rheumatoid arthritis	1[a]
Cervical disc	1[a]
Pneumoconiosis	1
No reported medical problem	18

[a]Not considered serious for present purposes.
[b]Only 2 considered serious.

of a malignancy was contributory to suicide in all four cases. Subject 9 had told a coworker he thought he had cancer of the throat. Subject 12 had confided to his nephew and drinking companion his belief that he had cancer of the stomach. Subject 27 told his wife he had leukemia. Subject 44 had rectal bleeding and told her sisters she thought she had rectal cancer. She refused to see a physician despite her family's urging. These subjects had last seen a physician 5, 6, 1, and 9 years, respectively, before their deaths. Subject 45 "might have thought he had cancer." In none of these cases was an autopsy performed. Subjects 27 and 44 had a second diagnosis of probable major depression. Subjects 9, 12, and 45 did not. One wonders how these patients might compare to 12 given a primary diagnosis of *Kanzerophobie* (cancer phobia) by Mitterauer (1981). Eleven of those were noted to have an additional diagnosis of major depression.

Dementia

Nine of our subjects had exhibited some degree of dementia. Four were severely afflicted. Subject 20 had progressively impaired memory and nightly arguments aloud with nonexistent others. He had no history of head trauma, only of severe and prolonged alcohol abuse. Subject 31 was identified 7 years before his death as having "considerable organic memory impairment." In the last year of his life he had problems with simple arithmetic and with comprehension. Subject 40, a day laborer, had suffered a skull fracture 7 years before his suicide and thereafter was unable to work as before. His memory became poor and he had trouble thinking.

Subject 42 suffered a fall in his tavern with unconsciousness and "probable concussion" 2 years before his death. Rather marked behavioral changes followed and he quit working 16 or 18 months later. A severe depression was simultaneously implicated in his disability. Of 5 subjects (1, 22, 29, 40, and 42) with a history of head injury, only 2 showed significant mental changes. Subject 15 was still experiencing post-ECT confusion as well as a resurgence of depression when he took his life. Subject 49 was seemingly delirious and behaving bizarrely for the last 2 weeks of her life. Finally, 23 of the 33 suicides (70%) in whom toxicological studies were performed had a legally intoxicating (≥ 0.1 g%) blood alcohol concentration. I think it likely that *the presence of serious medical illness is a contributor to the suicidal decision.*

LEGAL TROUBLES

These alcoholic suicides were not strangers to the law. More than half (54%) were reported to have had arrests. Most were alcohol related. Not many, however, were very recent. Subject 29 had served 19 years in prison for killing his first wife. Subject 38 had a long history of physical aggression, both in taverns and within the family. He started one too many rows at home and wound up in jail, where he hanged himself. Subject 11, repeatedly physically abusive of his wife, was under a peace bond since she separated from him 2 weeks before his suicide. Subject 38 was jailed at his wife's request because he was drunk and abusive. He took his life shortly after his release. Subject 4 had been charged with a hit-and-run vehicular offense 2 or 3 weeks before his suicide. He took his life the day before he was to have appeared in court on that charge. Subject 13 was about to be taken into custody for embezzlement of $5,000 and other possibly felonious behavior. Subject 24, a year before his death, had left the scene of a head-on automobile collision for which he was responsible. A suit for damages was pending but of unknown imminence. Subject 34, too, was involved in prolonged litigation over financial dealings. In addition, he had not satisfied a large obligation to the United States Internal Revenue Service. The immediacy of the problem was unclear. Finally, Subject 41 faced two small personal liability suits of doubtful significance. In three cases (Subjects 4, 13, and 38) it appeared that a legal matter was of immediate importance to the suicide.

PSYCHOACTIVE SUBSTANCE ABUSE

Drug abuse was not common or of common concern at the time this study was carried out. We asked specifically about hypnotics and about the informant's perception of abuse of medications and whether the subject or the informant had thought he took too much. Information about marijuana use was neither requested nor volunteered by any informant. While the inquiry could have been more searching, it did not turn up evidence of widespread psychoactive drug abuse such as that found more recently by Rich, Fowler, and Young. (1989).

Twenty-one (42%) of our alcoholic suicides were reported to have used psychoactive substances, only two of them definitely illegally. Subject 46, a 36-year-old single unemployed black male, had entered the federal narcotics treatment program in Lexington, Kentucky, at age 26 years. That did not end his intravenous use of narcotics, although he seems to have escaped further troubles with it. On hospital admission a year before his death, he was noted to have "needle tracks" (of recent intravenous use) on his arm. Toxicology did not include analysis for narcotics. Two subjects took elixir of terpin hydrate, an over-the-counter cough suppressant containing 40% alcohol, in large quantities. In one of these cases (Subject 31), the elixir was combined with codeine, making it a Class V controlled prescription drug. How the medication was obtained was unknown to our informant. He was also taking an unidentified hypnotic.

"Pep pills" were thought to have been recently abused by one subject (Number 8). In all, only 2 suicides had a history of using narcotics (Subjects 31 and 46), and 3 (Subjects 8, 17, and 22) of abusing other psychoactive substances. Psychoactive substance abuse appears to have been a rather minor matter at the time of this investigation (1969–1971).[4] In contrast, 48 of the 50 alcoholics were actively abusing alcohol right up to the time of their suicide.

COMMUNICATION OF SUICIDAL THOUGHTS

Robins, Gassner, et al. (1959) were the first to report that more than two-thirds of suicides had communicated their thoughts or intent to others. More alcoholics had done so than the rest. They also expressed a significantly greater variety of suicidal ideas. The present group, too, had expressed suicidal ideation more often than had nonalcoholics in the earlier study. Recency of onset of suicidal communication characterized the alcoholics in the earlier group; 73% had reportedly first conveyed their intent within the last year of their lives, 43% for less than 3 months. In the present series, only 23% of those communicating had *first* done so in the last year, and only 11% within the last 3 months. Thus communication regarding suicide was usual and had been going on intermittently for many months to many years. Only infrequently was it of recent onset.[5] Overall, at least one form of communication was reported in 88% of cases. This includes one case with only a suicide attempt.

Attempted Suicide as Communication

A suicide attempt, defined as any self-injurious act so characterized by the perpetrator or others, may be regarded as a means of communication of suicidal thinking. It was found to have occurred in 22% of the original series of 134 suicides. Among the alcoholics, 16% had taken that action (E. Robins, unpublished data). In the present study, 38% had done so. Other forms of suicidal communication were present in all but one case as well.

Barraclough et al. (1974) found a history of suicide attempt in 47% (7 of 15) of their alcoholic suicides, compared to 30% of their total cases. The comparable figure was 47% in Mitterauer's (1981) study as well. Berglund et al. (1984) identified a history of suicide attempt in 15% of 88 alcoholic suicides *on first hospital admission*.

Attempted suicide has long been recognized as a risk factor for future suicide (Ettlinger & Flordh, 1955; Ettlinger, 1964; Bohme, Schonfeld, & von Weltzien, 1982). Longer follow-ups of attempters—not restricted to alcoholics—suggest an annual risk of completed suicide among them to be somewhat under 1% per year after the first year, when it may be as high as 2% (Stengel, 1972, p. 251). Few studies have looked back more than 10 years. Schneider (1954) reported that of 355 patients who had attempted suicide, 9.6% had committed suicide over a 10-year observation period and 12.4% over 18 years. In the longest such investigation, Dahlgren (1977) looked up his original 229 suicide attempters (Dahlgren, 1945) after a mean of 35 years, obtaining information in 96% of his cases. Fourteen percent of the men and 8.8% of the women died this way. Of 18 alcoholics in his sample, 3 (16.7%) were suicides.[6]

It appears that suicide following suicide attempt approaches an asymptote of 12–13% on long follow-up, perhaps 15% for men and 10% for women. Those figures may be considered to be the lifetime risk of suicide among suicide attempters (not restricted to alcoholics). This is four to seven times higher than the lifetime risk I calculated for alcoholics irrespective of a history of suicide attempt (Murphy & Wetzel, 1990). Medically serious attempts in particular portend fatal outcome of a subsequent attempt (Ettlinger & Flordh, 1955; Rosen, 1976). *Suicidal communications—including attempts—by alcoholics are to be taken seriously.*

FAMILY HISTORY

Alcoholism

Sixteen subjects (32%) reportedly had an alcoholic father. In 3 more cases the father was described as a heavy drinker or possible alcoholic. In 5 cases, no family history at all was obtained. Including other relatives, alcoholism was reported to have been present in 27, or 59%, of families with any information. An additional 5 families included a "heavy drinker" or possible alcoholic.

In view of the fact that informants were inevitably secondary sources, and in most instances not blood kin, it is striking that the results are so strong. Diagnoses represent, for the most part, family tradition. The inquiry was systematic (Appendix B) but informants were not always informed. There was no difference in the proportion of alcoholic fathers of men with early onset alcoholism than in those with later onset.

Suicide

Five fathers had committed suicide and a sixth was believed by the subject (Case 35) to have done so. Suicide or probable suicide had occurred in the families of 10 (22%) of the 45 cases with information. These must be regarded as minimum figures. Mitterauer (1981) found nearly 50% underreporting of a family history of suicide by informants in his suicide study when compared to results of an earlier focused family survey that *included all of the same probands*. One out of six suicides (18%) in my series was said to have had a positive family history of self-destruction. Mitterauer's better-ascertained finding of 47 positive family histories among 94 exactly diagnosed cases (50%) (1981, p. 232) may be nearer the mark. Conservatively, I think that a family history of suicide may be an additional risk factor.[7] Our data are inadequate to assess its strength.

DISCUSSION OF THE FINDINGS

After continued alcohol abuse, the most striking feature of this group of alcoholic suicides was the level of psychiatric comorbidity (Table 8.1). At least 72% of the subjects had an accompanying affective disorder. It was temporally secondary to the alcoholism in most cases. Only 22% were without any identified psychiatric disorder complicating their alcoholism. Some 72% of the subjects had little or no social support; 38% were living alone. The isolation of living alone characterized all but 4 of the 13 subjects with recent interpersonal loss. Three had no more social support than tavern associates (Subjects 32, 43, and 47). Five didn't even have that (Subjects 6, 12, 20, 31, and 45). Only 1 of 13 with recent interpersonal loss had some remaining social support. The answer to the question "Why just now?" is at hand. The impact of acute loss is greatly magnified when there is little or no other social support left to cushion the blow.

Half of the subjects were unemployed at the time of their death. Loss of status or self-esteem from other avenues was noted in an additional 18% of the subjects. Serious health problems afflicted nearly half (46%). Four out of five had communicated thoughts of suicide. All but two were currently abusing alcohol.

While interpersonal loss is a sturdy, and by now well replicated risk factor for suicide in alcoholics, it does not act alone. Of those 13 subjects with identified recent loss of a close interpersonal relationship, depression was present in 8. There was poor

Table 8.5 Risk Factors for Suicide

Patient Number	Age at Suicide	Civil State	Living Circumstances	Social Support	Employment
1	50	m	wife, son	tavern, wife ±	unemployed
2	54	m	wife	work, wife ±	employed
3	35	m	alone 2 days	tavern, abused spouse	probably not but DK
4	52	m	wife, 2 minor children	tavern, co-workers, abused spouse	employed
5	57	div	alone	good	employed, come-down
6	49	sep 30 days	alone	0	employed
7	55	m	wife, 4 children	home ok, had friends	employed
8	57	m	wife	home poor, 2 close friends	0, lost or about to lose
9	48	m	wife	angry spouse tavern + 1 friend	employed
10♀	46	m	husband, daughter	5 friends (?)	employed
11	50	sep 2 wk	alone, motel	tavern	employed
12	69	m	wife	0, lost 1, 1 wk	retired 6 yr

Health Problems	Depressive Syndrome	Duration of Depression	Suicide Thoughts	Suicide Attempts	Most Important Reason for Suicide
0 [gout]	2°	1 yr	+	0	Inability to find employment; severe retarded depression
cirrhosis, seizure disorder [gout]	2°	3 mo	0	0	Deepening depression.
seizure, disorder 4 mo	2°	7 mo	+	+(2)	Wife left him; depressed. L
0	MAD 1° vs 2°	1 yr	+	+	Depressed; impending court hearing; shame; miserable marriage. TL
0	0 delusional disorder	N/A	+	0	Shame over having sunk to menial job.
CP, HT ASCVD	0		0	0	Fear of rehospitalization; inability to control drinking. L, TL
emphysema	prob 1° AD	4 mo, 1 previously	+	0	Major depression.
cirrhosis, DU	2°	2 mo	+	0	Feared psychiatric hospitalization; feared losing wife; depressed. TL
0 [thought he had throat cancer]	0	N/A	+	0	Drunk and angry; shot his wife; ? delusion of throat cancer. TL
0	2°	6 mo	+	+(2)	Depressed; alcoholic; feared husband would leave her. TL
cirrhosis	2°	6 mo	+		Marital separation; Depression. L
0 [thought stomach cancer]	0	N/A	+	0	Disrupted social and drinking relationship; belief he had cancer. L

Continued on next page

Table 8.5—*Continued*

Patient Number	Age at Suicide	Civil State	Living Circumstances	Social Support	Employment
13	29	s	alone 2 yr	0 × 1 wk	employed
14	54	w	with mother-in-law, 14 yo son	minimal mother-in-law, son	retired 8 mo
15	44	m	wife, 2 children	bar/tavern	employed
16♀	44	m	husband, daughter	husband distant, angry with daughter	unemployed 7 yr
17	30	m	wife, children	2 friends	employed (self)
18	35	s	alone 3 wk	none 3 wk except tavern	unemployed 3 mo
19	35	sep 3 yr	alone 1 day	girlfriend, tavern	employed
20	50	sep 3 wk	alone 3 wk	0	unemployed 2 yr
21	47	div 8 mo	alone 13 mo	0	part time
22	62	m	alone overnight	wife, children change < 1 day	employed
23♀	57	m	husband	0, husband ignored	housewife 30+ yr

Health Problems	Depressive Syndrome	Duration of Depression	Suicide Thoughts	Suicide Attempts	Most Important Reason for Suicide
DU	prob 2°	8 mo	+	+(3)	Major depression; major legal difficulty; interpersonal loss (boyfriend). TL
cirrhosis, emphysema	prob 2°	2 yr	+	0	Depression secondary to loss of wife; social isolation.
cirrhosis	2°	1 yr	+	0	Major depression; loss of provider role; self–disgust; fear of rehospitalization. TL
[TB history]	2°	5 yr	+	+(2)	Depression; fear of institutionalization. TL
0	2°	2 yr	+	0	Major depressive disorder; loss of wife's emotional support; severe chronic discomfort with practice of his profession.
0	0	N/A	+	0	Living alone; discouraged about unemployment; drunk.
"liver"	0	N/A	+	0	Girlfriend left him; drunk; feared responsibility, isolation. L
[DU history]	2°	0	+	0	Wife threw him out; no social support. L
[rheumatoid arthritis]	prob 2°	3+ mo	+	+	Depressed; alone; friendless; lost self-esteem; lost self-control. TL
[cerv disc]	2°	1 yr	+	0	Believed he had lost his wife; depressed. TL
HT, DU, emphysema	2°	3 yr	+	+	Depression; social isolation.

Table 8.5—*Continued*

Patient Number	Age at Suicide	Civil State	Living Circumstances	Social Support	Employment
24	37	sep 2½ mo	alone 2½ mo	tavern	employed
25♀	53	m	husband	none, husband avoided	never
26	48	m	wife, 3 children	0	unemployed 1+ mo
27	42	sep	alone 1 mo	taverns	employed
28	52	m	wife, stepson	0	employed
29	46	m	wife, stepdaughter	almost 0	employed
30	41	div	alone 13 mo	0	unemployed 10 mo
31	57	div	alone 2 wk	0	unemployed 8 yr
32	55	sep	alone 2–3 days	adequate	unemployed 18 yr
33	50	s	alone 2 mo	bars only	unemployed 1 yr

Health Problems	Depressive Syndrome	Duration of Depression	Suicide Thoughts	Suicide Attempts	Most Important Reason for Suicide
0	BAD	1 yr	+	0	Acute financial problems resulting from divorce proceedings; separation from wife (2–2½ mo); divorce notice (4 wk). TL
0	1° AD	> 3 yr	+	+(2)	Depression, greatly aggravated by alcoholic relapse.
pneumoconiosis, cirrhosis	0	N/A	+	0	Wife had ordered him to leave, saying she was filing for divorce. TL
DK [thought leukemia]	prob 2°	1 yr	+	+(2)	Separated 6 wk or less; belief he had leukemia (probably delusional); probable depression. L
diabetes	2°	6 mo	+	+	Depressed, secondary to demotion at work; failing health; mother's stroke. TL
0	0	DK	+	+(3)	Stepfather's death; possible depression. TL
DU, TB	2°	1 yr	+	+ several	Impending amputation; depressed; loss of status. TL
dementia	2°	change 3 yr "many yr"	+		Loss of social support and direction; depressed. L
tongue cancer, emphysema, cirrhosis	2°	2 yr	+	0	Feared impending surgery; major depressive disorder; wife left him. L
diabetes, PVD, cirrhosis	2°	5 yr	0	0	Depressed; alone; medically ill.

Table 8.5—*Continued*

Patient Number	Age at Suicide	Civil State	Living Circumstances	Social Support	Employment
34	45	m	wife, stepson	0	employed (self)
35	50	m	wife, daughter	bar/tavern	employed (self)
36	52	m	wife, son	good	retired 9 yr
37	50	m	wife, son	wife, son; OK	unemployed 3 mo
38	42	m	wife, 7 children	0	part time (self)
39	54	m	wife	reported good	employed part time
40	56	s	alone	bar/tavern, landlord	unemployed (medical) 5 yr
41	35	DK	alone, office	bar/tavern	employed
42(B)	63	m	wife, 13 yo adopted daughter	bar/tavern	unemployed 6 mo
43	46	sep 10 mo	male friend	2 friends	unemployed 4 mo
44 ♀	55	div	alone	minimal	unemployed 8 mo
45	45	m	wife 5 wk	angry spouse only	unemployed 4 mo

Health Problems	Depressive Syndrome	Duration of Depression	Suicide Thoughts	Suicide Attempts	Most Important Reason for Suicide
diabetes	2°	1 yr	+	+	Depressed; severe financial/legal problems; wife leaving. TL
0	2°	2 yr	+	0	Depressed; concern about finances—possibly delusional
multiple myeloma	2°	2 yr, change 3 mo	+	0	Dashed hope of recovery; depressed; worsening medical condition. TL
0	2°	1 yr	+	0	Depressed; unemployed
0	0	0	0	0	Confronted with loss of authority; shamed by jailing. TL
pulmonary emphysema	?	3 mo	0	0	Impairment of provider role; increasingly incapacitating medical illness; alcoholism out of control
brain damage, cirrhosis, HT	2°	5 yr	+	0	Humiliated; depressed; brain damaged.
0	0	N/A	+	0	Rejected erotic aspiration; drunk; obsessed. L
brain injury	prob 2°	1 yr	+	0	Alcoholism; dementia; depressed.
ASHD, MI	undiagnosed possibly BAD—depressed	2 mo	+	0	Rejection by girlfriend; alcoholic; depressed. L
[rectal bleeding; thought rectal cancer]	prob 2°	6 mo	+	+	Depressed; out of money; believed she had cancer.
[TB]	0	0	0	0	Loss of self-respect; feared wife leaving him (inferred) estranged from mother 5 weeks. L, TL

Table 8.5—*Continued*

Patient Number	Age at Suicide	Civil State	Living Circumstances	Social Support	Employment
46	37	s	parents	some	unemployed 10 mo
47(B)♀	32	s	father, sister, 2 yo son	decreased	unemployed life
48	42	m	wife, 2 daughters	almost 0	employed
49♀	40	m	husband, 8 yo daughter	almost 0	unemployed 9 mo
50	65	m	wife, son	wife, distant ? 1 other	unemployed 6 mo

Key: + = yes, plus; 0 = none; 1° = primary; 2° = secondary; AD = affective disorder; ASCVD = arteriosclerotic cardiovascular disease; ASHD = arteriosclerotic heart disease; (B) = black; BAD = bipolar affective disorder; cerv = cervical; CP = chronic pyelonephritis; div = divorced; DK = don't know; DU = duodenal ulcer; HT = hypertension; L = recent loss; m = married; MAD = major affective disorder; MI = myocardial infarction; mo = month(s); MR = mental retardation; N/A = not applicable; prob = probable; PVD = peripheral vascular disease; s = single; SCU = schizophrenia, chronic undifferentiated type; sep = separated; TB = pulmonary tuberculosis; TL = threatened loss; vs = versus; w = widowed; wk = week(s); yo = years old; yr = year(s).

social support in 10 cases, a lack of employment or of job stability in 9 cases, and serious medical illness in 6, in addition to the loss.

I will show in the next chapter that seven of the factors just discussed have important predictive significance for suicide when considered together. From the standpoint of risk, it appears that *the impact of these factors may be additive: the higher the number of such circumstances, the greater the risk.*

Health Problems	Depressive Syndrome	Duration of Depression	Suicide Thoughts	Suicide Attempts	Most Important Reason for Suicide
cirrhosis	prob 2°	2 yr	+	0	Depressed; low self-esteem because of inability to stop drinking and earn a living.
0	SCU, MR	N/A	0	+	Distraught over death of brother; lover distancing. L, TL
0	BAD 2° alcoholism	9 mo	+	0	Depressed; feared business failure.
0	prob 2°	1 yr	+	+ many	Alcoholic delirium; probable depression secondary to alcoholism.
0	2°	6 mo	+	+	Belittled by wife; financial problems; depressed.

9

Seven Risk Factors for Suicide in Alcoholics

> We envisage alcoholic suicide as a social phenomenon.
> W.C. Sullivan, M.D. (1900)

GENERAL CONSIDERATIONS

A Causal Nexus

Chapter 8 describes a number of life history features of our probands that seem unusually frequent in this group. Not a single suicide had escaped them all. They relate in various ways to one another, as illustrated in Figure 9.1. The features under consideration are in full capital letters, and the decimal figure beneath each one is the proportion of the 50 subjects in the study with that factor present at the time of suicide. The figure 1.0 beneath ALCOHOL ABUSE and also SUICIDE indicates that all subjects were affected. The figures along the arrow shafts represent the proportion of subjects in the group at the tail of the arrow who were also subject to the factor at the arrow's head. For example, the arrow running from ALCOHOL ABUSE to PHYSICAL ILLNESS carries a figure of .38. That means that 38% of the subjects developed a physical illness that I thought likely to have been a consequence of the abuse of alcohol. Those illnesses were hepatic cirrhosis, duodenal ulcer, seizure disorder, and dementia. I did not count pulmonary emphysema, diabetes, renal disease, or cardiovascular disease in that calculation, as their association with alcohol abuse is less direct. At the same time, half of the subjects were reported to have had a serious medical illness (Table 8.5), so the figure beneath PHYSICAL ILLNESS is .5.

PHYSICAL ILLNESS contributed to, or was associated with, unemployment in just over half (.52) of the cases. It was associated with DEPRESSION .8, that is, in 8 out of 10 cases. In general, the physical illnesses were of longer duration than the depression, but it would be overreading the data to assume causation in every case. A more obviously two-way interaction, albeit an indirect one, is that between POOR SOCIAL SUPPORT and DEPRESSION. Reading from left to right, the ratio is .72;

SEVEN RISK FACTORS FOR SUICIDE IN ALCOHOLICS

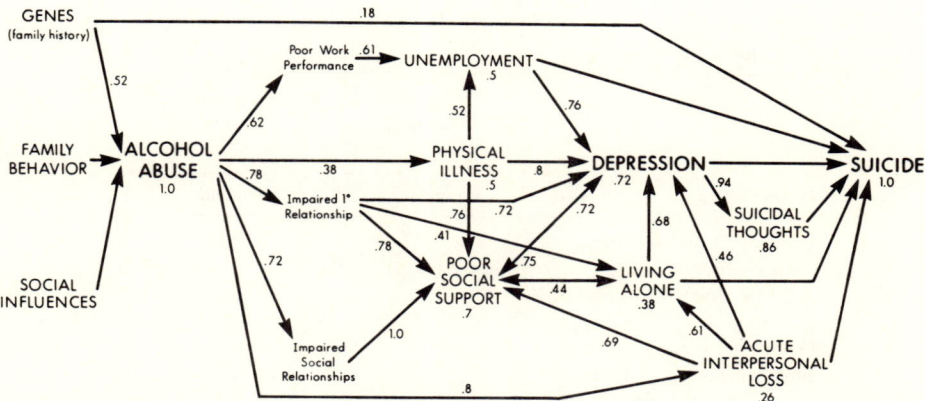

Figure 9.1 Interrelationship of common factors predictive of suicide. Experiences and behaviors in full caps are factors significantly related to suicide. The decimal figure beneath each is the proportion of my 50 alcoholic suicides having that characteristic at the time of suicide. Figures along the arrow shafts express the ratio of subjects having the characteristic at the base of the arrow having also that at its head. Causality is not assumed.

from right to left, it is .75. Depression can impair interpersonal relationships over a time scale of months to years.

The relationship of POOR SOCIAL SUPPORT with LIVING ALONE is reciprocal. The latter is usually (in 9 out of 10 cases) evidence of the former. I calculated the relationship of ACUTE INTERPERSONAL LOSS to POOR SOCIAL SUPPORT in a right to left direction because the loss was most often that of the last support. Other arrows might be drawn, but they would tend to clutter the diagram without contributing much. The arrows are unlabeled on their last segment, because the relationship of each to suicide is unity.

May these factors prove useful in identifying living alcoholics at high risk for suicide? To answer that question, we must first ask whether these features are unique to this sample or may they be more generally found among alcoholic suicides. If more general, it will then be necessary to determine whether they distinguish alcoholic suicides from living alcoholics.

REVERSE REPLICATION OF THE FINDINGS

Just as the present study was a replication of a portion of the earlier study of Dr. Eli Robins (Robins, Gassner et al., 1959; Robins, Murphy, et al., 1959; Murphy & Robins, 1967; Robins, 1981), data from that study may be used as a test of the stability of some of the findings of this one (Table 9.1). Owing to the use of more refined diagnostic criteria, two more suicides are identified as alcoholic in the 1981 book (Robins, 1981) than in the 1959 publications. I include only one of these, viewing the other (Subject 99) as undiagnosed. The comparison group, therefore, consists of 32 alcoholic suicides.

The findings are remarkably similar between the two studies, with a single exception. Psychiatric comorbidity was identified significantly less often in the first study.

Table 9.1 Comparison of Findings Between Alcoholic Suicides in Previous and Present Studies

Characteristic	Previous Study (Study 1) $N = 32$[a]		Present Study (Study 2) $N = 50$[b]	
	Frequency	%	Frequency	%
Currently drinking	31	97	49	98
Comorbidity[c]	16	50	38	76
Major affective disorder	13	41	36	72
Other	3	9	2	4
No or little social support	22	69	35	70
Employment: unemployed	21	66	25	50
Affectional loss: within 6 weeks	10	31	13	26
Threatened loss	7	22	17	34
Serious medical problem	16	50	26	54
Living alone	16	50	19	38
Talk or threat of suicide	26	81	43	86
Suicide attempt	7	22	16	32

[a]Robins, Murphy, et al, 1959; Robins, 1981.
[b]Murphy, et al, 1979.
[c]χ^2 Yates's correction = 4.77, 1 df; $P < 0.05$ for comorbidity. No other row differences approach statistical significance.

At the time of that investigation, our diagnostic criteria were not yet fully developed, so that not every criterion symptom currently in use was inquired about. In a number of instances, insufficient detail was recorded to allow a confident opinion regarding either presence or absence of a second diagnosis. The comorbidity estimate is thus a minimum figure. Even so, 41% of Robins's alcoholic suicides could be seen to have a definite or probable secondary depression, and at least half had some psychiatric comorbidity. If subjects with insufficient information are excluded from the comparison, the difference is not statistically significant. Family history of alcoholism and/or suicide were not as systematically recorded in Study 1 and cannot be compared.

In other respects, the depth of inquiry was quite comparable. Ninety-seven percent versus 98% were currently drinking. (One woman in Study 1 was not definitely known to be drinking. She was, however, intoxicated daily with barbiturates.) Social support was recorded in much the same detail in both studies. It appeared to be quite thin in 69%. Employment was well covered; it was shown that 66% of the alcoholic suicides were unemployed at the time of their death, compared to 50% in the present study. Serious health problems were noted in half of both series. Exactly half of Robins's alcoholics were living alone when they took their lives versus 38% in the second study. In both groups over 80% had talked of suicide.

As reported earlier (Murphy & Robins, 1967), 32% of the original sample of alcoholic suicides had experienced loss of a close interpersonal relationship in the last 6 weeks of their lives, compared to 26% in the present sample (Table 3.1). (The 32% becomes 31% with the addition of 1 case to the original 31.) Threatened loss was identified in 7 of Dr. Robins' cases, 22% versus 34%. Apart from comorbidity, there were no statistically significant differences between the findings of the two studies.

Thus, Study 1 (Robins, Murphy, et al., 1959), having yielded a predictor of suicide in alcoholics (Murphy & Robins, 1967) that was replicated in Study 2 (Murphy, et al., 1979), serves to validate further predictors of suicide identified in Study 2. Together, they show that the *high frequency of current drinking, psychiatric comorbidity, unemployment, poor social support, serious health problems, living alone, suicidal threats or communication, and recent interpersonal loss are part of the pertinent history characteristic of alcoholics who take their lives.*

These same factors have been recognized by other investigators as common among alcoholic suicides (Englebrecht, 1983; Kendell, 1983; Theret, Facy & Pascalis, 1989). These last authors state in the English summary of their review paper (in French):

> The main risk factors relate to the decrease of the socio-economic status,—loss of job and of income,—to the interpersonal loss—i.e. family bereavement or breach of relation,—to the existence of a suicidal ideation often communicated or of suicidal antecedents, to a degradation of the physical state or the presence of some affections like gastro-duodenal ulcer. *The identified factors are of little specificity.* It is difficult to assess their interrelations and their respective true values. The reliable prediction of a later suicide remains presently impossible. (emphasis added)

It is beyond argument that the prediction of an individual suicide is, and will remain beyond our grasp (Murphy, 1984). It may nevertheless be possible to sharpen our recognition of those alcoholics at substantially elevated risk of self-destruction by judicious application of new knowledge concerning the interrelationship of just these "factors . . . of little specificity" and several others.

ARE THE FINDINGS PREDICTIVE OR MERELY DESCRIPTIVE OF ALCOHOLIC SUICIDES?

The relationship of recent interpersonal loss to suicide in alcoholics is now well established (Murphy and Robins, 1967; Murphy et al., 1979; Rich et al., 1988). No studies employing comparable methodology have produced a contrary result. Such loss plays a role in one-fourth to two-fifths of the suicides of alcoholics and much less in other suicides. But what of our other putative risk factors?

Alcoholics in the Community

Our "factors of little specificity" require comparison with a control population of living alcoholics to show whether they are indeed lacking in specificity. Such a sample has been identified through the multisite Epidemiologic Catchment Area (ECA) study (Regier et al., 1984). The ECA study was conducted in five sites across the United States from 1981 to 1984 and included 20,291 persons age 18 years and older (Regier et al., 1990). A "second wave" re-interview was carried out 1 year after the first one with 84% of the original households responding. In St. Louis alone, a number of questions were asked in the second wave interviews that lend themselves to the comparisons we wish to make (L. Robins, unpublished data). Only those with full and complete interviews concerning persons still living in the household will serve.

Given the small numbers of blacks and of women in our two suicide studies, comparisons will be most meaningful if confined to white males. That is not to say that any significant findings could not pertain to women or minorities. It is simply a question of how representative 3 black men and 2 black women, or 10 white women can be. The scatter of descriptive characteristics would not lend itself to confident statistical handling. There were 67 white male alcoholic suicides in Studies 1 and 2. These will be compared to living white male alcoholics on the dimensions available for comparison.

White males from the ECA study who had a definite or probable diagnosis of alcoholism by our departmental research criteria (Table 2.3) (Feighner et al., 1972) make up the comparison population. A diagnosis of *definite* alcoholism requires one or more symptoms in at least three symptom groups; for a *probable* diagnosis, symptoms must be found in at least two symptom groups. These criteria were met by 106 ECA subjects. Comparison was possible on 7 of 8 features identified with suicide in Chapter 8 (Table 9.2). Only 44 (42%) of 106 living alcoholics reported having alcohol problems in the last 6 months. These 44 were taken as currently drinking, the remaining 62 as not. That is strikingly different from the low remission rates of *treated* alcoholics shown in Table 10.1 but not unusual for those never receiving treatment. Difference from the alcoholic suicides is large: $P < 0.0000$ - a probability of less than 1 in 10,000 of the populations being the same. Major depression comorbidity was 5% in the living versus 58% in the suicides: $P < 0.0000$.

Lack of social support was scored for those ECA subjects reporting having no one to trust or confide in. That statement was endorsed by 28 (26%) of the living alcoholics; 75% of the suicides had little or no social support ($P < 0.0000$). Interpersonal loss was not inquired about from the living men, so it can't be compared. Living alone and talk or threat of suicide differed at the same high level. Comparison on serious physical illness was affected by data collection. Nearly two-fifths of the alcoholic suicides had such a history. However, only hepatic cirrhosis and pancreatitis were

Table 9.2 Comparison of Frequency of Risk Factors in White Male Suicides and Living Alcoholic Controls from ECA Study

Characteristic	Alcoholic Suicides $N = 67$		Living Alcoholics 106		Probability[a]
	Frequency	%	Frequency	%	$P <$
Recent heavy drinking	65	97	44	42	0.0000
Major Depressive disorder	39	58	5	5	0.0000
Little social support	50	75	28[b]	26	0.0000
Recent interpersonal loss	23	34	—		
Unemployed	36	54	19	18	0.0000
Medical problem: liver, pancreas	11	16	7	7	0.080 (N.S.)
Living alone	30	45	18	17	0.0000
Talk/threat of suicide[c]	53	79	24	23	0.0000

[a]χ^2 with Yates's correction for all calculations.
[b]No one to go to for comfort.
[c]Reported suicidal communication versus self-report.

inquired about in the ECA study. On the narrowly defined hepatic-pancreatic dimension, the difference is not statistically significant. Overall, the experiences of the alcoholic suicides were markedly different than those of the living alcoholics.

The ECA population appears on the surface to be a highly appropriate control sample, and in nearly all respects it is. However, the subjects were, on average, 15 years younger than the suicides. Absence of exact data on years of drinking by the controls leaves open the possibility that some of them may have passed through as little as one-fourth of the years of risk. That fact could account for some of the very striking differences found.

The mean age of the living alcoholics was 35.98 years with a standard deviation of +15.24 years; the mean of the alcoholic suicides was 47.27 years with a standard deviation of +9.05 years. The greater standard deviation of the ECA sample reflects the fact that the living alcoholic group included many men younger than the youngest suicide and many men older than the oldest suicide. Both the means ($T= -6.11$, $P=0.0001$) and the standard deviations ($F=2.84$, $df=106,66$ and $P=0.0000$) were very significantly different. This population being otherwise suitable for these comparisons, we must look to statistical methods to compensate for age.

Statistical Adjustment

In the present study, logistic regression, a specific type of log linear analysis, was used (SAS Institute, Inc., 1988).[1] Logistic regression is similar to standard multiple linear regression and is appropriate when one or more of the predictor variables are binary (yes or no). It permits the contribution of each predictor to be assessed independently of the possible effects of other predictors. To ensure that age did not account for the differences between the two groups, age was entered in the model to remove its effects. Inclusion of age in the model means that all significant effects contribute independently of any age effect. A statistical test of significance of effects in the model was the likelihood ratio χ^2.

The result of this analysis (Table 9.3) shows current drinking ($P = 0.0000$), presence of major depression ($P < 0.0010$), suicidal thoughts or communication ($P < 0.0010$), poor social support ($P < 0.0023$), living alone ($P < 0.0146$), and unemployment ($P < 0.0474$) strongly predictive. Age does not emerge as significant in this

Table 9.3 Maximum Likelihood Analysis of Variance Table: 67 White Male Alcoholic Suicides versus 106 Living White Male Alcoholics

Source	df	χ^2	Probability
Current drinking	1	18.61	0.0000
Major depression	1	10.92	0.0001
Suicidal thoughts	1	10.76	0.0010
Age	1	0.19	NS
Poor social support	1	9.27	0.0023
Living alone	1	5.94	0.0148
Unemployed	1	3.93	0.0474

computation because of the narrow age range of the suicides and the very wide age range of the controls. Health data were too limited in the ECA study to permit meaningful comparison.

The Significance of These Findings

The strong difference between the groups on current drinking is owed to the fact that 62 of the living alcoholics in this comparison denied having had alcohol *problems* in the last 6 months. That was taken as the equivalent of no drinking, although actual abstinence was not determined. The finding is not a spurious one, however, as remission rates from early alcohol abuse show (Fillmore, Bacon, & Hyman, 1979; Helzer, Burnam, & McEvoy, 1991). (See also, discussion in Chapter 11.)

A 5% prevalence of current major depressive disorder in this community sampling of alcoholics was unexpected. Substantially higher rates are reported from studies of alcoholics admitted to hospitals and treatment centers (Berglund, 1984; Hesselbrock, Meyer, & Keener, 1985; Rounsaville, Dolinsky, Babor, & Meyer, 1987; Penick et al., 1988; Roy et al., 1991). However, the lifetime rate of depression/dysthymia was exactly the same (5%) in the ECA national sample of alcoholic men (but 19% in alcoholic women) (Helzer & Pryzbeck, 1988, Table 3, p. 222). Overall, temporally coexisting psychiatric comorbidity (*all disorders*) in the living alcoholics in the full ECA study was 24% in men and 32% in women. (DSM–III criteria are overinclusive regarding alcoholism: see Chapter 11.)

These ECA data reinforce our belief that whereas depression is an important factor in bringing alcoholics to treatment, it is not so characteristically a part of alcoholism in the community. Major depression, with or without the negative consequences of alcohol abuse, is the dominating risk factor for taking one's life. It accounts, in part, for the lifetime risk of suicide being nearly twice as high in previously hospitalized alcoholics as in the untreated (Murphy & Wetzel, 1990, and Chapter 11). It is an equally strong risk factor for suicide both in alcoholics and in the rest of the population.

Eighteen percent of living alcoholics with current drinking problems and 23% of the entire group of living alcoholics from the St. Louis ECA sample gave a history of having entertained thoughts of suicide. That is less than one-third of the prevalence of communication of such thoughts reported to have occurred in advance of suicides ($P < 0.0004$). The danger signaled by suicidal communication has been recognized for many years (Robins, Gassner, et al., 1959; Dorpat & Ripley, 1960; Barraclough et al., 1974). It is not simply a part of being alcoholic, but is associated with both increased distress and increased risk of suicide. Suicide attempts are about one-third as common as suicidal thoughts in living alcoholics; they have the same relationship to broadly defined suicidal communication in the alcoholic suicides.

Both living alone and being unemployed were much more frequent among the suicides (45% versus 17% alone; 54% versus 18% unemployed). Both are intercorrelated with drinking and poor social support, so they do not emerge in this model. Living alone has been shown to be highly correlated with suicide in alcoholics in the community (Gove & Hughes, 1980). Recent interpersonal loss as a predictor of suicide cannot be compared, as comparable data were not collected in the ECA study.

Risk Factors are Cumulative

The factors now under discussion were not characteristically acute. Suicidal communication was usually of several years' duration. Health had deteriorated gradually. So had economic and social functioning, as represented by unemployment, having little or no social support, and living alone. The terminal depression ranged in duration from 2 months to 5 years, with a mean duration of 18 months and a median of 1 year. The suggestion that depression is the consequence of losses such as these (Kendell, 1983), plausible on the face of it, is not well supported by the findings. It appeared more often to be the case that depression impaired functioning in a variety of areas, leading to poor work performance, further attrition of social support and the growing conviction that life was unlivable.

Since none of these potential predictors was particularly acute, the question "Why just now?" recurs. The answer to that question is twofold. None of the 19 men with a recent interpersonal loss reportedly had some social support to cushion the loss. On the other hand, only 11 (58%) of them were currently depressed. *Lack of interpersonal support is a more potent factor than psychiatric comorbidity in determining the alcoholic's response to interpersonal loss.* Other risk factors were present in every case.

Every one of the white male alcoholic suicides in our two studies had at least one of the potential suicide risk factors we have just been discussing. Only 3 had that few, while 3 men had two, 15 men had three, 19 had four, and 19 had five; 8 men had all six of the factors that can be compared. In contrast, only 1 of the living male alcoholics had as many as four of these factors and none had more than that. The probability of this inverse relationship occurring by chance is extremely small by χ^2 (1 df) = 123.8; $P < 0.0000$, or by T test, T, (106.8 df) = -15.823; $P = 0.0001$. The suicide's history is very different from that of living alcoholics.

A Numerical Gauge of Risk

Table 9.4 offers a numerical predictor of suicide risk. The presence of four or more of these factors in white male alcoholics would identify 46 of 67 suicides (69%) and yield

Table 9.4 Distribution of Risk Factors[a] in 67 Suicides and 106 Living Alcoholics: White Males

Number of Risk Factors per Subject	Alcoholic Suicides[b] $N = 67$	Living Alcoholics[b] $N = 106$
0	0	26
1	3	31
2	3	34
3	15	14
4	19	1
5	19	0
6	8	0

[a]The risk factors are current heavy drinking, current major depressive disorder, poor or no social support, unemployment, living alone, and suicidal thoughts or communication.
[b]χ^2, 6 df = 116.56; $P < 0.0000$.

1 false positive among 106 living alcoholic men. Given the problem of false positives in predicting rare events (Galen & Gambino, 1975; Murphy, 1984), it is interesting to see how this might work out with larger populations.

We have previously calculated the lifetime risk for suicide as about 2% for untreated and outpatient treated alcoholics in this country (Murphy & Wetzel, 1990; also Table 11.10). Weighting the living alcoholics so they will constitute 98% of the sample predicts 31 false positives among 3,283 living alcoholics while identifying 73% of the suicides, simply on the basis of having four or more of the cited factors. For alcoholics ever having had hospital treatment, the lifetime risk of suicide is calculated as 3.4%. The same type of weighted population projection predicts 21 false positives among 1,903 previously hospitalized living alcoholics using the same cutoff score of 4 or more of these factors. Given the kinds of intervention proposed in Chapter 10, these are very acceptable false positive numbers.

This Is Why Now

The findings of this study go a long way to explain "why just now?", both in the case of interpersonal loss and in alcoholic suicides generally. Interpersonal loss does not act as an isolated phenomenon but as the final link in a chain of events that flow from the alcoholism. But it is not a *necessary* link, being found in only 26% (Murphy et al., 1979) to 41% (Rich et al., 1988) of the suicides. The chain includes earlier losses, damaged and lost human relationships, damaged health, loss of role, both as a wage earner and as a companion, depression, and a mounting sense of infirmity, fatigue, and futility. Those with a recent loss had no fewer than 3 of the other risk factors. Only one (Case 47) had adequate social support.

The role of current heavy drinking is obviously very strong, but just how it acts is uncertain. Frequent reports that our subjects spoke of suicide only when drinking suggests that it both heightens dysphoria and lowers inhibitions, including the normal inhibition against taking one's life. Suicide attempts and communication of suicidal thoughts are warning signs of increasing risk.

A REPLICATION SAMPLE

As striking as the differences are between our alcoholic suicides and living subjects of the ECA study, a second comparison would be reassuring. Another data base was found within the Department of Psychiatry. Helzer et al. (1985) carried out a follow-up study designed to learn to what extent alcoholics coming to medical or psychiatric treatment facilities may return to stable moderate drinking. The 1,289 subjects of that investigation included (1) 228 medical and surgical patients from a 750–bed, predominantly private general hospital; (2) 260 patients from the inpatient psychiatry service of the same hospital; (3) 177 patients from the Washington University outpatient psychiatry service; and (4) 624 patients from the alcoholism treatment ward of a publicly funded local psychiatric hospital. Follow–up 5 to 8 years later was 81% successful (69 of 85) in a random sample of subjects known to have had further drinking problems.

It was 72% successful (324 of 449) with eligible subjects not known to have had further treatment for alcohol problems. The interviewed sample was 52.4% white and 78% male.

In this data base there were 142 living white male alcoholics with substantially complete data on matters of interest to us. Information was recorded regarding current heavy drinking, presence of major depressive disorder (Feighner criteria), history of suicidal thoughts or threat, current living circumstances, and employment. The health inquiry was limited to liver disease. Social support was not assessed, nor was recent loss.

Previous Findings Replicated

Current drinking (heavy drinking in last 6 months) was reported by 18% of the living alcoholics in this second sample compared to 97% of the alcoholic suicides with that history ($P < 0.0000$). Current major depressive disorder was found in 31% of the living alcoholics versus 58% ($P < 0.0002$). A history of suicidal thoughts was reported in 43% versus 82% ($P < 0.000$). Fewer were unemployed, 32% versus 54% ($P = 0.002$) or living alone; 30% versus 45% ($P = 0.031$). There was a reversal in prevalence of liver disease (40% versus 22%; $P = 0.070$), probably accounted for by the fact that 86% of the living subjects had been initially identified as hospital inpatients. The source of patients may also account for the relatively small difference in the proportion living alone. Symptoms calling for hospital admission when the patient lives alone might be handled at home when others are present.

This control group, selected for medical-surgical or psychiatric illness, had a higher prevalence of liver disease than did the suicides. Given their source, it may be supposed that they had similarly high rates of other serious illness as well. Yet, in the 5 to 8 years since identification, there were only 5 suicides among the men, amounting to less than 1% (0.0085) of the white males and only 2.7% of their total mortality for the period (T. Combs-Orme, personal communication, October 8, 1987). That is a very low rate compared to existing data concerning previously hospitalized alcoholics (Table 11.4). Given what we have just seen demonstrated regarding the differences between alcoholic suicides and their living counterparts, it cannot be assumed that these suicides were like the living. What we can say is that this relatively low suicide rate reinforces the finding that no *single* factor—such as physical illness—is sufficient to produce a suicide in a person afflicted with alcoholism.

Opposite to the ECA sample, this group of living alcoholics had a significantly higher mean age than the suicides (50.9 ± 12.6 years versus 47.3 ± 9.1 years; $T < 0.02$). The logistic regression analysis used in the earlier comparison to control for age difference generates Table 9.5, a maximum likelihood analysis of variance. Current drinking emerges as most significantly differentiating the living from the dead. Major depression is not a discriminator, and unemployment just misses statistical significance ($P < 0.0522$). History of suicidal threats and thoughts is significantly different ($P < 0.0064$), but living alone fails to reach statistical significance. Given their high frequencies, there is substantial intercorrelation among the factors under consideration (Figure 9.1). The presence of one factor may predict the presence of another. The 2

Table 9.5 Maximum Likelihood Analysis of Variance Table: 67 White Male Alcoholic Suicides versus 142 Living White Male Alcoholics

Source	df	χ^2	Probability
Age	1	19.01	0.0000
Current drinking	1	46.37	0.0000
Suicidal thoughts	1	7.42	0.0064
Unemployed	1	3.77	0.0522
Living alone	1	1.09	NS
Major depression	1	0.94	NS

factors are then said to be intercorrelated. In the type of data analysis employed, the emergence of one significant factor may suppress the emergence of an intercorrelated one. That was the case for the nonsignificant items: unemployment, living alone, and depression. Each was significantly greater among the suicides and should not be ignored. This type of analysis says nothing about the *clinical* importance of these seemingly downgraded factors.

Poor social support not having been inquired about, there is one less factor available for comparison. The risk factor table that is generated (Table 9.6) again shows a different pattern of distribution between the suicides and the living for the factors under consideration. A cutting score of 3 or greater (owing to one less item for comparison) correctly identifies 76% of the alcoholic suicides and would falsely identify 19% of the living alcoholics as candidates for suicide. Poor social support, absent from this comparison, appears to be a highly discriminating risk factor.

This second sample of living alcoholics was not characterized by reported absence of recent alcohol problems, as had been true of 58% of the first sample. They were only *not known* before interview *to have been free of such problems*. The study from which this sample was drawn found few instances of evolution to moderate drinking under good control. Fifteen percent had become abstainers, 4.6% occasional drinkers, and 1.6% moderate drinkers (Helzer et al., 1985, Table 4). Nevertheless, 82% denied current problems with drinking. Continued drinking with attendant problems is reemphasized as a risk factor for suicide in alcoholics.

Table 9.6 Distribution of Risk Factors[a] in 67 Suicides and 142 Living Treated Alcoholics: White Males

Number of Risk Factors per Subject	Alcoholic Suicides[b] N = 67	Living Alcoholics[b] N = 142
0	0	31
1	4	46
2	12	38
3	19	16
4	23	9
5	9	2

[a]The risk factors are current heavy drinking, current major depressive disorder, unemployment, living alone, and suicidal thoughts or communication.
[b]χ^2 5 df = 75.71; $P < 0.0000$.

Table 9.7 Maximum Likelihood Analysis of Variance Table: 65 Still-Drinking White Male Alcoholic Suicides Versus 69 Still-Drinking Living White Male Alcoholics

Source	df	χ^2	Probability
Suicidal thoughts	1	11.21	0.0008
Major depression	1	7.19	0.0073
Unemployed	1	6.73	0.0095
Age	1	4.96	0.026
Living alone	1	0.06	NS

Because only a minority of the two control samples acknowledged recent problems associated with drinking, the question is raised whether the differences from the suicides that we have just seen may simply reflect the experience of the nonabusing majority. I therefore compared the 65 still–drinking suicides with still–drinking controls of the two sets on the remaining dimensions (Table 9.7). Unavailable for comparison are poor social support (not asked of the second control group) and poor general health (not asked of either group). Current drinking was a selection factor for the comparison. Living alone did not differ in frequency between suicides and still–drinking controls ($\chi^2 = 3.52$; $P > 0.05$). Age differs, the living alcoholics being substantially younger than the suicides.

Although the foregoing comparisons were carried out for white males only, the black men and the women showed exactly the same pattern as seen here regarding risk factors. The lowest number of risk factors was three (four cases), the highest, seven (one case). For the entire sample of 82 alcoholic suicides the distribution of these factors is given in Table 9.8. Eighty-three percent of the suicides had four or more.

One further concern must be examined: Are these risk factors specific to alcoholics, or are they characteristic of suicides generally? This question can be answered by comparing their distribution in alcoholic suicides to the 1959 study of suicides with a primary depression (E. Robins, unpublished data). Neither continued drinking nor cur-

Table 9.8 Distribution of Seven Risk Factors in 82 Alcoholic Suicides

Number of Risk Factors Per Subject	Number of Subjects
0	0
1	1
2	5
3	11
4	19
5	27
6	11
7	8
	82

Table 9.9 Distribution of Risk Factors in Alcoholic Suicides and Suicides with Primary Depressive Disorder

Number of Risk Factors[a] per Subject	Alcoholic Suicides $N = 82$	Depressive Suicides $N = 63$
0	1	11
1	8	13
2	18	15
3	27	15
4	17	5
5	11	3

[a]Risk factors are communication of suicidal thoughts, little or no social support, unemployment, serious medical illness and living alone. Current depressive episode and current drinking are selection factors for the compared groups and so cannot be counted.
T = 4.50; df = 140; $P < 0.0000$

rent depressive episode can enter the tabulations because they define the groups to be compared. (In the tabulations, housewives are counted as employed.) With those restrictions, it is seen (Table 9.9) that despite some overlap, the distributions are indeed distinct. Interpersonal loss has already been shown to distinguish these two groups.

Nor is the depressive episode responsible for the other risk factors. Suicidal communication is characteristic of depressives, but even more so of alcoholics who take their lives. The rate was 84% in alcoholic suicides and only 65% in primary depressives from the Robins study (Robins, Gassner, et al., 1959), and 88% in the replication study. Communication was both more frequent and of longer duration in the alcoholics in both studies. Drinking was a consequence of depression in no more than four or five of the alcoholic suicides. It was usually the other way around. Loss of social support is not particularly characteristic of depressives. When it does occur, it is more likely to be through widowhood than marital conflict or dissolution. The serious medical conditions associated with depression are different from those in alcoholics; familial and age-related, not due to habitual intoxication and self-neglect. Unemployment among the alcoholics came early (mean age 48.0 years at death) and was nearly always performance related. Among the depressives it was related to illness, age, and normal retirement. Fifty-four percent of the unemployed depressives were 65 years old or more; the youngest was 53 (mean age at death 66.2 years). Only two (4%) of the alcoholics were 65 or older. Living alone was traceable to interpersonal conflict in the alcoholics; to bereavement in depressives. The advent of depression is a highly dangerous event for alcoholics, but it does not act alone. Nor can it be held accountable for the other subacute and chronic features cited here as risk factors for suicide in alcoholics.

CONCLUSIONS

I have demonstrated that a number of subacute or chronic features found prevalent in one set of alcoholic suicides (Murphy et al., 1979) were similarly prevalent in another set investigated some 12–15 years earlier (Robins, 1981). These features—current drinking, major depressive disorder, little or no social support, unemployment, serious medical illness, living alone, and suicidal communication—have been observed by others as well (Engelbrecht, 1983; Kendell, 1983; Theret et al., 1989) to be associated with suicide in alcoholics. I have further shown that the frequency of all but one of these features is significantly greater among alcoholic suicides than among living alcoholics. Despite a lack of comparable data regarding medical illness in living alcoholics, I see no reason to discount the contribution of that factor.

There may well be factors other than those identified here that lower the barrier to self destruction and predict heightened risk. These were the ones cited in the literature and those we found most strikingly frequent and most frequently associated with suicide. They are not often found singly; they occur in numbers and are cumulative (Tables 9.4 and 9.8). The clear implication of these findings is that every physician should, at frequent intervals, assess the existence and level of each of these factors. As they accumulate, the risk of suicide grows. As few as four of them may serve to identify four–fifths of those at highest risk for suicide (Table 9.8). Three would identify 93% of those at high risk, but at a cost in increased false positives.

Excessive drinking is the behavior that drives most, if not all, of the factors under consideration. Therefore, every measure must be taken to bring about and support abstinence. Since abstinence is the goal of treatment for alcoholics, whether at serious risk of suicide or not, false positives are not necessarily a problem. It is better if both the recognition of the alcoholism and the push for treatment come earlier.

But drinking is not by any means the sole focus of treatment. The strong role of concomitant depression must be kept always in mind. It is easy to diagnose and is readily treatable, with a high rate of recovery that is probably independent of the diagnosis of alcoholism. Its centrality to suicide prevention is underscored by the fact that no alcoholic in either Study 1 or Study 2 who had a prior episode of depression was without that diagnosis at his or her terminus. That was also true for those in our original study (Robins, Murphy, et al., 1959; Robins, 1981) who had *only* a diagnosis of major depression. *The recognition and vigorous treatment of major depressive disorder is the cornerstone of suicide prevention, with or without the presence of alcoholism.*

10

What Can Be Done About Suicide in Alcoholics?

> . . . . by being better diagnosticians, by being more aware of the dangers or disguises of depression, we in general medicine and in general practice can do more to lower the suicide rate than the psychiatrists themselves.
> C. A. H. Watts, M.D. (1961)

SPONTANEOUS REMISSION

A number of studies have shown that some alcoholics remit spontaneously (Cahalan, 1970; Armor, Polich, & Stambul, 1978; Saunders, Phil, & Kershaw, 1979; Vaillant & Milofsky, 1982; Fillmore & Midanik, 1984; Helzer, Burnam & McEvoy, 1991), that is, without benefit of professional (medical or psychiatric) or organizational (Alcoholics Anonymous) intervention. What seems to characterize these remitters includes relative youth and relatively short history of alcohol abuse (mean 7.5 years). Some claim to drink socially under good control, rather than requiring abstinence (Saunders et al., 1979). Those who effectively moderate or abandon their habit credit social change, usually positive, for their behavior change. A supportive marriage, job change to one entailing lower stress or lower exposure and "maturity" are prominently mentioned, but concern over both physical and financial deterioration have been important in a minority (Saunders et al., 1979, p. 257). Despite the limited effectiveness of medical treatment of this disorder, it is highly inappropriate for the physician to adopt or recommend a posture of "wait and see." That has already proved futile prior to the consultation.

THE REMAINDER

There is evidence that abstinence, even in rather severe alcoholics, can arrest morbid processes and abolish the excess mortality of alcoholism (Barr, Antes, Ottenberg, & Rosen, 1984). It is the cornerstone of socioeconomic rehabilitation. Vaillant and Milofsky consider abstinence to be a means, not an end (1982, p. 132), social rehabilitation being the goal. But social rehabilitation of alcoholics is rarely achieved except in a state of abstinence. When it is, the preceding social deterioration, like the accompanying alcohol abuse, has been relatively mild (p. 131).

Suicidal Alcoholics Are More Likely to See a Physician

The ECA data show that 18% of those they identified as alcoholics had a history of hospitalization for any mental health reason. Eight to 14% of the living alcohol abusers with symptoms in the last 6 months had been in contact with caregivers (Robins et al., 1988, p. 15). Alcoholics well along the path to suicide are several times more likely to have contact with health care professionals than are more loosely defined alcohol abusers.

Thirty-eight percent of our alcoholics had been hospitalized for symptoms related to their alcoholism. The same proportion had seen a psychiatrist at some time, but only 6 (12%) had ever participated in an alcohol rehabilitation program. Although treatment was ultimately unsuccessful, sobriety of a few months to 2 years was reported in a few cases. More importantly, 82% had seen some physician, whether medical doctor or osteopath, in the course of the year in which they died. Exactly half had had physician contact in the last month, 22% in the last week. *Suicide is a clinical problem*—medical in a broad sense.

For that segment of the alcoholic population that does come into contact with physicians, it is important that their caregivers learn to recognize the disorder in its various presentations and try to get every alcoholic into treatment (Kranzler & Babor, 1990). The effort may succeed. If the patient won't accept referral, the spouse or significant other may benefit from participation in Alanon, an organization sponsored by Alcoholics Anonymous to provide emotional support and education for spouses and children of alcoholics. As a result, they may cease to be "enablers"—those who, by apparently well-intentioned actions, facilitate the drinking behavior of the alcoholic (see Case 45). Changed behavior on the part of spouses and significant others is believed to propel some alcoholics into treatment.

Since very few suicides are without a recognizable psychiatric illness in the final few weeks and months of their lives, it is substantially true that psychiatric illness is a necessary, although not an altogether sufficient cause. What is sufficient will depend on the individual and his or her history; it includes those factors discussed in Chapter 9.

The Diagnosis Is Too Often Missed

Physicians have been shown to have blind spots, characteristically where the patient or his condition is perceived as violating the "Protestant Ethic." Not restricted to Protestants, this ethic might better be described as the Middle-Class Value System, strongly endorsed by the great majority of physicians (Klein, Najman, Kohrman, & Munro, 1982). Alcoholics violate these values by their behavior, which is viewed as self-indulgent, improvident, and willfull. Worse, they are often poorly cooperative with treatment. It is not surprising, therefore, that Klein et al. found alcoholism/alcoholics negatively perceived by over half (55.8%) of 450 Michigan general practition-

Table 10.1 Abstinence Rates in Follow-Up Studies of Hospital-Treated Alcoholics

Reference	N Followed Up	Follow-Up Duration (yr)	Abstinent N	Abstinent %	Moderate N	Moderate %	Severe N	Severe %	Mortality N	Mortality %
Gabriel (1935), Austria	1,058	1–12	311	29	157	14	590	55	148	14
Ellerman (1948), Denmark	159[a]	1–9	40	25			119	75	18	11
Prout et al. (1950), United States	85	1–8	25	29	30	35	22	26	8	9
Nørvig & Nielsen (1956), Denmark	181[a]	3–5	39	22	57	32	43	24	42	23
Davies et al. (1956), United Kingdom	49[a]	2	15	30	15	30	19	39	1	3
Selzer & Holloway (1957), United States	83	6	18	22	9	11	56	67	18	21
Pokorny et al. (1968), United States	101[a]	1	22	22	23	23	63	63	5	5
Gillis & Keet (1969), South Africa	797	1–5	113	14	176	22	414	52	95	12
Gillies et al. (1974), Canada	968	1	123	13	604	62	241	25	0	
Sheehan et al. (1981), United States	61	3	29	48					4	7
Barr et al. (1984), United States	503	2	134	27	14	3	302	60	?	
Ornstein & Cherepon (1985), United States	1,210[a]	2	106	9	49	4	1005[b]	83	50	4
O'Sullivan et al. (1988), Ireland	249[c]	1½–2	96	39	94	38	59	24	0	
Shaw et al. (1990), United States	91	1	42	46	22	24	27	30	0	
Imber et al. (1976),[d] United States	83[a]	3	8	10					10	12

[a]Present author's reconstruction. Includes 8 living subjects refusing follow-up, assumed "severe."
[b]Includes 290 subjects unclassified for lack of information.
[c]Patients without personality disorder.
[d]Untreated alcoholics.

ers. Among other physicians as well, and for the same reasons, alcoholism is not a favored disorder. One consequence of that distaste is failure to make the diagnosis (Barchha, Stewart, & and Guze, 1968; Persson & Magnusson, 1989).

Not frequently volunteered as disliked by Klein's respondents, the diagnosis of depression is nevertheless often overlooked. Many depressed and/or alcoholic patients are treated, their suicidal ideation and/or depression recognized and addressed. The suicides that occur despite medical attention are largely of patients who have fallen through the diagnostic net. Psychopathology or risk has gone undetected; the depression went unrecognized, suicidal thoughts were not inquired about (Murphy, 1975). It is my hope that wider knowledge of the findings presented here will lead to greater clinical alertness and appropriate action.

Detoxification/Rehabilitation Results are Unimproved?

There seems to have been little improvement over the past 50 years in outcome for those alcoholics whose symptoms bring them to inpatient treatment. Treatment studies reported from 1935 to 1957 showed abstinence rates ranging between 22% and 30% (weighted mean 27.7%) on follow-up of 2 to 12 years. Similar studies reported in the last 22 years show abstinence rates from 9% to 48% (weighted mean 15.88%). These means are calculated on the studies cited in Table 10.1. I did not review all treatment follow-up studies in the literature. Those who have done so have not found a basis for crediting longer treatment with better outcome (Finney, Moos, & Chan, 1981; Miller & Hester, 1986; Longabaugh, 1988; Kranzler & Babor, 1990). The search for pretreatment predictors of favorable outcome has failed to yield replicable findings as well (Ornstein & Cherepon, 1985). In any medical sense, our treatment of substance abuse disorders is largely nonspecific. Lacking an understanding of the neuropsychobiology of addictions, can we expect it to be otherwise? Perhaps the next decade will bring enlightenment. Meanwhile, current efforts are not without benefit. They simply are far less powerful and predictable than we would like.

TREATMENT CONSIDERATIONS

Blaming Isn't Useful

A ubiquitous problem for the medical as well as the psychiatric practitioner in dealing with alcoholics is the perception that alcohol abuse and its consequent behaviors are voluntary and willful. That interpretation leads to a judgmental attitude that may result in neglect and avoidance. Apart from lawyers, no one benefits from blaming the alcoholic. That is not to say that the drinker isn't ultimately responsible, but only that blaming is counterproductive (Rose, 1988).

No one becomes an alcoholic altogether on his or her own initiative. There is strong evidence for a genetic factor of susceptibility for at least some alcoholics (Goodwin, 1979, 1985; Cloninger et al., 1981; Schuckit, Li, Cloninger, & Deitrich, 1985; Pickens et al., 1991). Environment, too, plays a role. Assumptions about motivation are therefore premature and probably mistaken.

It helps to think of alcoholism as a chronic, relapsing illness analogous to rheumatoid arthritis. Relapse—"falling off the wagon"—is most usefully regarded as a common *symptom* of the disorder, an integral part of its natural history, rather than as willful noncompliance and an occasion for disapprobation.

Steps taken by the treating physician to help the alcoholic establish or reestablish sobriety as quickly as possible will be more helpful than even the least bit of scolding. An accepting and helpful attitude may also cement a relationship that, in the eyes of the relapsed alcoholic, he has violated by his fall from sobriety. I advise telling the drink-sodden and ashamed alcoholic patient, "This is no time to reject treatment. You won't need me when you are well, but right now we must work together to get you back on the track." Punitiveness and blaming simply arouse defensiveness. That being the case, it will be more effective to work with alcoholics in search of ways to help them *a step at a time*. Disulfiram (Antabuse) may help the patient maintain sobriety. Small steps can lead to bigger ones. Too large a step results in a fall.

Treat the Depression

Of the predictors of suicide in alcoholics identified by the present study—continued drinking, being depressed, having little social support, having a history of suicide thoughts, experiencing interpersonal loss or threatened loss, living alone, being unemployed, being medically ill—only one is directly remediable by health professionals. Depression, found in nearly three-fourths of the suicides, is not characteristic of alcoholics in general but of a relatively small proportion of them. It is often what brings them to treatment for their alcoholism. Having done so, it must not be overlooked.

Treatment of depression is the cornerstone of successful treatment of alcoholism in about three-fourths of the cases. The depression may not be severe, but it is an added burden. The pessimism, in some cases the hopelessness, that are common symptoms of depression stand in the way of a strong commitment to sobriety. Depression lends a degree of believability, even of inevitability, to feelings of discouragement and helplessness that must be combated. Since depression can be expected to respond to conventional measures, these should be pursued vigorously.

Cognitive Behavioral Therapy

Cognitive behavioral therapy (CBT) (Rush, Shaw, & Emery, 1979) has been shown to be as effective as antidepressant medication in treating outpatients with uncomplicated major depression of moderate severity (Rush, Beck, Kovacs, & Hollon, 1977; Blackburn, Bishop, Glenn, Whalley, & Christie, 1981; Murphy, Simons, Wetzel, & Lustman, 1984; Elkin et al., 1989). I am unaware of any clinical trials of cognitive therapy in treating alcoholism. An analogous study compared outcome of drug counseling alone to that of counseling plus either CBT or "supportive-expressive" psychotherapy with opiate addicts (Woody et al., 1983). The psychotherapies produced significantly better results than drug counseling alone. Not only was depression improved, a number of other dimensions improved as well. Surprisingly, the more severely affected patients psychiatrically benefited most from the addition of psychotherapy (Woody, McLellan,

Luborsky, & O'Brien, 1985). If the analogy holds, more may be expected of CBT than has been shown.

Whereas CBT has the advantage of being nonchemical, it is more expensive than pharmacotherapy in terms of professional time. Weekly sessions of 50 minutes for 12 to 20 or more weeks are common. Administered one to one, it is somewhat costly, although cheaper than psychodynamic psychotherapy. Cost may limit its use. However, when the cost of medication and the greater duration of pharmacotherapy are taken into account, along with the potential for lasting remission with CBT (Blackburn, Eunson, & Bishop, 1986; Simons, Murphy, Levine, & Wetzel, 1986), the cost differential may not be a primary consideration. There is some evidence of similar effectiveness for group format CBT (Covi & Lipman, 1987). Treatment programs that wish to preserve an across-the-board "no chemicals" philosophy should find CBT indispensable in view of its impressively documented efficacy in the treatment of depression.

Pharmacotherapy

Less expensively administered and no less effective is our steadily growing pharmaceutical armamentarium. The older tricyclic compounds of the imipramine series (Tofranil, Norpramin, Surmontil) and those related to amitriptyline (Elavil, Pamelor, Vivactil) as well as doxepin (Sinequan) offer a spectrum of sedative and activating characteristics and differences in effects on neurotransmitters that call for informed choices. Their uses, advantages, and disadvantages are generally well understood by psychiatrists and widely discussed in the literature (Klein, Gittelman, Quitkin, & Rifkin, 1980; Richelson, E., 1989). This knowledge is accessible, and the information needs to be better understood by other physicians.

The newer heterocyclic compounds are sometimes useful but are not usually first-line choices. The obsessional alcoholic may be specifically benefited by fluoxetine (Prozac) or clomipramine (Anafranil). They are potent serotonin reuptake blockers. Fluoxetine has the advantage of not overstimulating appetite. It is reported to have a very wide safety margin on overdose (Cooper, 1988), a matter of some significance in the actively or potentially suicidal patient. One must keep in mind, however, the occasional effect of suppressing orgasmic response (Musher, 1990). The possibility of a paradoxical compulsive suicidal urge, which was recently reported (Teicher, Glod, & Cole, 1990), is probably not different in either frequency or intensity from that seen with the older antidepressants.

Lithium carbonate can provide a boost to the effectiveness of any of these drugs and has antidepressant potential in its own right as well (Schou, 1986). For the alcoholic with accompanying bipolar affective disorder, lithium carbonate will generally be the bedrock of clinical management. Concerns about its long-term effects on the kidney are probably needlessly exaggerated (Waller & Edwards, 1989; Hetmar, Povlsen, Ladefoged, & Bolwig, 1991), but periodic assessment of renal function is advisable.

Monamine oxidase inhibitors (MAOIs) often are effective where the tricyclic antidepressants fail (Tollefson, 1983). When ineffective, it may be because the manufacturer's dosage recommendations are too conservative. Peripheral edema and afternoon drowsiness are infrequent but potentially troublesome side effects. Opinions differ on the danger of alcohol ingestion to the patient taking an MAOI antidepressant. Is it only Chianti that is risky, or all red wines, or red wines and beer as well? Tyramine (an amino acid precursor of serotonin) is the dangerous ingredient. These MAOIs do require some dietary restrictions in order to be reasonably safe, but the manufacturers are probably excessively cautious in their warnings. The spontaneous use of nonprescription cough and cold remedies by the patient poses a substantial risk of provoking a hypertensive crisis and perhaps an intracranial bleed (Bazire, 1986). Nasal decongestants such as ephedrine, metanephrine, and pseudonephrine must be clearly warned against. Whether the alcoholic can be relied upon to follow any restrictive regimen must be decided case by case.

Despite package insert warnings, most experienced clinicians have found at least occasional beneficial use from the combination of an MAOI and a tricyclic antidepressant (TCA) (Lader, 1983; Razani et al., 1983; Lippmann, 1986). Amitriptyline and trimipramine seem to be the safest TCAs, imipramine the least safe in combination with an MAOI (Marley & Wozniak, 1983). Great caution and deliberateness are required in transiting between an MAOI and fluoxetine or clomipramine (Feighner, Boyer, Tyler, & Neborsky, 1990). Combined administration is out of the question (Beaumont, 1973).

Some benzodiazepine compounds marketed as anticonvulsants are finding an increasing and often unique role as antidepressants. Carbamazepine (Tegretol) has the longest track record of this class of compounds. Alone or in combination with a TCA, it has rendered many treatment-resistant depressions responsive. As a class, the benzodiazepines are best known as anxiolytics or mild sedatives. Most of them can produce a chemical dependency. The alcohol abuser is psychologically (and perhaps physiologically) disposed to abuse euphoriants of all classes. One must therefore undertake the prescribing of any benzodiazepine compound to an alcoholic with the greatest circumspection and full control of the medication supply. The shortest acting members of this group have the greatest abuse potential. Withdrawing alprazolam (Xanax) after long use can present very serious problems, including seizures, and requires *extremely* gradual dose reduction (Noyes et al., 1986).

We still don't know, in any individual case, if the antidepressants work because they right some upset in neurotransmitter balance or because our optimistic expectancy does that, or because the systematic trials of various medications buy time until the depression remits—or gives us the vehicle to work our positive attitude on a negatively thinking patient. In any event, I believe it is important to present a positive attitude without offering false or unfounded assurances. Psychotherapeutic support is never misplaced in treating alcoholics.

Most depressions encountered in the course of alcoholism treatment will be manageable in outpatient care. However, alcoholism is not a protection from the most severe endogenomorphic depression. Suicidal urges can become increasingly compelling. Not only hospital admission to a maximum security psychiatric service, but electroconvulsive therapy (ECT) is called for in that event. It can be lifesaving. ECT can also interrupt the delirium of alcohol withdrawal (Roberts, 1963; Dudley & Williams, 1972).

Getting the alcoholic to enter a psychiatric hospital for treatment is often difficult. It usually requires help from the spouse or family. In view of the several suicides in our series that may have been hastened or precipitated by that prospect, it had best be accomplished with utmost dispatch and with tight supervision between the decision and its execution. Once admitted, it is important that the patient stay long enough for full detoxification as well as other indicated treatment. The suicide rate is highest shortly after hospital discharge, which may mean that discharge often comes too early.

SUICIDE PREVENTION EFFORTS

Ettlinger (1975) undertook to keep in periodic contact with a large group of persons discharged from the Sodersjukhuset in Stockholm after a serious suicide attempt. All were unconscious on admission, following an overdose of medication. They were given follow-up appointments at intervals after discharge and encouraged to come in for consultation. The mortality experience of this group of 670 suicide attempters, 276 men and 394 women, was compared to that of 681 similar patients admitted to the same unit over the 3-year period before the start of the increased contact study. These control patients had not been offered posthospitalization support. A 5-year follow-up failed to show a difference in overall mortality or in the occurrence of suicide between these two groups.

A one-third sample of each sex was taken from both the study sample and controls for more intensive study. About one-third of the men and 6% of the women in each subsample were alcoholics. Overall, there was no between-group difference in the mortality over the observation period. "The men in group S [experimental] who had a record of crime or drunken behavior had a significantly lower suicide mortality than those without a record" (Ettlinger, 1975, p. 124). This is the only prospective study of suicide prevention specifically involving alcoholics that I have found. Although not overwhelmingly successful, it does seem to demonstrate some value in increased social support.

RISK PREDICTION IS NOT SUICIDE PREDICTION

I do not claim that any of our findings can predict an individual suicide. Elsewhere (Murphy, 1984) I have discussed the very potent reason why that is so. It has to do with the rarity of the phenomenon of suicide and the statistical properties of infrequent events (Galen & Gambino, 1975). As Alex Pokorny (1983) has pointed out:

> We do not possess any item of information or any combination of items that permit us to identify to a useful degree the particular persons who will commit suicide, in spite of the fact that we do have scores of items available, each of which is significantly related to suicide.

I have identified here no less than seven observational items that were significantly more often found in alcoholics who took their lives than in two control groups of living alcoholics. In common psychological parlance, these are "predictors." They have a heightened association with the phenomenon in question. Their individual occurrence, albeit at much lower frequency among the very much more common living alcoholics, promises high false positive rates in any attempt to *predict* individual suicides (Murphy, 1972). My data show that as the number of such predictors found in a given individual increases, so does the probability of suicide (Tables 9.4 and 9.6).

The presuicidal syndrome in our alcoholics developed over a period of months or years, although recent escalation was common. Only interpersonal loss was relatively acute. Excessive drinking was more or less continuous over many years; major depression was not often of very recent onset; medical illnesses were chronic; suicidal communication was usually repetitive, over a long period of time; living alone was of long duration almost as often as it was recent. Some interpersonal support systems had undergone an abrupt worsening, but almost always on a background of progressive deterioration. The same was true of unemployment. As *risk factors,* they acquire significance in *cumulative* fashion. The physician can monitor the progression of risk by counting their accumulation.

Treat the Underlying Illness

Abstinence can reverse the deterioration process, but is difficult to induce. There is evidence that sobriety will be accompanied by a lower mortality, both generally and by suicide (Barr et al., 1984). But as our study shows, alcohol is not the only problem. Nearly three-quarters of our alcoholic suicides had developed a complicating depression—a potent risk factor for suicide. That comorbidity seems to have been recognized only rarely and never to have been appropriately treated by attending physicians, despite half of the suicides having been seen within a month, well within the time frame of the depressive episode.

Depressive disorder is usually responsive to treatment.[1] Vigorous intervention at that level was never seen in this series, an omission that has been noted more widely (Murphy, 1975; Barraclough, Jennings, & Moss, 1977; Åsgård, 1990). A careful search for depressive disorder, repeated periodically, will reveal this complication in a substantial number of alcoholics. *The recognition of depression, followed by vigorous treatment, could prevent many suicides, both of alcoholics and others.* Watts's (1961) observation, heading this chapter, is as true today as it was in 1961, and it was entirely true, if widely disregarded, then.

Physician Awareness, Physician Readiness

The physician's failure to identify and effectively treat depressions is remediable, as described by Rutz, von Knorring, and Walinder (1989):

> In 1983–1984 the Swedish Committee for Prevention and Treatment of Depression (PTD Committee) introduced an educational program for all general practitioners (GPs) on the Swedish island of Gotland. The primary goal was to increase knowledge about diagnosis and treatment of patients with affective disorders. The effects of the educational programs were evaluated in detail; GPs identified more patients with depressive disorders and treated them more accurately. The suicide rate on Gotland . . . dropped the year after the educational programs were introduced. This was a statistically significant deviation both from the long-term trend on Gotland and from the trends in Sweden as a whole.

I have argued earlier (Murphy, 1984) that it would be very difficult to demonstrate a clear effect of physician reeducation on the nationwide suicide rate. By choosing a community of limited size to receive focused attention, Rutz et al. have amply demonstrated that *education of physicians in the community directed to more accurate diagnosis and more appropriate treatment of depressive disorders can and does reduce the frequency of suicide.* This should be no less true for depression complicating alcoholism than for uncomplicated depression.

Effective treatment of any disorder is enhanced by its early recognition. As difficult as alcoholism is to treat, it is not totally unyielding. Nearly all of its negative consequences can then be reversed. Untreated, alcoholics will die prematurely, some of them by suicide. Of the seven recognizable components of the presuicidal syndrome identified here (Chapters 8 and 9), the most readily remediable is depression. We must all shed our blinders and recognize alcoholism as a common disorder. We must courageously ask about suicidal thoughts and acts. Most important, all physicians must become alert to the diagnosis of depressive disorder and comfortable and skillful in treating it. It *will* make a difference.

11

What Is the Lifetime Risk of Suicide in Alcoholism?

Important to the full understanding of suicide is the question of what proportion of persons suffering from the various psychiatric disorders may be expected to die by their own hand. In other words, What is the proportional risk that a sufferer from depressive disorder, alcoholism, or schizophrenia will become a suicide? That is the lifetime risk.

EXISTING ESTIMATES OF LIFETIME RISK OF SUICIDE

Follow-up studies of persons diagnosed as suffering from affective disorders have been interpreted as suggesting a lifetime risk of about 15% for that outcome (Guze & Robins, 1970).

Little data-based literature exists on the question of lifetime risk of suicide in alcoholism. Lemere (1953) asked his alcoholic patients to recall the manner of death of their deceased alcoholic relatives over two generations. Based on 500 deaths reported, 11% were by suicide. Obvious potential biases in such a study include the uncertainty of diagnosis at a distance, the possibility of selective recall affecting the completeness of the family history, and selecting for severity by starting with affected probands.

Miles (1977) plotted the proportion of deaths by suicide against the proportion dead in 12 follow-up studies of alcoholics, along with Lemere's data and those of a mortality study without a known population base (Mečiř & Brežinová, 1960). He asserted that these data demonstrated a lifetime risk of 15% for suicide in alcoholics.

Why These Figures Are Too High

Murphy & Wetzel (1990) have addressed this question from a much larger data base. First, we examined the data from follow-up studies of alcoholics having an overall

---

An earlier and more detailed version of this chapter appeared in the AMA *Archives of General Psychiatry,* Vol. 47, pp. 383–392, 1990, as The Lifetime Risk of Suicide in Alcoholism, by G. E. Murphy and R. D. Wetzel. Copyright 1990, American Medical Assocation.

LIFETIME RISK OF SUICIDE IN ALCOHOLISM

mortality greater than 30% (Table 11.1). We argue that a conservative estimate of lifetime risk might be derived by assuming that no more suicides would occur until all of the probands were dead. (This is a reasonable undertaking, as most suicides occur early in the follow-up period. Those that come later have their effect diluted by rapidly increasing deaths from other causes.) Using the number of suicides already identified as the dividend and the number in each entire population as divisor, the result would be the minimum suicide rate that could obtain: there could not, in the long run, ever be fewer suicides than there were already. The proportion dead by suicide ranges from 8.5% to 2%, with a median of 5%.

Since there is considerable numerical difference between the results, the studies are presented in Table 11.1 not chronologically as in other tables, but in descending order of calculated suicide rate. The annual rate of death by suicide (male, female, or combined) for each country of origin at the midpoint of the follow-up is given in the last column on the right of the table. As can be seen, there is a fairly good rank order correlation between the calculated rates for the studies and their contemporaneous national rates (Pearson product moment correlation 0.84, $P < 0.01$; Spearman rank order

Table 11.1 Minimum Rate of Suicide Among Alcoholics Dead in Follow-Up Studies with More Than 30% Dead

Reference	Source of Probands	N	Minimum Percentage Dead by Suicide	Contemporaneous Population Rate[a]
Wieser & Kunad (1965), Federal Republic of Germany	Psychiatric hospital admissions	153	8.5	19.2[b]
Ciompi & Eisert (1969), Switzerland	Psychiatric hospital admissions	1,386	7.1	23.9[c]
Berglund (1984), Sweden	Psychiatric hospital discharges	1,312	6.7	22.3[d]
Nicholls et al. (1974), United Kingdom	Psychiatric hospital discharges	865	5.3	11.2[b]
MacKenzie et al. (1986), United States	Psychiatric hospital discharges	79♂	5.1	18.6[e]
Helgason (1964), Iceland	Population cohort	241	5	12.4[f]
Hyman (1976), United States	Brief outpatient alcohol rehab	48♂	4.2	15.4[b]
Sundby (1967), Norway	Psychiatric hospital discharges	1,693	3.8	8.7[c]
Smith et al. (1983), United States	Psychiatric hospital admissions	100♀	2	6.5[g]

[a]Pearson product moment correlation with percentage dead by suicide = 0.817; $P = 0.0072$.
[b]World Health Organization (1968).
[c]World Health Organization (1956).
[d]World Health Organization (1971).
[e]U.S. Department of Health, Education and Welfare, *Vital Statistics of the United States* (1979).
[f]United Nations, Department of Economic and Social Affairs. (1951).
[g]U.S. Department of Health, Education and Welfare (1973).

correlation 0.833, $P < 0.01$), despite two outliers, small studies of men only. The calculated lifetime risk of suicide is seen to vary with the national rate, a finding in keeping with what is known of national suicide rates. Even the highest calculated figure is substantially lower than the estimates cited above.

We (Murphy & Wetzel, 1990) next examined the credibility of a 15% lifetime risk of suicide in alcoholics based on the U.S. suicide statistics. For that operation, we needed to know the number of suicides in the population and the proportion of suicides that are alcoholics. We also needed to know the mean duration of abusive drinking that precedes suicide, that is, the number of years at risk.

Lacking any data-based estimate of years of alcoholism preceding suicide, we calculated the mean duration from onset of excessive drinking to suicide on the basis of the 67 male and 9 female alcoholic suicides on whom we had the requisite information from two studies (Murphy et al., 1979; Robins, 1981). The resulting figure was 20.5 years (mean) for males and 14.0 years for females. Combining the data gave a duration of risk of 19.49, with 95% probability limits of 18.7 and 21.0 years. For convenience, we used 19 years as the mean. That is the "lifetime" from which suicide risk is calculated.

All of the published retrospective community studies of suicide are presented in Table 2.1. Excepting the recent reports of Mitterauer (1981), Kapamadžija, Biro, and Sovljanski (1982), Rich, Young, and Fowler (1986) and Arató, Demeter, Rihmer, and Somogyi (1988), which give inclusive, rather than hierarchical diagnoses, the mean proportional contribution of alcoholics is 25%. The range is 5% (Åsgård, 1990, women only) to 31% (Beskow, 1979, men only.) The lowest figure for a both-sex sample, 15% (Barraclough et al., 1974), that from the United Kingdom, was obtained in an area of older, retired persons, where depression could be expected to be frequent and alcoholism rare. The highest, 31% from Beskow (1979) is undiluted by women, who have a much lower suicide rate (see Table 7.1 and Discussion, Chapter 7). Among the studies employing multiple diagnoses, that with the highest proportion of alcoholics, 54%, is from the United States (Rich, Young, & Fowler, 1986) and is also the largest sampling. The diagnosis of alcoholism was based on DSM-III (APA, 1980) criteria for alcohol *abuse,* which are markedly overinclusive. Additionally, this figure includes all subjects given a diagnosis of alcohol abuse, whether primary or secondary to another diagnosis. Rediagnosing the cases using research criteria (Feighner et al., 1972) identified 29% as alcoholic (C. L. Rich, personal communication, May 10, 1989). This figure can also be calculated from their Table 4.)

There were 30,407 officially identified suicides in the United States in 1988 (United States Department of Health and Human Services, 1990), the last year for which complete figures are available. From the range of outcomes in Table 2.1, between 15% (Barraclough et al., 1974) and 54% (Rich et al., 1986) of those suicides could have been alcoholics, accounting for 4,561 to 16,420 of the 30,407. Consider these the outer limits of the problem we are working with. The National Council on Alcoholism (NCA; 1987) claims an estimated 10.5 million alcoholics in the United States in 1985 (Williams, Stinson, Parker, Harford, & Noble, 1987). Over a 19-year period, the drinking "lifetime" we calculated as ending in suicide, assuming the same proportions each year, there would have been between 86,659 and 311,976 suicidal deaths of alcoholics. This represents between 0.82% and 3% of the

NCA estimated number of alcoholics, far below the 11–15% previously estimated lifetime risk.

To look at it another way, consider that the 54% of the suicides of 1988 were alcoholics under the maximum estimate of Rich et al. (1986). If this number (16,420) were 15% (Miles' estimate) of the alcoholics dying in 1988, and the same 15% rate had prevailed for the 19-year "lifetime" of those alcoholics, the number of alcoholics at risk would have been only 2,079,867 (16,420 × 19 ÷ 0.15). The lowest estimate, that of Barraclough et al. (1974), would project an absurdly low alcoholic population at risk of 577,727 persons (4,561 alcoholic suicides × 19 years ÷ 0.15). The number of alcoholics in the population at risk of suicide appears to be greatly overestimated. Moreover, as shown in Chapter 9, only a fraction of all persons loosely identified as alcoholics are seriously at risk.

The recurrent question of whether national suicide figures are reliable, semireliable, or gross underestimates is not germane. Retrospective suicide studies (Table 2.1) are all based on officially identified suicides, so the base is the same as the official statistics for the region studied. Only if there were a very large differential bias against recognizing the deaths of alcoholics as suicide would ascertainment be a critical variable. There is no a priori reason to assume that to be the case. Three studies, one Scottish (Ovenstone, 1973), one English (Holding & Barraclough, 1978), and one American (Brent et al., 1987), bear on the question of whether missed cases differ from those identified. According to the best information available, they do not. (See discussion in Chapter 2.)

FOLLOW-UP STUDIES AS A DATA BASE

Having shown that current estimates of lifetime risk of suicide in alcoholics are impossibly high, we derived more believable figures from a data base of 46 follow-up studies of alcoholics from 14 countries published in four languages, reporting both suicide and total mortality in a population of stated size over a specified time period. One-third of them are from the United States. Both sample size and length of follow-up vary widely. Space considerations dictate that I omit much of the discussion included in "The Lifetime Risk of Suicide in Alcoholism" (Murphy & Wetzel, 1990). Moreover, my continuing search for new data unearthed 13 additional studies emcompassing four additional countries, adding materially to the conclusions. The newly added studies are identified by an asterisk in the tables. Three recent studies from Japan permit a risk calculation for that country not included in the previously published paper.

Suicide rates vary widely by nationality and culture. Most European and Scandinavian countries have much higher suicide rates than the English-speaking countries: the United States, the United Kingdom, Canada, Australia, New Zealand, and Iceland. Although approaching the U.S. suicide rate today, both Scotland (when considered separately from England and Wales) (Barraclough, 1972) and Norway (Bolander, 1972) have long recorded substantially lower rates. The Netherlands has a continuing low rate. Owing to these differences in suicide rates, the high, medium, and low suicide rate countries are considered separately.

Treated and Untreated Alcoholics

Most published follow-up studies of alcoholics begin with consecutive hospital admissions or discharges. It is safe to say that alcoholics admitted for treatment are not representative of all alcoholics. In the ECA study, where alcohol abuse (DSM-III criteria) was diagnosed in 13% of the population, only 18% of them had a history of hospitalization for any mental health reason (L. McEvoy, personal communication, April 11, 1988). In contrast, 38% of our alcoholic suicides had had such an admission. Thus the great majority of alcoholics escape treatment, and the untreated are likely to be less severely affected than those treated.[1] Different risk figures should be generated by samples of alcoholics having inpatient, outpatient, or no formal treatment. At the level of inpatient treatment there is no justification or need to distinguish types or durations of programs (Longabaugh, 1988).

SUICIDE RISK FROM FOLLOW-UP STUDIES

Annual and lifetime risk of suicide were calculated in the following manner. The number of subjects in a follow-up study multiplied by the length of the follow-up in years gives the number of person-years at risk of suicide for that particular study. The number of suicides within the follow-up period divided by the person-years at risk multiplied by 100 gives the *annual* percentage of subjects dead by suicide. That figure, multiplied by 19 years—the mean duration of alcoholism leading to suicide calculated from our data—yields an approximate lifetime risk for suicide. The larger the number of studies and of subjects, the more reliable the result is likely to be.

I consider first those studies in which treatment did not play a part in accession. Next, we look at follow-ups from outpatient treatment. Finally, risk for probands identified from inpatient admissions is calculated. Although it is unlikely to be the case that no patient identified at a lower level of attention went on to a higher level, internal evidence in the various studies suggests that few had done so within the follow-up period.

The United States and Intermediate Risk Countries

Table 11.2 shows the just described calculations for studies of (presumably) untreated alcoholics. Only two follow-ups of this class were found. The United States study is of an industrial population (Pell & D'Alonzo, 1973), uncertainly diagnosed by company physicians. The other is from a longitudinal survey of the entire population of Iceland (Helgason, 1964), which has a suicide rate similar to that of the United States.

Studies of alcoholics treated in outpatient settings yield an annual suicide rate of 0.120% and a lifetime rate of 2.29% by the same method (Table 11.3). These figures are just slightly higher than the published ones, owing to my late discovery of a study from New Zealand (Lambie et al., & Johnson, 1983) in which the patients were "usually involved in out-patient treatment and only very occasionally was in-patient treatment necessary" (R. Johnson, personal communication, March 4, 1991).

LIFETIME RISK OF SUICIDE IN ALCOHOLISM

Table 11.2 Annual and Lifetime Rate of Suicide[a] Among Untreated Alcoholics: Intermediate Rate Countries

Reference	N	Years Follow-Up	Person-Years	Suicides
Pell & D'Alonzo (1973), United States	848	5	4,240	2
Helgason (1964), Iceland	241	42[b]	10,122	12
Total	1,089		14,362	14

[a]14 suicides ÷ 14,362 person-years = 0.0975% annual rate; 0.0975% × 19 years = 1.85% lifetime risk.
[b]Actual follow-up period 47 years. Probands were 13–15 years old at intake. Subtracting 5 years from the observation period ensures that the entire population is within the age of risk of alcoholism.
Note: From G. E. Murphy and R. D. Wetzel. The Lifetime Risk of Suicide in Alcoholism. *Arch. Gen. Psychiatry,* 1990, *47*:385, Table 3. Copyright 1990, American Medical Association.

The majority of follow-ups of alcoholics have identified their probands from psychiatric hospital admissions or discharges. Cumulated figures are given in Table 11.4 for the 14 U.S. studies (3 newly added), 5 from the United Kingdom, and 1 each from Canada, Iceland, and (newly) New Zealand. A yearly suicide rate of 0.179% is found. The lifetime risk of suicide among alcoholics who have been hospitalized comes to 3.4% (0.179% × 19 years). This is much lower than currently quoted estimates. The roughly 20% increment in risk progressing from untreated to outpatient treated alcoholics and a nearly 50% increment from these to alcoholics having inpatient treatment is consistent with the expectation of a gradient of severity of alcohol problems in relation to the level of treatment received.

Scandinavian and European Risk Estimates

Most of the Scandinavian and European countries have substantially higher suicide rates that those just considered. While alcoholism rates are not uniform across these countries, Beskow's (1979) data for males and Hagnell and Rorsman's (1979) for both sexes (Table 2.1) suggest that the proportional contribution of alcoholism to the suicide

Table 11.3 Annual and Lifetime Rate of Suicide[a] Among Outpatient–Treated Alcoholics: Intermediate Rate Countries

Reference	N	Years Follow-Up	Person-Years	Suicides
Choi (1975), United States	863	1.5	1,294	2
Hyman (1976), United States	48	15	720	2
Martin et al. (1985a, b), United States	67	12	804	4
Schmidt & deLint (1972), Canada	6,478	7.5	48,585	51
*Lambie et al. (1983), New Zealand	1,068	1.5	1,602	4
	8,524		52,305	63

[a]63 suicides ÷ 52,305 person-years × 100 = 0.120% annual rate; 0.120% × 19 years = 2.29% lifetime risk.
*Newly included study.
Note: Expanded from Table 3, in G. E. Murphy and R. D. Wetzel. The Lifetime Risk of Suicide in Alcoholism. *Arch. Gen. Psychiatry,* 1990, *47*:385. Copyright 1990, American Medical Association.

Table 11.4 Annual and Lifetime Risk of Suicide[a] for Alcoholics Identified by Inpatient Treatment: Intermediate Rate Countries

Reference	N	Years Follow-Up	Person-Years	Suicides
U.S. Studies				
Prout et al. (1950)	85♂	4.5[b]	382	1
Selzer & Holloway (1957)	86	6	516	1
Hastings (1958)	23	8[b]	184	1
Tashiro & Lipscomb (1963)	1,692	3[b]	5,076	6
Pokorny et al. (1968)	101♂	1	101	0
Schuckit & Winokur (1972)	45♀	3	136	0
Schuckit & Gunderson (1974)	4,755♂	3.5	16,642	16
Costello & Schneider (1974)	400	6[b]	2,400	3
Polich et al. (1981)	781♂	4	3,124	13
Smith et al. (1983)	100♀	11.5[b]	1,150	2
Combs-Orme et al. (1983) (2 references)	1,289	7.5[b]	9,668	10
*Barr et al. (1984)	456	2	912	6
*Ornstein & Cherepon (1985)	1,210♂	2	2,420	3
*Mackenzie et al. (1986)	79♂	8	632	4
Non-U.S. Intermediate Rate Countries				
Davies et al. (1956), United Kingdom	50	2	100	1
Kessel & Grossman (1961), United Kingdom	218	6*	1,308	11
Rathod et al. (1966), United Kingdom	105♂	2	210	2
Dubourg (1969), United Kingdom	76♂	1.75	133	1
Nicholls et al. (1974), United Kingdom	865	12.5	10,812	46
deLint & Levinson (1975), Canada	143	5	715	3
Thorarinsson (1979), Iceland	2,863♂	13*	37,219	45
*Wells & Walker (1990), New Zealand	616	9*	5,544	3
Total	16,047		99,384	178

[a]178 suicides ÷ 99,384 person-years × 100 = 0.179% annual rate; 0.179% × 19 years = 3.40% lifetime risk.
[b]Mean duration of follow-up.
*Identifies a newly included study.
Note: Expanded from Table 4, in G. E. Murphy and R. D. Wetzel. The Lifetime Risk of Suicide in Alcoholism. *Arch. Gen. Psychiatry*, 1990, 47:385. Copyright 1990, American Medical Association.

rate in Sweden is not materially different from that in the United States. We will assume the same for the other countries included.

No studies of untreated populations were found. Dahlgren's very large follow-up of Swedish males known to the Temperance Board of the province of Malmöhus (Table 11.5) includes "not only institutional cases, but all the individuals who have come before a Temperance Board, warned, superintended or treated in an institution" (1951, p. 298). By no means have all alcoholics admitted for treatment been reported to the Temperance Board, and only a minority of those reported are hospitalized. This rather mixed group resembles outpatients more than inpatients.

Little if any treatment was afforded the alcoholic probands in Öjesjö's (1981) longitudinal population study of Lundby, Sweden (Hagnell & Öjesjö, 1975), or those in Fremming's study of the population on the Danish island of Bornholm (1951). Both are general population surveys. Nielsen, Juul, and Munk-Jorgensen (1987) report a

Table 11.5 Annual and Lifetime Risk of Suicide[a] in Less-Than-Inpatient–Treated Alcoholics: Scandinavian/European

Reference	N	Years Follow-Up	Person-Years	Suicides
Dahlgren (1951), Sweden	10,588	4.5[b]	47,646	63
Öjesjö (1981), Sweden	96	15	1,440	3
Fremming (1951), Denmark	61	36	2,196	2
*Nielsen et al. (1987), Denmark	408	6.7[b]	2,724	18
Total	11,153		51,006	86

[a]86 suicides ÷ 51,006 person-years × 100 = 0.169% annual rate; 0.141% × 19 years = 3.20% lifetime risk.
[b]Mean duration of follow-up.
*Identifies a newly included study.
Note: Expanded from Table 5, in G. E. Murphy and R. D. Wetzel. The Lifetime Risk of Suicide in Alcoholism. *Arch. Gen. Psychiatry,* 1990, *47:*386. Copyright 1990, American Medical Association.

follow-up of two Danish samples of alcoholics receiving outpatient treatment that was missed in the earlier publication. The annual suicide rate for alcoholics in these four studies (Table 11.5) comes to 0.169%. Assuming that our 19 years at risk holds for Europe and Scandinavia, the lifetime risk is 3.20%, nearly 50% higher than that for nonhospitalized alcoholics from countries with intermediate suicide rates. The population is a mixed one. It may cautiously be considered to represent nonhospitalized Scandinavian/European alcoholics.

To the six Scandinavian and European follow-up studies of inpatient treated alcoholics is added a study from South Africa (whites) (Gillis, 1969), which also has a high suicide rate (Table 11.6). The annual suicide rate of alcoholics is calculated as 0.284%, with a lifetime risk of 5.3%.[2] This is one and one-half times that for countries with intermediate and low suicide rates. It is also more than one and one-half times the comparable risk for nonhospitalized Scandinavian/European alcoholics.

Countries with Low Suicide Risk

Only one follow-up study of an outpatient treated sample of alcoholics was found from a low suicide rate country (van Dijk & van Dijk-Koffeman, 1973). Small as the population is—200 males followed up after 4 years—it yields a satisfactory result (Table 11.7). The annual rate of suicide was 0.125% and the lifetime risk 2.38%, very close to that found for intermediate rate countries (2.29%).

Inpatient treated alcoholics in low suicide rate countries yield an annual suicide rate of 0.179% and a lifetime risk of 3.4% (Table 11.8). The risk rates for these countries are virtually the same as those calculated from comparable studies in countries with intermediate suicide rates. Perhaps there is a lower limit to lifetime risk of suicide in alcoholics, regardless of the population's suicide rate. Alternatively, both hospital admission and outpatient treatment may be less easily achieved in relatively poor countries, thus selecting for greater severity. In any event, the results rest heavily on a single small outpatient study and on a large inpatient study (Sundby, 1967), albeit a careful one.

Table 11.6 Annual and Lifetime Risk of Suicide[a] in Inpatient–Treated Alcoholics: Scandinavian/European

Reference	N	Years Follow-Up	Person-Years	Suicides
Gabriel (1935), Austria	1,109	7[b]	7,763	30
*Lesch et al. (1986), Austria	444	5.5[b]	2,442	13
Ellerman (1948), Denmark	159	5[b]	795	1
Nørvig & Nielsen (1956), Denmark	181	4	724	15
Wieser & Kunad (1965), West Germany	153	10[b]	1,530	13
Ciompi & Eisert (1969), Switzerland	1,386	30	41,580	98
Gillis (1969), South Africa	802	3.5[b]	2,807	11
Salum (1972), Sweden	1,005	7.5[b]	7,538	33
Lindelius et al. (1974), Sweden	257	7.5[b]	1,918	10
Medhus (1975), Sweden	83♂	9	747	4
Dahlgren & Myrhed (1977), Sweden	200	9[b]	1,800	4
Berglund (1984), Sweden	1,312	20.5[b]	26,896	88
*Lindberg & Ågren (1988), Sweden	4,872	11.5[b]	56,028	119
Total	6,717		158,470	439

[a]439 suicides ÷ 158,470 person-years × 100 = 0.277% annual rate; 0.277% × 19 years = 5.26% lifetime risk.
[b]Mean duration of follow-up.
*Identifies a newly included study.
Note: Expanded from Table 6, in G. E. Murphy and R. D. Wetzel. The Lifetime Risk of Suicide in Alcoholism. *Arch. Gen. Psychiatry,* 1990, 47:386. Copyright 1990, American Medical Association.

Japan

Three recent reports from Japan of substantial size and duration present an irresistible opportunity to extend the present methodology to the Far East. Higuchi (1987) followed up 272 women and 281 men admitted for treatment of alcoholism in Tokyo. Ohara et al. (1989) learned of 257 deaths in a mean interval of about 6 years since discharge of 1,021 patients from an alcoholism treatment ward in Hamamatsu. Nunomura, Shingae, Ikeda, Ohta, and Miyagishi (1989) conducted a 1- 12½-year followup of 1,195 alcoholics admitted to Sapporo Ohta Hospital for treatment of alcoholism. Table 11.9 shows an annual suicide rate of 0.215% and a lifetime risk of 4.09% for the Japanese. This falls midway between the rates of the high suicide rate countries and the others.

Table 11.7 Annual and Lifetime Risk of Suicide[a] in Outpatient–Treated Alcoholics: Low Suicide Rate Countries

Reference	N	Years Follow-Up	Person-Years	Suicides
van Dijk/van Dijk-Koffeman (1973), Netherlands	200	4	800	1

[a]1 suicide ÷ 800 person-years × 100 = 0.125% annual rate; 0.125% × 19 years = 2.38% lifetime risk.

LIFETIME RISK OF SUICIDE IN ALCOHOLISM

Table 11.8 Annual and Lifetime Risk of Suicide[a] in Inpatient–Treated Alcoholics: Low Suicide Rate Countries

Reference	N	Years Follow-Up	Person-Years	Suicides
*O'Sullivan et al. (1988), Ireland	300	1	300	0[b]
Sundby (1967), Norway	1,693	29.5[c]	34,951[d]	65
Bratfos (1974), Norway	478	10	4,780	1
Haver (1986), Norway	55♀	6.5[c]	358	2
Vallance (1965), Scotland	68	2	136	2
Beaubrun (1967), Trinidad	45	7	315	3
Total	2,857		40,840	73

[a] 73 suicides ÷ 40,840 person-years × 100 = 0.179% annual rate; 0.179% × 19 years = 3.4% lifetime risk.
[b] S. K. O'Sullivan, personal communication, February 22, 1989.
[c] Mean duration of follow-up.
[d] Author's figure.
*Newly included study.
Note: Expanded from Table 7, in G. E. Murphy and R. D. Wetzel. The Lifetime Risk of Suicide in Alcoholism. *Arch. Gen. Psychiatry*, 1990, 47:386. Copyright 1990, American Medical Association.

Table 11.10 organizes these calculations by level of treatment and suicide rate categories. The data base is quite extended, both temporally and geographically. The results of the calculations show a satisfyingly logical progression. Rather than a single suicide risk for all alcoholics everywhere, these figures reflect both a progressive risk with increasing evidence of psychopathology and a differential rate for countries with high versus those with medium and low suicide rates. It is clear that earlier risk estimates are both conceptually unsound and mathematically untenable. It is also clear that the risk of suicide in alcoholics is a function of the culture in which they live.

Table 11.9 Lifetime Risk of Suicide[a] in Inpatient–Treated Alcoholics: Japan

Reference	Source	N	Years Follow-Up	Person-Years	Suicides
*Higuchi (1987), Japan	Hospital admission for alcoholism treatment	553[b]	6.5[c]	3,594	11
*Ohara et al. (1989), Japan	Alcoholism treatment ward discharge	988[b]	6[c](?)	5,928	14
*Nunomura et al. (1989), Japan	Hospital admission for alcoholism treatment	1,195	6.4[c]	7,648	12
Total		2,736		17,170	37

[a] 37 suicides ÷ 17,170 person-years × 100 = 0.215% annual rate; 0.215% × 19 years = 4.09% lifetime risk of suicide.
[b] Recalculated data base.
[c] Mean follow-up, years.
*Newly identified study.

Table 11.10 Summary of Calculated Lifetime Risk of Suicide by Treatment Status and Background Suicide Rate

	High Suicide Rate Countries (%)	Intermediate Suicide Rate Countries (%)	Low Suicide Rate Countries (%)	Japan (%)
No treatment		1.85		
Outpatient treatment	3.20	2.29	2.38	
Inpatient treatment	5.26	3.40	3.4	4.09

PROBLEMS WITH RECENT PREVALENCE ESTIMATES

The National Council on Alcoholism (NCA) estimates 10.5 million alcoholics in the United States. This figure was calculated by Williams et al. (1987) based on a 1979 NIAAA survey reported by Clark and Midanik (1982). The criteria are essentially those of DSM-III. This method will produce an overestimate of the prevalence of the disorder (Fillmore & Midanik, 1984).

The Epidemiologic Catchment Area (ECA) Study (Regier et al., 1984), conducted between 1980 and 1982, concluded that a mean of 13.5% of the population aged 18 years and older surveyed in five ECA sites had suffered, on a lifetime basis, from alcohol abuse/dependency disorders according to DSM-III criteria (Robins et al., 1988, Table 1, p. 17). The U.S. population 18 years and above was 162,790,845 in 1980 (United States Department of Commerce, 1985). The ECA prevalence figure of 13.5% produces an estimate of 21,977,000 alcoholics, more than double the already inflated figure of the National Council on Alcoholism (1987).[3]

ALCOHOLICS AT RISK OF SUICIDE

Having demonstrated the untenability of even the lower of these two estimates, we now approximate the population of alcohol abusers at risk for suicide, using the figure of 25% of suicides attributable to alcoholics. Twenty-five percent of the 30,407 officially identified suicides for the year 1988 equals 7,600 such deaths. We found that roughly one-third of our 50 alcoholic suicides had a history of inpatient treatment (Murphy et al., 1979). One-third of the 7,600 alcoholic suicides (7,600 ÷ 3 = 2,534) divided by the annual rate of suicide calculated for previously hospitalized alcoholics from Table 11.6 (0.179%) yields an estimate of 1,415,643 hospital-treated alcoholics. The remaining two-thirds of the alcoholic suicides (7,600 − 2,534 = 5,066) divided by the annual suicide rate for nonadmitted alcoholics calculated for untreated plus outpatient treated subjects from Tables 11.2 and 11.3 (0.112%) gives an estimated 4,515,333 nonadmitted alcoholics. The total, 5,930,975, would be roughly *the number of alcoholics in the population at some risk of suicide*. This figure is little more than half as large as the NCA (1987) estimate of the prevalence of alcoholism.

Not All Alcohol Abuse Is Alcoholism

In two longitudinal samples, Fillmore et al. (1979) found a much higher remission rate from alcohol abuse in a 4-year follow-up of men aged 21 to 29 at intake than among men 40 to 49 at index examination. Their data indicate a high prevalence of abusive drinking among younger men, which is likely to diminish markedly over time. Paradoxically, the likelihood of abandonment of this behavior was greater among those reporting higher levels of alcohol consumption and attendant problems. This finding is echoed by Vaillant and Milofsky (1982). In their long follow-up, young male alcohol abusers who later achieved sustained abstinence were significantly more likely to have shown alcohol dependence than had those who continued to drink (χ^2 with Yates's correction = 10.76; $P < 0.01$ [present author's calculation].)

In contrast to the high levels of chronicity of alcohol abuse in those who come to treatment, Helzer, Burnam & McEvoy, (1991) found in the ECA follow-up study remission rates in the neighborhood of 50% for both blacks and whites, males and females identified as ever having met DSM-III criteria for alcoholism. Remission was defined as no alcohol problems in the past year. Lifetime prevalence rates of alcoholism were significantly higher in those under 45 (both men and women) than in those older. Remissions accumulate linearly, starting at 36% in the youngest age group of males, and have doubled by age 65 and older. The young who might be identified as alcoholic in a population survey withdraw increasingly from that category. Mostly, they do so without coming to professional attention (Vaillant & Milofsky, 1982; Helzer et al, 1991).

Addictive drinkers among the young are shown to have a substantially higher remission rate than do mere abusers of alcohol (Fillmore et al., 1979; Vaillant & Milofsky, 1982), so the core group that will contribute to suicide is not readily identifiable early. But if half of the untreated (or minimally treated) alcoholics remit, then the lifetime risk of suicide in the remainder is not greatly different from that of treated alcoholics.

These studies show in part why the earlier numbers don't work. A period of alcohol abuse not meeting conservative diagnostic criteria is a poor predictor of longitudinal course. On the other hand, Guze et al. (1988) showed that 84% of a group of alcoholics diagnosed by conservative criteria (Feighner et al., 1972) would still be so diagnosed 6–12 years later by raters blind to the initial diagnosis. Thus conservative diagnosis, requiring both a syndrome and a substantial number and variety of symptoms, better defines the population at risk of suicide. These or similar criteria were used to diagnose alcoholic suicides in our two studies (Robins, Murphy, et al., 1959; Murphy et al., 1979; Robins, 1981).

COMORBIDITY AS A RISK FACTOR

Survey Data

Psychiatric comorbidity—one disorder complicating or complicated by another—is just now receiving serious attention. Comorbidity with alcohol abuse is common. Helzer and Pryzbeck (1988) report that 47% of alcohol abusers identified in the ECA study had a second diagnosis and that alcoholism was particularly likely to coexist with other diagnoses. The strongest associations were with other substance abuse (men, 19%; women, 31%) and antisocial personality disorder (men, 15%, women, 10%). Major depression was one and one-half times more frequent in alcoholics than in nonalcoholics. It was found in 5% of the male and 19% of the female alcoholics. Psychopathic or antisocial personalities are prominently mentioned in association with alcoholism (Fremming, 1951; Helgason, 1964; Vallance, 1965; Kendell & Staton, 1966; Ciompi & Eisert, 1969; Dubourg, 1969; Berglund, 1984; Ross, Glaser, & Germanson, 1988).

Complicating depression plays a crucial role in the suicide of alcoholics, as discussed more fully in Chapters 8 and 9. Other substance abuse is seen more frequently now than in the past. It shortens the career from onset of substance abuse to suicide, regardless of which comes first (Rich et al., 1989, Table 4). When the less common contributors to suicide are considered, such as antisocial or other personality disorders and Briquet's Hysteria (Feighner et al., 1972), alcoholism or other substance abuse is almost invariably present as well (Robins, 1981, pp. 347–348; Rich et al., 1989, p. 80; Runeson, 1990, p. 563). Thus we may say that *suicide in alcoholism is largely dependent on the supervention of a depressive episode, whereas in the personality disorders suicide is conditioned upon substance abuse* (and possibly depression as well).

THE MEANING OF LIFETIME RISK OF SUICIDE IN ALCOHOLISM

Based on our calculations regarding *untreated* alcoholics, one could say that their lifetime risk of suicide (1.85%) is only slightly higher than that in the general population (1.3%). But we know that the greatest part of the general population is not at risk at all. Fewer than 5%—perhaps 1–3% of suicides—are not identifiably psychiatrically ill (Robins, Murphy et al., 1959; Dorpat & Ripley, 1960; Barraclough et al., 1974; Beskow, 1979; Hagnell & Rorsman, 1979; Chynoweth, Tonge, & Armstrong, 1980). Even the sometimes overinclusive DSM-III diagnoses of the ECA data do not identify above one-third of the population age 18 and older as having a psychiatric illness in their lifetime. Excepting simple phobias, which have not been shown to contribute to suicide, less than 25% of the population was identified as *ever* affected (Robins et al., 1984), whereas nearly all of the deaths by suicide are in the psychiatrically ill population.

Allowing that 5% of suicides are not psychiatrically ill, that group would account for $0.05 \times 30,407$ suicides (for 1988) = 1,520 suicides not accounted for by the psychiatrically ill. Seventy-five percent of the U.S. population, by ECA estimate, comprises the "not psychiatrically ill." This percentage of the 1988 U.S. population age 18 and over amounts to 136 million persons (0.75×182 million) (United States Department of Health and Human Services, 1990). The annual suicide rate for that population is then 1,520 nonpsychiatrically ill suicides $\div$ 136,000,000 = 0.0000111, or 0.00111%. We estimate 25% of the 30,407 suicides to have been alcoholics: 7,602 alcoholic suicides.

Taking our calculated 5,930,975 conservatively diagnosed alcoholics at risk, the ratio is $0.00128 \div 0.0000111 = 115$. Alcoholics as a whole are seen to have 115 times the suicide risk of the nonpsychiatrically ill population. This is a clearly conservative estimate compared to our risk calculations for hospital-treated alcoholics. A 3.4% lifetime risk of suicide sounds small, but that group would be at roughly 300 times greater risk than the nonill population.

The alcoholic who becomes truly abstinent is probably protected from suicide to a great extent, at least so far as the role of alcoholism itself is concerned. Unfortunately, only 1 study out of the 56 found with pertinent data addresses this question with adequate methodology (Gabriel, 1935). It suggests that that is the case. The protection is not perfect, however, as an occasional case shows (Vallance, 1965; Rathod, Gregory, Blows, & Thomas, 1966). In our studies (Robins, Murphy, et al., 1959; Murphy et al., 1979; Robins, 1981), all but 3 diagnosed alcoholics were recently active abusers of alcohol with current problems from it. A small number had stopped drinking for a few days before their suicide. It appeared in general that a severe depressive episode was the cause of not drinking, rather than abstinence having been decided upon.

ALCOHOLICS AT GREATEST RISK

Suicide risk is not uniform across all inebriates, or at all times in any of them. It is certainly higher in conservatively diagnosed alcoholics (Feighner et al., 1972) than in the broader group of DSM-III alcohol abusers. Risk varies curvilinearly with age, the peak period being in the 40s, and directly with duration and severity of alcohol abuse. It is greatly increased by the supervention of a depressive episode, social isolation, and loss of emotional support, as well as by medical illness, unemployment, and continued drinking. Finally, it has been shown (Murphy & Robins, 1967) and replicated (Murphy et al., 1979; Rich et al., 1988) that disruption of a major interpersonal relationship signals a period of heightened risk of suicide in the alcoholic.

12

Some Final Thoughts on the Final Act

RISK FACTORS FOR SUICIDE

Following the well–replicated finding of recent loss of a close interpersonal relationship as a predictor of suicide in alcoholics (Murphy & Robins, 1967; Murphy et al., 1979; Rich et al., 1988), this more detailed study of the data collected for that replication (Murphy et al., 1979) has helped us gain a better understanding of why the loss had such a forceful impact. It had nearly always occurred in a setting of diminished or absent social support. A last link to others had failed, generally as a consequence of the alcoholic's heedless disregard for its value to him or her. But it wasn't the lack of social support alone that sealed the alcoholic's doom. There was an accumulation of other, more chronic concerns. Some were more, some less directly traceable to the long-established habit of alcohol abuse. Most importantly, the habit continued. Serious physical illness, social isolation (living alone), unemployment or underemployment, and psychiatric comorbidity, especially major depressive disorder, reduced the quality of life. Suicide was not a new idea to many of these individuals. Thoughts of that nature had previously been voiced by all but a few. Nor were they often of recent origin. But it wasn't only those with a recent loss who were so afflicted; these same historical and behavioral features characterized the remaining three–quarters of the alcoholic suicides just as strongly.

None of these factors is unexpected in long–term alcoholics. In contrast to interpersonal loss, they were rarely acute. But occurring in numbers, particularly four or more, they sharply distinguish alcoholic suicides from living alcoholics. These data suggest to the clinician a numerical approach to suicide risk assessment. Simply counting the number of specified risk factors that have accumulated will show how far the patient has moved from the norm of living alcoholics to that of the suicides. I believe this is a substantial new contribution to the assessment of suicidal risk. The recognition of the supervention of a depressive syndrome on the alcoholism provides the best and most imperative motivation to clinical action.

IS SUICIDE AN IMPULSIVE ACT?

Various authors have suggested that because alcohol is a disinhibiting substance, acute intoxication releases the latent self-destructive drive, resulting in impulsive suicide. The often unstated implication is that in the absence of acute intoxication, these suicides would not have occurred (Welte, Abel, & Wieczorek, 1988). In 10 of my cases the interval between the presumed precipitant and the suicide was a matter of only a few hours. Some prior communication of suicidal thinking had been reported in 6 of these cases. Another subject has spoken of having no hope and of being a burden, but not of suicide as such. In 2 cases the *only* suicidal communication had occurred within hours of the fatal act. They are not considered to have had earlier thoughts of that nature. Thus the final act usually had a historical substrate. On the other hand, communication had not been as recent as within a week in half of the cases. Some light may be shed on the question of impulsivity by review of the 10 cases with acute precipitation.

Subject 3 was drunk when his wife took their children and left. She came back with the police to try to get him into the hospital, but she was unsuccessful. After she left, he talked with both his aunt and his psychiatrist on the telephone before taking his life. In the last year he had spoken several times of killing himself, but only when drunk. His blood alcohol concentration was 0.09 g%, just below the legally defined level of intoxication, and below what he probably achieved daily..

Subject 9 was drinking heavily; he was argumentative, and flourishing a revolver. After visiting his ex–wife. he returned home, still waving the pistol. His wife locked him out until he put it out of sight. Later he became enraged over her food preparation and emptied the pistol at her. Out of ammunition, he went out and bought more, lay down beside her and shot himself. Alcohol may have released his hostility, but he had plenty of time to reflect on the choice of suicide. He had spoken increasingly of it in the last few months of his life.

Subject 18 was out of money and out of a job, but our poorly informed informant did not know of his having symptoms of depression. He shot himself shortly after having been brought home drunk from a tavern. As he was only visiting St. Louis to look for work, his having a pistol with him raises a question of premeditation. He was not reported to have spoken of suicide in the last 2 years.

Subject 22 had threatened suicide 1 or 2 days before he did it, in reference to his belief that his wife was having an affair. Drunk, he argued with her over food preparation and choked her. She left overnight, returning the next day to find him dead. How immediately after her leaving he ended his life is unknown. The act was clearly precipitated by her leaving. His BAC was 0.30 g%—very intoxicated.

Subject 24 was already quite depressed. He found he couldn't get money he needed from his wife. Several days later he was found dead. Toxicology wasn't performed, as no blood could be obtained. Whether he was drinking is unknown. In the last 2 months he had spoken of "no hope" and of being a burden, but not specifically of suicide.

Subject 26 had been jailed overnight after a drunken assault on his daughter. He was sober in the morning when his wife told him to pack his things and go. Packing, he drank an entire bottle of whiskey, then shot himself. He had several hours to reflect on the implications of his wife's rejection. Three weeks earlier he had described to his priest a specific suicide plan, but not the one he followed.

Subject 36, suffering from multiple myeloma, failed to get favorable news from his doctor that morning. Later, during an argument with his wife over a trivial matter, he broke it off and shot himself. His BAC was 0.21 g%. He had talked openly of suicide at least weekly for many months; he had openly stated he would not die in a hospital bed but would shoot himself. Perhaps the alcohol did release him to do it, but not without reason or forethought.

Subject 38 had been drinking heavily most of the day. He became loud and threatening in the late evening and his wife had him jailed. There, he hung himself. He had at least some hours to reflect on his abrupt loss of status. His BAC was 0.201 g%. There was no record of prior direct mention of suicide.

Subject 39 had crippling emphysema. He left work early and drank. When he returned home, his wife remonstrated with him. He went and got a gun and shot himself. His BAC was 0.21 g%. There had been no prior communication of suicidal thoughts that we learned of.

Subject 40, brain damaged and unemployable, lost his little money at the liquor store and was rebuffed by the clerk. He opened a blood vessel in his wrist with his pocket knife and quietly exsanguinated on the front steps of the boarding house where he had lived for many years. Was he drunk? Probably no more than usual. Toxicology was not done. He had made mention of cutting his throat on a number of occasions when drunk.

Subject 47, a mildly retarded, schizophrenic black woman, took her life on the same day her brother was shot and killed. On hearing the news, she became agitated and continued in that state for many hours. She then spoke of "joining" her brother. After drinking to the point of intoxication (BAC 0.12 g%), she went to her lover's office in his home, where she knew there was a pistol, and shot herself. (The family's view was that she went there for solace and was killed by the man or his wife.) Planning had obviously occurred over several hours. The significance of a medically trivial suicide attempt 2 weeks earlier is obscure.

Of these and the remaining cases, I see only the acts of Numbers 39 and 40 as truly impulsive. That of Subject 24 may have been. Only Subject 40 was without a recent buildup of disturbing events. Based on careful study of this series and the 32 alcoholics in Robins's study, I conclude that suicide in alcoholics is not often impulsive. It is the culmination of an accumulation of negative circumstances, not just a matter of being drunk. In adults generally, suicide is a planned act; warning may or may not be given. In adolescents, it may be impulsive, but data are meagre.

IS SUICIDE AN AMBIVALENT ACT?

The British psychiatrist Erwin Stengel held a prominent place in the study and discussion of suicide in the middle years of this century. He is generally credited with pointing out the separate but overlapping characteristics of suicide attempters and suicides

(Stengel, 1960). He strongly asserted the belief that every suicide is an ambivalent act:

> Uncertainty of outcome is not a contamination of the genuine suicidal act, but rather one of its inherent qualities. (Stengel, 1973, p. 78)

To further emphasize the point, he says:

> If determination to achieve a fatal outcome was the main criterion of suicidal and homicidal acts, only a few would qualify. (p. 79)

This opinion would not be worth mentioning were it not that it seems to have acquired a certain currency. That some indecision precedes self-destruction is clearly evidenced by the fairly long time span over which suicides have communicated their suicidal thoughts before the final act. Terminating one's existence is such a weighty matter that it could hardly be otherwise. As clinicians, we receive reports from our patients of "gambling with death"—usually taking hands off the steering wheel while driving at high speed. Such events are not rare in the course of depression. They may not be all that rare in youth, with their characteristic delusion of invulnerability. But when one studies actual suicides, one can hardly fail to be impressed by the highly purposive way in which most of these acts are carried out.[1] There is nearly always evidence of planning: choosing the method, usually one with little chance of failure, securing the means, ensuring against interruption. Little or nothing is left to chance. Clearly, ambivalence has been resolved, not set aside. Suicides have *wanted* to die—or to cease to live, which comes to the same thing.

Persons suffering from a major depression commonly develop a nihilistic perception of the future. It looks bleak or "black" to them. Things will never get better, or will surely get worse. This is a state of hopelessness, and it is very dangerous (Beck, Steer, Kovacs, & Garrison, 1985). Not every depression reaches that point, but if it does, and if the depression remits rather than suicide ending it, any subsequent depression is likely to be attended by hopelessness as well (Beck, Brown, Berchick, Stewart, & Steer, 1990).

Alcoholics, too, may have the perception that the future is hopeless. To a large extent, it is a manifestation of a depressive syndrome that has supervened. To some alcoholics, the future appears not hopeless, but intolerable. In light of what has already occurred, it may be a fairly realistic perception—given their seeming inability to quit drinking. But the hopelessness and the intolerability are reversible cognitive assessments. The clinician's job is to reverse those assessments—not by argument, but by treating the illness that gave rise to them.

PERSONALITY DISORDER AND SUICIDE

Two Scandinavian studies have identified "personality disorders" (PD) as contributing to suicide. Beskow (1979) made a principal diagnosis of PD in 7% of his 271 male suicides. More recently, Runeson and Beskow (1990) diagnosed borderline personality disorder (BPD) in 16 of 58 consecutive suicides between the ages of 15 and 29 years. All but 2 were in association with substance abuse/dependence, antisocial personality disorder (ASPD), and/or major depression. Personality disorders are being diagnosed with increasing frequency since the introduction of criteria for these diagnoses—particularly BPD—in DSM-III (APA, 1980).

I am highly skeptical of the "personality" diagnoses,[2] apart from the well-established antisocial personality disorder. BPD has not been shown to follow a characteristic course over a number of years of follow-up. Other diagnoses emerge: major depressive disorder, bipolar affective disorder, schizophrenia, ASPD, substance abuse disorders, even no psychiatric diagnosis (McGlashan, 1983; Pope, Jonas, Hudson, Cohen, & Gunderson, 1983). What this means, in plain terms, is that the diagnosis of BPD does not entail a prognosis. The outcome on follow-up is quite varied. Lacking both a demonstrated construct validity and predictive validity for a diagnosis of BPD, I think the most meaningful diagnosis that can be made in the presence of a clinical picture suggestive of BPD is that of the other, better established diagnosis that is present in all but a small minority of cases. That diagnosis is adequate to account for all or nearly all of the observed symptoms. Familiarity with the protean manifestations of major depressive disorder will clarify much of it.[3]

PSYCHOACTIVE SUBSTANCE ABUSE AND SUICIDE

Rich et al. (1986, 1988) found a much higher frequency of polysubstance abuse among their suicides than had previously been seen. Alcoholism was infrequently found alone; it was commonly associated with abuse of other psychoactive substances. Such comorbidity was much more common in younger than in older suicides, suggesting a temporal trend. Although it is tempting to dismiss this association as a California phenomenon or one of U.S. coastal cities more generally, polysubstance abuse does appear to be increasing across the nation. A recent Minnesota study of alcoholism in twins (Pickens et al., 1991) with mean age of onset between 22 and 28 years ($\pm$ 10 to 11.6 years) found a lifetime history of other drug abuse and/or dependence in 39% to 48%. The ECA study found other substance abuse associated with alcoholism in 28% of living men aged 18–29 years and in 7% of those aged 30–59 years (Robins et al., 1988). This is undoubtedly a growing trend.

The comorbidity of alcohol and other substance abuse in Rich's cases appeared to shorten by about one-third the interval between first abuse and suicide as compared to uncomplicated alcohol abusers in Rich's study. Might we therefore expect to see substance abuse increase its proportional contribution to the suicide rate? A nonsignificant increase is found in the Rich et al. series. Conservatively diagnosed substance abuse was identified in 29% of their cases (Rich et al., 1989, Table 4), compared to a mean of 25% for most of the earlier studies. Whether this marks a general trend or simply random variation remains to be seen. The prevalence of depressive disorders is also on the increase (Klerman et al., 1985), but so far, suicide is not. Its alarming rise among the young in the 1960s and 1970s (Murphy & Wetzel, 1980) has slowed, and the birth cohorts affected early have not carried an increased risk into later decades (Wetzel, Reich, Murphy, Province, & Miller, 1987).

The similarity of the psychodynamics among various sorts of substance abusers is attested to by the identical impact of recent loss (Rich et al., 1988). Risk factors identified in the alcoholics in this book may therefore be expected to be generalizable

SOME FINAL THOUGHTS ON THE FINAL ACT

to those with polysubstance abuse. Clinical management, however, may prove to be increasingly difficult, at least until the nature and mechanism of substance abuse/addiction is better understood.

THE FUTURE

Psychopathophysiology of Addiction/Dependence

It is usually the case that understanding the pathophysiology of a disorder leads rapidly to effective clinical management. Psychopathophysiology will more nearly cover the substance abuse problem. We don't seem to be much nearer to it, but who can predict when the breakthrough will come or what it may tell us? The pursuit of that goal is certainly important.

Replication of the Present Work

Replication and possible extension of the findings and conclusions presented here would be most welcome. Follow-up of the living alcoholics used as comparison populations in Chapter 10 might prove interesting. A simple search through the state's death records would not be particularly revealing, however, as those records do not contain the necessary data—the medicopsychosocial status of the suicides *at the time of their death*. For that, nothing short of personal interview with surviving family members will suffice. Were I still engaged in academia, that would be my next step. There are other suitable data bases in existence and to come, however, and other investigators to recheck the conclusions. It is always important to replicate promising findings.

Physician Education

We already know a good deal about suicide that can be used to prevent its occurrence. There can be little doubt that that knowledge is in daily use. But the roughly 50% of suicides who have had recent physician contact shows that it isn't used enough. They have usually been underdiagnosed and undertreated (Barraclough et al., 1974; Murphy, 1975). The work of Rutz et al. (1989) demonstrates that physician education focused on recognition and treatment of depressive disorders can make a positive difference in physician awareness and response, *and thus save lives*. Given the role of depression in the suicide of alcoholics, it can be expected to make a difference there as well.

FINALLY

An investigation such as this one, seeking to identify common factors in suicide, is inevitably reductionist. Subtleties are ignored in favor of more broadly defined issues. Each suicide is unique and highly personal, but much like others in a broader view. The mounting problems of these alcoholics are shared with the living. It is easier to say why these men and women took their lives than to explain why many more did not. I like to ask prominent psychiatrists why they think so *few* do it. One responded, "It's against nature." Of course it is, or there would be few of us left. A more satisfying response was that of Dr. Alex Pokorny: "I think it's a behavior that isn't psychologically available to everyone" (personal communication).

What makes that behavior "available"? I think of "releasors". A family history of suicide is one such. Although only 20% of our suicides were reported to have had a family history of suicide, Mitterauer (1990) has shown that information from a single informant is likely to greatly underestimate the true rate. This same author has presented compelling evidence that it isn't simply inheritance of high risk psychiatric disorders. But whether there is a "suicide gene" as a releasor or simply behavioral "permission" remains to be discovered. Lacking a family history of suicide, one can hardly grow to maturity without knowing of someone taking his or her life. How that information is taken in might be critical. (Case 21 is illustrative.)

A history of a prior suicide attempt entails a lifetime risk of subsequent suicide, around 12% (Dahlgren, 1977). Apparently, a willingness to imperil one's life in that particular way may persist. In assessing suicidal risk, the clinician would be well advised to ask not only about current and past ideation and family history, but also about the patient's attitude toward suicide, the circumstances under which he/she would consider it, the basis for that thinking, and reasons to *not* do it. It is my clinical impression that citing negative impact on others shows connectedness and is strongly protective. The low level of connectedness in the present sample of suicides is in keeping with that view.

APPENDIX A

DSM-III-R Diagnostic Criteria

CRITERIA FOR PSYCHOACTIVE SUBSTANCE DEPENDENCE

A. At least three of the following:
   (1) substance often taken in larger amounts or over a longer period than the person intended.
   (2) persistent desire or one or more unsuccessful efforts to cut down or control substance use.
   (3) a great deal of time spent in activities necessary to get the substance (e.g., theft), taking the substance (e.g., chain smoking), or recovering from its effects.
   (4) frequent intoxication or withdrawal symptoms when expected to fulfill major role obligations at work, school, or home (e.g., does not go to work because hung over, goes to school or work "high," intoxicated while taking care of his or her children), or when substance use is physically hazardous (e.g., drives when intoxicated).
   (5) important social, occupational, or recreational activities given up or reduced because of substance use.
   (6) continued substance use despite knowledge of having a persistent or recurrent social, psychological, or physical problem that is caused or exacerbated by the use of the substance (e.g., keeps using heroin despite family arguments about it, cocaine-induced depression, or having an ulcer made worse by drinking).
   (7) marked tolerance: need for markedly increased amounts of the substance (i.e., at least a 50% increase) in order to achieve intoxication or desired effect, or markedly diminished effect with continued use of the same amount.

   NOTE: The following items may not apply to cannabis, hallucinogens, or phencyclidine (PCP):
   (8) characteristic withdrawal symptoms.
   (9) substance often taken to relieve or avoid withdrawal symptoms.
B. Some symptoms of the disturbance have persisted for at least one month, or have occurred repeatedly over a longer period of time.

American Psychiatric Association. *Diagnostic and Statistical Manual of Mental Disorders, third edition, revised.* Washington, DC. Copyright 1987, American Psychiatric Association.

CRITERIA FOR PSYCHOACTIVE SUBSTANCE ABUSE

A. A maladaptive pattern of psychoactive substance use indicated by at least one of the following:
   (1) continued use despite knowledge of having a persistent or recurrent social, occupational, psychological, or physical problem that is caused or exacerbated by use of the psychoactive substance.
   (2) recurrent use in situations in which use is physically hazardous (e.g., driving while intoxicated).
B. Some symptoms of the disturbance have persisted for at least one month, or have occurred repeatedly over a longer period of time.
C. Never met the criteria for Psychoactive Substance Dependence for this substance.

APPENDIX B

Suicide Interview

Code No.: _____

Name _____
               Last   First   Middle

Maiden name _____

Address _____

      How long lived there? _____

Phone _____ Did S have telephone where he last lived? _____

Place of exam _____

Examiner _____ Birthplace _____

Date of exam _____ Age _____

Time of exam _____ Birthdate _____

Date of act _____ Sex _____

Date of death _____ Marital state _____

Date of inquest _____ Religion _____

Coroners No. City _____ Race _____

              County _____ Note _____ To whom _____

Parent Name   Parents Address and Phone

_____

Father's birthplace: U.S. ____ Foreign ____ Mother's birthplace: U.S. ____ Foreign ____

Father's occupation _____ Mother's occupation _____

_____

Children's Names (2 or 3)	Children's Address

Spouse's Name _____

Spouse's Address and Phone _____

Whom was patient living with? (Description of household)

Name	Age	Sex	Relation to patient
_____			
_____			
_____			
_____			
_____			
_____			
_____			

Address and Telephone (If different than that above given for patient) _____

_____

Was this his usual living arrangement _____ or a change _____ ?

If change, how recent? _____

Reason _____

_____ Did he take his meals there? How many meals a day? _____

_____ Did he sleep there?

Relatives (3) (Local relatives or those he saw most often)

Name	Relation	Address
_____		
_____		
_____		

Informant's name _____

Informant's address _____

Relationship to patient _____

SUICIDE INTERVIEW

How often did you see him? _____

How long had you known him? _____

The Act

Tell me about what happened (Probe)

Why do you think he did this? (Probe)

What have others said about why he did this?

_____ Did you have an idea something was the matter with him?
What was it? (Probe)

_____ Did he think he was ill?
What did he think the illness was?

_____ Was he under a doctor's care?

    Doctor's name _____ M.D. or D.O. _____

    Where located _____

    Type of practice (i.e., medical, psychiatric, etc.) _____

When had he last seen a doctor?

    _____ Same day

    _____ < one week

    _____ < one month

    _____ < three months

    _____ < six months

    _____ < one year

    _____ how much longer

Why did he go to the doctor (specific complaint or diagnosis—Get details!)

_____ Had he seen any other doctor in the past year? (Get same information as above)

_____ Did he try to get help in any other way?

_____ Had he ever seen a psychiatrist or someone else for nervous trouble?
    (Get same information as above)

_____ When did this present trouble begin? (months)

_____ Was he like his usual self just before this time?

SUICIDE INTERVIEW

Was this trouble entirely new for him or was it a worsening of the way he generally was?

_____ Entirely new

_____ Recurrence after being well

_____ Worsening

_____ Can't tell

_____ Informant denies any trouble

Did he talk to anyone about (dates)

_____ 1. Committing suicide

_____ 2. Say he would be better off dead

_____ 3. Wanting to die

_____ 4. Refer to methods of committing suicide

_____ 5. Make dire predictions—what _____

_____ 6. Say that informant (or family) would be better off if he were dead

_____ 7. Refer to dying before or with spouse

_____ 8. Talk about putting affairs in order

_____ 9. Other _____

To whom did he talk about these things? (Get details for each, including verbatim statements)

Over what period of time?

At any time in the year preceding his death would you say or did someone else say he was

_____ 1. Depressed

_____ 2. Disgusted with self

_____ 3. Disgusted with the world

_____ 4. Felt worthless

_____ 5. Blamed himself unduly for his own or family's troubles

_____ 6. Angry

_____ 7. Spiteful

_____ 8. Frustrated in a love relationship

_____ 9. Felt he was a burden

_____ 10. Felt neglected

_____ 11. Was this an attempt to force attention to himself or his illness?

In the year preceding his death, did he: (Note if informant or examiner believes it was important in relation to suicide.)

	When occurred
_____ 1. Have any job trouble? (Fired, quit, demoted, lower income, or promoted, higher pay, more responsibility)	
_____ 2. Lose someone close to him by death? (Spouse, parent, sib, close friend—describe closeness and effect)	
_____ 3. Become divorced?	
_____ 4. Become separated? (When, why, which one left?)	
_____ 5. Have marital friction short of separation? (Fights, infidelity, unwanted or illegitimate pregnancy)	
_____ 6. Fight with parent, other close relative? Become estranged?	
_____ 7. Have serious financial trouble? In debt? (Describe)	

SUICIDE INTERVIEW   265

| | When occurred |

_____ 8. Have trouble with the law?

_____ 9. Hurt or kill anyone?

_____ 10. Sue anyone or get sued?

_____ 11. Have to change his living arrangements?

_____ 12. Think he was about to lose someone or something important to him? (Separation threatened, serious illness, etc.)

   Was it a realistic fear?

_____ 13. Live alone or in an institution?

_____ 14. Have a feeling of disgrace or shame?

_____ 15. Make a suicide attempt?

_____ 16. Have a physical illness?

_____ 17. Have any other kind of trouble? (Describe)

Was he ever in a hospital? (If yes, get details then ask about other hospitalizations)

Date	Name of hospital	Place	Reason	Type of hosp. (S, M, P)

_____ Previous suicide attempts of patient (Fill in number)

When	How	Why

_____ Did he ever have a nervous breakdown? (Details)

_____ If yes, did he recover?

SUICIDE INTERVIEW

FAMILY DISEASE

	Relation (Blood relation only)	Inclusive dates	Treatment
____ Nervous breakdown			
____ Alcohol			
____ Mental hospital			
____ Nervous			
____ Like patient's			

Suicides in family (Method, date, illness like patient's) (If this had happened would you have known?)

	Successful	Attempt
____ Father		
____ Mother		
____ Brother		
____ Sister		
____ Grandparent		
____ Uncle		
____ Aunt		
____ Child		
____ Spouse		
____ Friend or other close person		

Symptoms (Find out if only in relation to drinking or if chronic)

	Date began	Before present episode	Part present episode
___ Dyspnea			
___ Palpitation			
___ Chest pain			
___ Dizziness			
___ Headache			
___ Anxiety attacks (apprehension, impending death, palpitation, shortness of breath, weakness, trembling)			
___ Fatigue			
___ Visual blurring			
___ Crowd trouble			
___ High-strung			
___ Cry easily			
___ Feelings hurt easily			
___ Moody person			
___ Sensitive person			
___ Always sickly (majority of life)			
___ Outbursts of rage			
___ Did he read or talk about suicides or accidental deaths or other violent deaths			
___ Did he try to avoid hearing about or seeing violence in any form—either in the papers, movies, or TV			
___ Fears (heights, streets, dark public conveyances, leaving home)			

SUICIDE INTERVIEW

	Date began	Before present episode	Part present episode
___ Obsessions (injure someone)			
___ Compulsions (handwashing, locks, gas)			
___ Preoccupation (with any subject)			

Now in the past few days, weeks, or months did any of these occur or had he ever had them before this?

                                                    When

___ Weight loss

___ Anorexia

___ Insomnia

___ Fatigue

___ Constipation

___ Inertia

___ Indecision

___ Loss of interest

___ Joylessness

___ Sadness

___ Reduction in sex drive

Diminished social relationships

   ___ See friends less

   ___ Less movies

   ___ Less TV

When

____ Less cards

____ Less sports

____ Less reading

____ Job disability (housework, family care)

____ Generally less active

____ Looked depressed

Delusions (Summary)

____ Sin

____ Guilt

____ Worthlessness

____ Somatic

____ Poverty

____ Did he have any ideas you considered unusual for him or that you considered mistaken even though he wouldn't admit his mistake?

____ Did he believe he had committed some sin?

____ Did he believe he was worthless or no good?

____ Did he believe he was bad for his family and they would be better off without him?

____ Did he believe he had lost most or all of his money?

____ Did he worry about being poverty-stricken?

____ Did he believe he had lost his memory?

____ Did he fear he was losing his mind?

____ Hallucinations (complain of voices calling him bad names or saying he was not good)

SUICIDE INTERVIEW

<u>When</u>

____ Statement of being sad

____ Statement of black future (without hope, nothing good will ever happen again, etc.)

____ Statement of being guilty

____ Statement of being no good

____ Suicidal ideas

____ Statement of being in the way or a burden

____ Had he ever had a nervous breakdown that was in any way similar to this?

____ Did he seem to have any trouble thinking?

____ Did he talk less?

____ Did he have any thoughts out of the ordinary?

____ Did he believe somebody was deliberately annoying him, trying to scare him, or was after him?

____ Did he believe someone was trying to harm him?

____ Did he believe someone was trying to kill him?

____ Had he talked about or acted as though he felt like hurting someone?

____ Had he threatened someone?

____ Had he talked about or acted as though he felt like killing someone?

____ Had he ever killed anyone or tried to?

____ Had he thrown something at a person?

____ Did he behave strangely in any way?

____ Had his memory gotten poor?

<u>When</u>

____ Did he know the date?

____ Could he find his way around by himself?

____ Did you trust him out of the house without a companion?

____ Could he read and understand things as well as ever?

____ Did he have any difficulties with simple arithmetic, such as having trouble making change?

____ Any other symptoms?

____ I know that most people find it hard to talk about their sex life, but since this may be very important, I would like to know if you knew anything about his sex life that may have disturbed him or led to his suicide.

School History

____ Grade reached

____ Truancy

____ Fighting

____ Expulsion

____ Suspension

Homes

____ Length of time in St. Louis or St. Louis County (Years)

SUICIDE INTERVIEW

Current or Most Recent Occupation

_____ Kind of job held (be specific). (If S was a housewife get this information from husband or son or father)

Name of Company _____

Address _____

Phone _____

Work History—Past 10 years
(For most recent jobs and for jobs in past two years be sure to get exact income)

Week	Month	Year
a. less than 60	less than 250	less than 2,999
b. 60–99	250–399	3,000–4,999
c. 100–149	400–599	5,000–7,499
d. 150–199	600–799	7,500–9,999
e. 200–299	800–1,199	10,000–14,999
f. more than 300	more than 1,200	more than 15,000

Date	Job	Where	Income	Why left

_____ Any income from pensions? (How long and how much)

_____ Any income from compensation—VA, job, due to injury or illness? (How long and how much)

_____ Most money ever made?

_____ If unemployed at time of suicide, what was usual source of support?

_____ In general, did he do okay on his jobs?

_____ Did he ever drift from job to job? When?

___ Was he ever fired? How many times?

___ Did he ever quit a job because of difficulties with boss or fellow employees? How many times?

    ___ (Did she ever have to stop taking care of children and house? How many times?)

___ Did he ever neglect his children?

___ Total number of jobs

___ Total length of working life

___ Was he ever not working for a long period of time (more than 6 months) for any reason—illness, didn't want to work, couldn't find a job? How many times? How long each time?

Date	Reason

Marital History

Current marital status
___ Married   ___ Bigamy

___ Divorced

___ Separated

___ Legal separation

___ Desert

___ Widow

___ Never married

___ Common law

SUICIDE INTERVIEW

Marriage No.	Inclusive Date	How ended	Reason for incompatibility: difficulties in present marriage if married and living with spouse

___ Have there been separations in this current marriage?
Details:

Children; Stepchildren; Foster Children

Rank	Sex	Marriage No.	Date of birth	Date of death	Date permanently left home	Why left home

Parental Home (Fill in age of patient)

	Time	Mother	Father
___ Divorced			
___ Separated (time)			
___ Died			
___ Jailed (time)			
___ Physical illness (time)			
___ Mental illness (time)			
___ Alcoholism			

____ Was he brought up in a foster home? (Dates)

____ Was he brought up in an institution such as an orphanage? (Dates)

____ Was he brought up by relatives or friends? (Dates)

Alcohol

____ Did he ever drink?
How often: Daily ____ ; Less than daily but more than weekends ____ ;
Weekends only ____ ; Benders only ____ .

____ Did his family every object to his drinking?

____ Did anyone else tell him he was drinking more than was good for him?

____ Did he ever get into trouble at work because of drinking? (fired, late, warned)

____ Did he ever have trouble with auto driving (speeding, accident, etc.) because of drinking?

____ Was he ever arrested, even for a few hours, because of drinking and/or peace disturbance?

____ Did he ever get in fights while drinking?

____ Did he ever go on benders? (Forty-eight hours of drinking associated with default of obligations.)

____ Did he ever drink before breakfast?

____ Did he think he drank too much?

____ Did he feel guilty about his drinking?

____ Did you think he drank too much for his own good?

____ Did he ever lose friends on account of drinking?

____ Did he ever want to stop drinking and couldn't?

____ During the past 6 weeks, did he drink more than usual? ____
                                         less than usual? ____

____ During the past 6 months, did he drink more than usual? ____
                                         less than usual? ____

SUICIDE INTERVIEW

____ How much did he drink each day (or each week)? (Amt./time period)

____ Did he ever have DTs, shakes, liver trouble, fits on account of drinking?

____ Drinking at time of suicide?

____ At what age did he start heavy drinking?

____ Were there times in his life when he did not drink at all?

If so, when did he stop? (age or dates) _____

When did he start again? _____

Evaluation of alcoholic status:

    ____ Chronic alcoholic
    ____ Heavy drinker
    ____ Mild drinker (Normal social drinking)
    ____ Teetotaler

Arrests

____ Did he ever have trouble with the police?

____ Was he ever in reform school?

	Date	Sentence	Time served	Where
____ Was he ever arrested for traffic violation				
____ Drinking				
____ Disturbing the peace				
____ Fighting				
____ Robbery				
____ Burglary				
____ Forgery				
____ Other				

Drugs

____ Did he take drugs for sleeping?

____ Every night?

____ During the day?

____ Was he ever addicted to dope?

____ Did he ever want to stop taking drugs and could not?

____ Did he think he took too many drugs?

____ Did you think he took too many drugs?

Evaluation of drug status:

____ Addict
____ Took too many
____ Took occasionally
____ None

Military

____ Dates in service?

____ Overseas, combat, decorations?

____ Kind of discharge?

____ Ever court martialed in service?

Social Life

____ Would his friends come to his house?
____ Would he go to their houses?
____ Both
____ Other (Describe)

____ How many really close friends did he have?

Where did he have the main part of his social life?

____ His home
____ Friends' homes
____ Relatives' homes
____ Bar or tavern

SUICIDE INTERVIEW 279

____ With fellow employees after work
____ Church
____ No social life

Home

____ Number of rooms (identify and list every room, including bathrooms)

____ Own own home (Age of home)

____ Rent home or apartment (Amount of rent)

____ Roomer

____ Institution

____ Live with relatives or friends

Summary

    ____ Living alone in house
    ____ Living alone in apartment
    ____ Living alone in room
    ____ Living with friends
    ____ Living with relatives, including siblings
    ____ Living with spouse
    ____ Living in an institution
    ____ Living with parents or children

Condition of home

    ____ Good
    ____ Fair
    ____ Poor

____ Census tract of residential neighborhood

____ From what you say there was no reason for suicide and yet there must be a reason? (Probe)

Reliability of Informant

    ____ Very
    ____ OK
    ____ Questionable

Other Informants

No.	Name	Address and Phone	Relation to Patient	How Close per week	How Close per month	How Long (years)

Information:

Present illness, including previous episodes of same illness, if any, in prose:

SUICIDE INTERVIEW

Diagnosis:

    ____ 1. Primary affective disorder, depressed

    ____ 2. Primary affective disorder, manic

    ____ 3. Schizophrenia

    ____ 4. Chronic brain syndrome

    ____ 5. Toxic psychosis

    ____ 6. Mental deficiency

    ____ 7. Alcoholism

    ____ 8. Drug addiction

    ____ 9. Homosexuality

    ____ 10. Anxiety reaction

    ____ 11. Hysteria

    ____ 12. Obsessive-compulsive reaction

    ____ 13. Sociopathic personality

    ____ 14. Undiagnosed psychiatrically ill

    ____ 15. Undiagnosed, don't know if sick or well

    ____ 16. Criminality   ____ a. Secondary depression

    ____ 17. No disease

Degree of confidence

    ____ Very
    ____ Moderate
    ____ Slight

Glossary

Affective disorder: Depressive disorder; can include mania, manic-depressive disorder.
Agitation: Marked restlessness, inability to sit still or remain in one place. The opposite behavioral pole of psychomotor retardation.
Anorexia: Loss or lack of appetite.
Anxiolytic: Antianxiety medication.
Bipolar: Manic-depressive disorder. Mood changes from high to low or the reverse. About one-fifth as common as unipolar or simply depressive disorder.
Comorbidity: The simultaneous occurrence of two or more psychiatric illnesses—such as alcoholism and depression. One is said to complicate the other.
Delirium: Clouding of consciousness severe enough to affect perceptions of reality. Hallucinations (usually visual) are likely to occur and are often frightening. Judgment is severely impaired, and acts are "senseless."
Diabetes mellitus: The medical term for what is commonly known simply as diabetes.
Dyspnea: Shortness of breath; difficulty breathing.
Emphysema: *See* Pulmonary emphysema
Endogenomorphic: Having the *form* of an endogenous depression. The distinction between endogenous (arising from within) and reactive (externally provoked) depressions has not proved to identify discrete groups of patients. The "endogenous," or melancholic, symptoms of marked lack of pleasure (anhedonia), feeling worse in the morning, early morning awakening, psychomotor agitation or retardation, significant anorexia or weight loss, and absence of premorbid personality disturbance have been found to define severity, not etiology.
Hematemesis: Vomiting blood.
Hepatocellular disease: Hepatic (liver) cirrhosis. Scarring and shrinkage of the liver with impaired function, usually resulting from prolonged abuse of alcohol. Exposure to toxic chemicals as well as viral hepatitis also can produce this result.
Melena: Blood in the stools (much more serious than bleeding hemorrhoids, but usually painless).
Ménière's syndrome: An affliction of the inner ear causing vertigo (dizziness), nausea, vomiting, and ringing in the ears. May be episodic.
Mental status exam: A systematic approach to assessing intellectual functioning. It includes observation and testing of mental content, flow of thought and speech, orientation as to date and place, hallucinations, delusions, mood, ability to calculate, recall, reason, repeat test words, insight and judgment. Both testing and recording the results are properly part of any psychiatric assessment.
Organic brain syndrome: The result of structural damage to the brain, whether gross or mi-

croscopic. Impairment of memory and of recall are the most common early signs. With further damage, orientation and judgment as well as calculating ability and reality testing are affected. Acute intoxication affects mental functioning in these ways and is reversible as the intoxicant is metabolized and/or excreted. What we are concerned with here is the chronic form, which can result from chronic alcohol abuse, other toxins, certain metabolic, infectious and degenerative processes, or head injury.

Organic mood syndrome: The symptoms of major depression sometimes arise on the basis of an organic brain syndrome, but more often without it. When there is evidence of organic brain dysfunction, the source of an ensuing depression is uncertain.

Pathophysiology: The physiology or mechanism underlying the pathology—essentially how a disease produced its effects.

Pneumothorax: Air in the chest outside of the lung. It may result from a perforating wound of the chest wall or of the lung, and greatly reduces the expansion of the lung.

Proband: A subject in a study, also referred to in the scientific literature, especially the Germanic and the Scandinavian as a *propositus*. I use the term sometimes to distinguish my experimental subjects, the suicides of this study, from the living subjects with whom I am comparing them.

Psychomotor retardation: An involuntary slowing down of nearly all biological—including mental—functioning, occurring in some severe depressions. The psychomotor-retarded individual speaks slowly, moves slowly, thinks and responds slowly, and may be virtually immobile for long periods of time.

Psychopathophysiology: The impact of the psyche or mental processes on the disease picture.

Pulmonary emphysema: A degenerative disorder of the lungs in which the walls of the tiny air sacs break down, reducing effective surface for gas exchange. Oxygen exchange is gradually and irretrievably lost. Tobacco smoking is a major cause.

Semi-comatose: Responsive to painful stimuli but not to verbal stimuli. Next step is coma—complete unconsciousness.

Notes

Chapter 2

1. The first study of a large number of consecutive suicides from a sociological as well as a diagnostic standpoint was that of Robins and his associates (Robins, Gassner, et al., 1959; Robins, Murphy, et al., 1959; Robins,1981). All deaths in the City of St. Louis and St. Louis County between May 15, 1956, and May 15, 1957, that were ruled suicide by the respective coroners were systematically investigated by personal interview. There were 134 such deaths in that time period. Data were gathered by means of a prepared interview, following a printed protocol to ensure that the same questions were asked of each respondent. In 119 cases a primary interview was obtained with a close relative or friend of the victim. In 13 cases relatives refused to be interviewed and 2 suicides were transients in St. Louis. Additional interviews were obtained with other relatives, friends, job associates, landladies, bartenders, policemen, and personal physicians for a total of 305 interviews, averaging over 2 hours in length. Ancillary interviews were obtained concerning all of the 15 persons for whom a primary informant was unavailable. Police records, social service records, and hospital records were sought and examined as well. The interview protocol is reproduced as Appendix B. The point at issue here is that 23% of the total sample and 28% of those given a specific psychiatric diagnosis or none were diagnosed as suffering from chronic alcoholism. Three suicides were apparently clinically well.

2. In a similar study, Dorpat and Ripley (1960, 1962) investigated 114 consecutive suicides in King County (greater Seattle), Washington, between July 1, 1957, and July 1, 1958. No knowledgeable informant was available in 6 of the 114 cases, so the diagnostic distribution was based on 108 cases. Diagnostic criteria were unstated. The authors diagnosed alcoholism in 27% of their sample. Thirty percent were considered to have been suffering either from "psychotic depression" or "psychoneurotic depression." A surprisingly high 12% were given a diagnosis of schizophrenia. Sixteen percent were thought to be psychiatrically ill but could not be further diagnosed. The authors state: "Not one patient was found to have been without psychiatric illness" (1960, p. 353).

Palola, Dorpat, and Larson (1962), referring to the same King County study, diagnosed 34 (31%) of the suicides as alcoholic. Specified criteria for a diagnosis of alcoholism were having at least three of the following items: "(a) considering a morning drink to be a necessity; (b) staying drunk on workdays; (c) neglecting food in favor of drinking; (d) needing more alcohol to achieve the same effect; (e) feeling anxious about having enough to drink; (f) feeling indifferent to brand or type of beverage alcohol; (g) sneaking drinks; (h) solitary drinking; (i) protecting alcohol supply; (j) drinking non-beverage alcohol." These criteria identified a few more suicides as alcoholic than was done by Dorpat and Ripley (1960) earlier. Inasmuch as the Palola et al. reference is rarely cited and not widely available, I have retained the figure of the original report for reference.

3. Barraclough, Bunch, Nelson, and Sainsbury (1974), employing a systematic interview based on ours, investigated 100 coroner-ascertained suicides among residents of the County of West Sussex and the County Borough of Portsmouth, U.K. Twenty-five suicides occurring in West Sussex in 1966 and 1967 comprised a pilot sample and 75 consecutive suicides occurring in both areas in 1968 completed the series. Clinical diagnosis was by consensus of three psychiatrists independently reviewing the records. The authors made a principal diagnosis of depression in 70 cases (70%), of alcoholism in 15%, and of schizophrenia in 3%. Seven victims were judged not mentally ill, although one of them had a history of a previous suicide attempt and previous psychiatric treatment.

Although diagnostic criteria for alcoholism were not explicitly stated, descriptions of the symptoms, behaviors, and problems of those diagnosed alcoholic strongly suggest that they would readily meet current DSM-III-R criteria. Conducted in an area of southern England favored by retired persons, the population tends to be skewed in an elderly direction. This fact probably accounts for the higher proportion of diagnoses of depressive disorder and the lower proportion with alcoholism in comparison with the other studies reviewed here.

4. Jin-Inn Teoh (1974) studied 30 cases of suicide occurring in the Kuala Lumpur district of Malaysia in 1972. Investigation was by personal interview conducted with surviving relatives in the home of the deceased shortly after the death. There were 20 males with a median age of 35 years, and 10 females, median age 29.5 years. Ages of the suicides ranged from 14 to 83. In that ethnically mixed country, Chinese contributed most, 11 males and 8 females. Ten East Indians (9 male) and one Sikh completed the 30 cases. One Malay suicided during this period, but he was from Malacca and no relatives were available. The ethnic distribution of the suicides is similar to that for the period of 1965–1970, but the ethnic makeup of Kuala Lumpur is not given. Suicide rates differ a good deal from one ethnic group to another in West Malaysia. For 1970, these rates were 23.3/100,000 Indians, 8.1/100,000 Chinese, 1.1/100,000 Malays, and 14.4/100,000 others. Islamic religion (Malays) was suggested as protective. Being poor, single, and male characterized nearly half of the suicides.

This exotic study reached the conclusion that only 14 (47%) of the 30 suicides were due to mental illness—a wide departure from Western findings. The 14 "mentally ill suicides" were diagnosed as follows: schizophrenia, 5 cases; endogenous depression, 5 cases; chronic alcoholic, 4 cases; and chronic anxiety neurosis, 1 case. I suspect that a differently oriented investigation would have yielded a much higher prevalence of psychiatric disorder, although a similar figure of 35.5% with psychiatric illness was reported by Chia and Tsoi (1972) for Singapore. Ethnicity, religion, culture, and perhaps local psychiatric assumptions as well, make the findings incommensurable with the other studies cited here.

5. Taking the view that the suicide *pattern* in women is different from that in men, Beskow (1979) elected to study only suicides in males in Sweden, part urban, part rural. The urban population studied was "a systematic two-thirds sample" of "all male Swedish citizens, 15 years of age or more, who were registered in the city of Stockholm including 'inner suburbs,'" who died between April 15, 1970, and April 14, 1971. The rural population "consisted of all male Swedish citizens, 15 years of age or more, registered in three counties in the north of Sweden," who died between January 1, 1970, and December 31, 1971, and were officially classified as suicides. The total sample comprised 271 suicides, 161 urban and 110 rural. The interview, conducted with relatives, was semistructured and open-ended. Supplementary information was sought from employers, other informants, and official sources as well. Diagnosis was hierarchical: "The syndrome which over the years dominated the mental disorder was given priority. . . . Addictive alcoholism and drug dependency had priority over the other disorders. Paranoid-schizophrenic and psycho-organic syndromes had priority over affective. Affective

syndromes had priority over neurotic syndromes, personality disorder and crisis reactions" (p. 77–78).

Alcoholism was diagnosed in 39% of urban and 18% of rural male suicides, 31% overall. When drug dependence is added to these, a total of 37% of the Swedish male suicides were diagnosed as substance abusers. Affective disorders accounted for 20% of the suicides among urban males and 38% of those among rural suicides, for a combined figure of 28%. Allowing for comorbidity, the total proportion of depressive syndromes was 45% in both the urban and rural samples. The proportion of alcoholics identified as having a concomitant depressive syndrome was also 45%. Personality disorder was the principal diagnosis in 7%.

The reader must keep in mind that this was an all-male population. Alcoholism rates, and probably other substance abuse rates as well, are always higher in men than in women in the Western world. Despite this, Beskow's figures are somewhat diluted by the two-fifths of his total sample that were drawn from rural areas where alcoholism and other substance abuse appear to have been substantially less prevalent.

6. In a 25-year follow-up of an entire Swedish community's population, "The Lundby Project," Hagnell and Rorsman (1979) found 28 suicides, 23 among men and 5 among women. Suicides represented 5.8% of the deaths among men and 1.5% of the deaths of women. Alcoholism was found as an antecedent to suicide in 18% of cases, depression in 50%. The incidence of alcoholism among the suicides was double that found in an age- and sex-matched control group twice the size of the suicide group and in a group of 25 persons from the same study population who died nonviolent deaths at ages matched to the suicides. Diagnoses in this study, particularly those of a chronic nature, may be considered reliable, in that each of the subjects had been personally interviewed by psychiatrists on one or two previous occasions (Öjesjö & Hagnell, 1980).

7. Chynoweth, Tonge, and Armstrong (1980) interviewed relatives and/or close friends of a consecutive series of 135 suicides occurring in Brisbane, Australia, between March 1, 1973, and February 28, 1974. Multiple sources of information were used. The interview schedule was based on that used by Barraclough et al. (1974), which, in turn, owed much to the pioneering study of Robins (1981). Of the 135 suicides, 44 (33%) were identified as suffering primarily from a depressive illness. The second group, 34 subjects, was characterized as "physically ill" on the basis that they "had been attending for treatment of a physical disorder within a year of death and/or postmortem [examination] revealed clear evidence of organic disease." In this group, 17 subjects were additionally found to have been suffering from depression, while 7 were further noted to have drug dependence.

Thirty subjects (22% of the total sample) were identified separately as dependent on drugs or alcohol—23 on alcohol alone, 3 on barbiturates, and 4 on both. Thus 20% were alcohol dependent, with or without other substance abuse. There was some additional diagnostic overlap, so that "for the whole group a depressive disorder was found in 74 (55%), a physical disorder in 70 (52%) and drug [including alcohol] dependency in 46 (34%)." The miscellaneous group included schizophrenia, 4%; personality disorder, 3%; not ill, 2 subjects, including one 12-year-old boy; and "other," 12%. Overall, "thirty-four percent of the men and 33% of the women had been heavy drinkers, whether or not there were any associated problems resulting from the use of alcohol" (Chynoweth et al., 1980, p. 41).

8. Mitterauer (1981) obtained interviews with relatives and/or attending physicians in 94 of 121 suicides occurring in the province of Salzburg, Austria, during 1978. He classified them according to a multidimensional diagnostic system unfamiliar in this country (Berner & Kryspin-Exner, 1977). Diagnoses were made on four dimensions: (1) developmental disorders; (2) abnormal stress reactions; (3) preexisting organismic modification; (4) acute organismic disorders. Comparison with the other studies cited here along conventional diagnostic lines is somewhat problematic. Diagnoses are multiple, rather than hierarchical. However, 30 cases (30.3% of 99 considered adequately investigated) were given a primary diagnosis of chronic alcoholism. Of

these, 28 (93%) were said to have had "a depressive condition" as well. Of 24 alcoholic cases in which the appropriate information was obtained, 17 (70.8%) had suffered loss of a significant other within 6 *months* of the suicide. A figure for the last 6 weeks is not given.

Thirteen individuals were drug dependent in addition to other diagnoses. Twelve cases were given the diagnosis of "cancer phobia" (*Kanzerophobie*), 11 having the additional diagnosis of endogenous depression. In all, it appears that 59 suicides (63%) received a diagnosis of endogenomorphic depression. A diagnosis of schizophrenia was made in 5 cases, "organic psychosyndrome" in 23. Paraphrenia and paranoid "axis syndromes" were diagnosed in 18 cases.

9. Kapamadžija, Biro, and Sovljanski (1982) studied 100 consecutive suicides occurring over a 2-year period in the southern part of the territory of Backa, around the city of Novi Sad, in northeastern Jugoslavia. The population is 86% Serbian and 15% Hungarian, with Hungarians contributing 28% of the suicides, compared to 55% by Serbs. Jugoslavia, overall, has a fairly high rate of suicide; that of the Autonomous Region of Vojvodina is higher. Alcoholism is a national problem of considerable significance.

The investigation combined sociopsychiatric and pathomorphologic analyses with anatomical autopsy. Psychiatric diagnoses were multiple rather than hierarchical, so that 61% of the suicides received a diagnosis of depression and 41% a diagnosis of alcoholism. Criterion symptoms for the diagnosis of depression seem to be similar to those of Feighner et al. (1972), except for guilt and specified duration. Five or more of seven key symptoms seem to authorize a *definite* diagnosis of depression, given in 41% of cases. A definite or probable (four depressive symptoms) diagnosis of depression could be made in 61% of cases. Twenty-three percent of the suicides were alcoholics of the addictive type and 18% nonaddictive, to give the total of 41%. Ten percent received a diagnosis of schizophrenia. Organic brain syndromes were identified in 30%. Comorbidity cannot be assessed from this report.

10. Rich, Young, and Fowler (1986), investigated 204 consecutive suicides in San Diego County, California by the method pioneered by Robins (1981; Robins, Murphy, et al., 1959) commencing in November 1981. This yielded 150 consecutive suicides aged 30 and older and 54 cases under age 30. From that point on, they studied only the consecutive suicides under age 30 until the end of June 1983. By then they had collected 133 consecutive young cases. Retrospective diagnoses were made using DSM-III criteria, which permit multiple diagnoses. Thus although 54% of the young (under 30) suicides and 55% of those older received a diagnosis of alcohol use disorder, it must be borne in mind that the young group received 2.14 diagnoses per person and the older group 1.89 diagnoses per person. Moreover, the DSM-III criteria overdiagnose alcoholism, as demonstrated in Chapter 11.

Using the diagnostic criteria of Feighner et al. (1972), Rich found the proportion of strictly diagnosed alcoholics (with or without drug abuse) to be 29% for both those under 30 and those older; a figure close to the mean (25%) of the earlier studies, Kapamadžija et al. (1982) excepted. (C. L. Rich, personal communication, May 10, 1989).

11. Arató, Demeter, Rihmer, and Somogyi (1988) investigated 200 suicides occurring in Budapest, Hungary, in 1985. They carried out a semistructured interview with "the closest family member or friend" and classified the victims according to Research Diagnostic Criteria (RDC; Spitzer, Endicott, & Robins, 1978). Major depression was diagnosed in 58%, minor depression in 5.5%. Eight percent had chronic alcoholism alone and an additional 12% had both alcoholism and affective disorder. The authors did not attempt to determine which was primary. Schizophrenia was diagnosed in 8% and schizoaffective disorder in 1%. Fourteen percent were considered to have had neither physical nor mental illness, a larger proportion than we or others have found. Physical illness without psychiatric comorbidity was found in 5%, bringing the total without psychiatric illness to 19%!

The diagnosis of affective disorder seems to have been given precedence over at least alcoholism. I have given the alcoholism diagnosis precedence, a choice that the findings in Chapters 8 and 9 justify for present purposes. The suicide rate in Hungary in 1985 was stated to be

47/100,000 persons, nearly four times that in the United States and twice that in Denmark, the second ranking country in this grisly ordering. Such a high rate suggests a degree of social acceptability that may find its reflection in suicides without identifiable psychiatric illness.

12. The most sophisticated retrospective study of a community sample of suicides yet reported is that of Åsgård (1990). He carried out personal interviews with relatives in 93 of the 101 suicides committed by Swedish *women* in Stockholm in 1982. (Åsgård gives his sample size as 104, but 3 cases were not investigated for administrative reasons.) A comparison sample of 159 male suicides, as well as living female and male controls, was similarly studied but not extensively described in this report. Police reports, autopsy reports (102 cases!), toxicological reports (101 cases), and full records of both hospital and outpatient diagnosis and treatment, along with other parish registry data, augmented the interview data base.

These records were reviewed prior to contacting family informants (Åsgård, 1990, p. 26) and undoubtedly sharpened the focus of the inquiry. Psychiatric diagnoses were made according to the RDC of Spitzer et al. (1978) based on the SADS (Schedule for Affective Disorders and Schizophrenia) interview (Spitzer & Endicott, 1975). As with pre-1980 studies, diagnoses are hierarchical, with one diagnosis per patient. For present purposes, diagnoses of the final month seem most pertinent.

Depressive disorder was diagnosed in 59%, with 35% considered "major," 20% "minor," 2% "intermittent," and 2% schizoaffective. A manic disorder was diagnosed in one case, bringing the total with affective disorder to 60%. Schizophrenia was diagnosed in 3%, alcoholism in 7%, drug/narcotic use disorder in 5% (separate from alcoholism), generalized anxiety disorder in 4%, adjustment disorder in 14%, and organic mental disorder in 3%. The author found it impossible to conclude a diagnosis in 5%, not the same as a finding of no psychiatric disorder. He makes the point that adjustment disorder (DSM-III criteria) was diagnosed in the presence of identifiable stress *and the absence of another psychiatric diagnosis* (Åsgård, 1990, p. 27). "On a lifetime basis, 16 [16%] were considered alcoholics but 9 had stopped drinking before suicide" (p. 42). How long before their suicides they had stopped drinking was not stated. Alcoholism is less common in women than in men throughout the world.

13. A recent feature article in the (Little Rock) *Arkansas Gazette* (February 17, 1991) lists principal occupations of the coroners of the state's 75 counties as follows: mortician (32); physician (8; one retired); paramedic/EMS tech (8); funeral director (less training than a mortician) (7); "fulltime coroner" (3); machine operator (2); ambulance service owner, bail bondsman, body shop/wrecker service owner, dentist, foreign-language teacher, grocery store owner, health supply retailer, insurance agent, jeweler and pawnshop/motel operator, nurse, nursing home operator, radio station owner, saw filer, truck stop/care owner, and X-ray technician (1 each). Not for nothing does Arkansas call itself "The Opportunity State."

14. Brent et al. (1987) found the overlooked cases to have been more often by violent means ($P < 0.0001$) with efforts to conceal the activity ($P = 0.0006$) and, paradoxically, to have made a prior statement of suicidal intent ($P < 0.0001$). In all of these respects, they are *like* a majority of adjudicated suicides.

15. In a copyrighted story dated January 13, 1991, investigative reporters Martha Shirk and Bill Smith of the *St. Louis Post-Dispatch* offered the following:

". . . the affable coroner of _____ County and the man responsible for determining the cause of dozens of deaths each year, says it wouldn't be hard to get away with murder in his county.

"Kill your husband or wife, make it look like an accident and buy one of his fanciest caskets, he suggests.

"'What hurt do I do putting someone's body in a nice casket and not asking any questions?,' he said. 'I'm not saying it's happened like that, but it could.'

"_____ , who runs two funeral homes and a real estate business, believes his approach is by no means unusual.

" 'Most of this state's coroners are funeral directors,' he said. " 'I doubt if you're going to raise a lot of hell about a death if you're looking at a $6,000 or $7,000 funeral.' "

With that level of laxity, some suicides are bound to be missed, but not in any systematic way. It would appear that the major underestimation will be of homicide.

Chapter 3

1. We were unable to locate any family or other informant in five instances. In two of these cases, there was no informant found by the coroner's team. Blood alcohol concentration was 0.02 g% in one of these, 0.12 g% in the other. A history of heavy drinking was recorded at inquest in a third case. We would have secured interviews in the two last-mentioned cases if we could have, but no potential informant could be identified. In two further cases it was unclear to me from the records (20 years later) how we concluded alcoholism was not present.

2. Only occasionally did we secure a second primary interview. It was not because we thought additional information might not be helpful (or feared it would be confusing). In the earlier study, I had found both contacting and interviewing the bereaved to grow increasingly difficult, even aversive. I was not certain that the inquiry was necessarily benign in every case. My interviewers were at about the same training level as I had been. As time consuming as each contact was, I did not find it easy to ask these unpaid volunteers to do more.

3. A legitimate question can be raised as to inherent bias in using suicidal thoughts as one of the eight diagnostic criteria for a diagnosis of depressive disorder, given that the entire data base consists of suicides. To minimize that objection, I was careful not to assume prior thoughts based on the outcome. I scored the item positive only when there was a positive interview report specific to that question.

4. Should onset of alcoholism be dated from the first presence of the full set of diagnostic symptoms, from the beginning of daily drinking, of withdrawal symptoms, or of drinking to secure relief? I used five criteria, in roughly hierarchical order, to date onset: date of first social, legal or medical complication; onset of daily drinking; evidence of loss of control; drinking described as a problem; drinking for symptom relief (i.e., to relieve tension or fatigue). Sometimes the informant's knowledge of onset of any of these indices was only approximate. Age of onset of alcoholism was less clear in some cases than in others.

5. In any study of alcoholic suicides to be done in the future, a more detailed inquiry into patterns and changes in patterns of interaction, as well as evidence of closeness or distance from significant others would well repay the effort.

6. Drinking at the time of suicide increased the likelihood of a subject being considered for inclusion. It proved to be a good predictor of alcoholism. Although BAC was determined in only two-thirds of suicides, half of the alcoholic suicides in whom toxicologic studies were performed had a BAC greater than 0.10 g% versus 22% of nonalcoholics studied.

Chapter 4

1. Hasin, Grant, and Endicott (1990) recently reviewed some earlier longitudinal data on a community sample of men, among whom 180 were identified either as alcohol abusers ($N = 71$) or alcohol dependent ($N = 109$). At 4-year follow-up, 24% were still abusers, 30% dependent, and 46% of the abusers were judged remitted. Of the 109 originally dependent, 46% were still so, 15% were judged only abusers, and 39% remitted. The results were taken to indicate that "alcohol abuse often has a course distinct from that of alcohol dependence."

Confounding this conclusion were two important factors. One was that the inquiry, carried out 16 years earlier, had not included all of the current criteria for these two diagnoses. In the face of that lack, the authors chose to apply only to the diagnosis of abuse the criterion of continued use despite problems or danger. This criterion is a *sine qua non* of any definition of pathological substance use. Restricting its application must inevitably have shifted an unknown number of subjects from the dependent to the abuse category. The remission rates are surprisingly high, and one could wish for more detail. Overall, I think the outcome suggests some flow from abuse to dependence, but with no difference in remission rate. The two categories probably simply reflect a difference in severity within a pathological behavior.

2. Cloninger (1987) proposed a serotonin deficit to be implicated in low harm-avoidance and alcohol-seeking behavior (i.e., early onset of abusive drinking).

Buydens-Branchey and associates (Buydens-Branchey, Branchey, & Noumair, 1989; Buydens-Branchey, Branchey, Noumair, & Lieber, 1989) studied levels of blood serotonin and its precursor, tryptophane, in 218 male alcoholic military veterans admitted to a Veterans Administration detoxification unit. Patients with severe medical illness, a recent history of abuse of narcotics or other psychotropic drugs, a diagnosis of schizophrenia, mania, or a preexisting (i.e., primary) depression were excluded. Alcoholics with onset of excessive drinking before age 20 ($N = 66$) were compared to those with later onset ($N = 152$). Early onset alcoholics were three times more likely to have been depressed at the time of investigation ($P < 0.001$), four times as likely to have attempted suicide ($P < 0.001$), and more than twice as likely to have been incarcerated for violent crimes ($P < 0.001$) as those with later onset. Eighty-eight percent of their early onset alcoholics met DSM-III criteria for antisocial personality disorder (ASPD), compared to 25% of those with a later onset alcoholism (Buydens-Branchey, Branchey, & Noumair, 1989). They comment that "the simple variable of age at alcoholism onset has allowed the differentiation of two subgroups of patients who differ markedly in their clinical picture" (p. 230). Buydens-Branchey, Branchey, Noumair, and Lieber (1989) found in a subgroup of their patients that tryptophane, a serotonin precursor, was significantly lower ($P < 0.001$), as was the ratio of tryptophane to competing amino acids (tryptophane ratio) ($P < 0.001$) in those alcoholics who had exhibited the most severe forms of psychopathology (violence and/or depression) compared to those whose behavior was less deviant. These findings appear to support Cloninger's hypothesis, at least in extreme cases. They also suggest areas for further research into the neuropathophysiology of some alcoholics and their families.

Chapter 5

1. Schuckit's group (Irwin, Schuckit, & Smith, 1990) examined Type 1 and Type 2 characteristics versus age of onset in 171 primary alcoholics hospitalized for treatment. They found that age at onset of alcoholism (age at which the subject first met DSM-III criteria for alcohol abuse or dependence) was significantly associated with more severe alcohol and other drug and childhood criminality problem histories, as well as meeting criteria for a diagnosis of antisocial personality, compared to subjects with later onset. These findings were independent of Type 2 score, which failed to discriminate indices of severity. They propose that "the type 2 prototype might represent a separate diagnosis, antisocial personality disorder, and not alcoholism itself" (p. 320). In another study (Schuckit, Irwin, & Mahler, 1990) this group failed to find significant correlations between Type 2 characteristics in fathers with early onset alcoholism and their sons. They came to the same conclusion as their colleagues. It is regrettable that we were unable to confirm a diagnosis of antisocial personality disorder in any of our subjects.

Chapter 8

1. The finding of a preceding affective disorder in 4% of a group of alcoholics is probably well within normal expectation. In Robins's (1981) description of the individual case histories in his 1957 study (Robins, Murphy, et al., 1959), 63 suicides were diagnosed as having a major

depressive disorder, depressed phase. Four of these cases meet our diagnostic criteria for alcoholism and three for probable alcoholism as well. In two additional cases of definite alcoholism, it was uncertain whether the inebriety was primary or secondary in a temporal sense. The choice of primary diagnosis when two or more are present is not always clear-cut either in research or in clinical practice.

2. Even between studies that employ similar diagnostic criteria by virtue of a common tradition (Woodruff, Guze, Clayton, & Carr, 1973; Cadoret & Winokur, 1974; Fowler, Liskow, & Tanna, 1980), the identified prevalence of depression ranges from 12% (Fowler) to 55% (Woodruff). Both source of patients and sample size are relevant to the differences in findings. Ross, Glaser, & Stiasny, (1988) diagnosed major depression in 19% of 260 alcoholic men and 22% of 241 alcoholic women applying for assessment or treatment at a largely outpatient substance abuse clinic. Lifetime rates for major depression were 23% and 28%, respectively. One must not take these data as representing the universe of alcoholics. It is likely that relatively few alcoholics come to treatment in the absence of an affective disorder (Woodruff, Guze, & Clayton, 1973; Robins et al., 1988).

Nakamura, Overall, Hollister, & Radcliffe (1983) identified "at least moderate depressive symptoms" in 22 (25%) of 88 male veteran admissions to an alcohol dependency treatment program. Assessment was by Hamilton Rating Scale for Depression (HRSD; Hamilton, 1960) scores $\geq$ 20, not by clinical diagnostic criteria. Only 4 patients (4.5%) met this criterion after 4 weeks of treatment. Overall, Reilly, Kelley, and Hollister (1985) assessed 73 private patients in an alcohol treatment center. "None received a clinical diagnosis of depression." A score of 55 or greater on Zung's (1965) Self-Rating Depression Scale was considered to represent "depression." Forty-five percent of these patients had Zung scores that high on admission, and only 10% remained that "depressed" after 4 weeks of treatment. It is of interest that the only item of a 32-item Drinking Behavior Inventory that correlated with persistent "depression" was "disruption of close personal relationships."

Brown & Schuckit (1988) found "clinically significant levels of depression" (same criterion as Nakamura et al., 1983) in 42% of 177 male alcoholic veterans of military service on admission to a Veterans Administration Hospital. By the fourth week of their stay, only 6% were scored at or above the same HRSD level. Neither the Zung nor the Hamilton depression scale is properly a diagnostic instrument. They were designed to rate the *severity* of clinically diagnosed depression.

3. Hagnell & Wretmark (1957), Knop & Fischer (1981), and Berglund (1984) have all commented that peptic ulcer disease often antedated the onset of alcoholism. That was true in only one of our five cases (Subject 20). In the present study, peptic ulcer disease does not appear to be an unusual risk factor for suicide. Pulmonary emphysema was as frequent (Table 8.4). Three follow-up studies of patients with a history of duodenal or gastric ulcer have found an excess of suicides among them (Krause, 1963; Westlund, 1963; Viskum, 1975). Krause found a greater proportion of suicides among those who underwent surgical correction than among those treated medically. That difference was not confirmed by Westlund or by Viskum. Alcoholism as a risk factor was not examined separately by any of these authors. Considering only postsurgical ulcer sufferers, Knop and Fischer (1981) found that suicide was more frequent than expected ($P < 0.001$). Psychiatric morbidity also was greater than expected ($P < 0.05$), with alcoholism the most frequent diagnosis ($P < 0.001$). Alcoholism, having been diagnosed in 8.4% of their 1,000 patients, was associated with half (50.7%) of the 67 suicides in their study (p. 350). Berglund (1984) found suicide to have been three times more frequent among alcoholics with a history of peptic ulcer than among those without such a history ($P < 0.001$). He did not find that surgical intervention increased the risk of suicide.

4. In the recent study of Rich et al. polysubstance abuse was found to be more common than abuse of either alcohol or another drug alone. That this is a fairly recent phenomenon is

shown by the relative infrequency of psychoactive substance abuse other than alcohol in their suicides age 40 and older. It was much more often seen in the young group. Non–alcoholic substance abusers showed the same high frequency of recent interpersonal loss as found among the alcoholics. Without knowing the general prevalence of polysubstance abuse, it is difficult to assess its impact on the national suicide rate. Rich et al. (1989) estimate it to be of considerable magnitude. Many things have changed since completion of my study. Among them may be the drug culture, especially that of large coastal cities.

5. It is difficult to know how prevalent suicidal communication is among alcoholics in the community. Whitehead (1972) investigated the presence or absence of suicidal thoughts in 147 male alcoholics recruited from a prison and from inpatient and outpatient venues. While 55 of his subjects (37%) acknowledged having had such thoughts, 92 denied it. Suicidal thinking is thus not found to be characteristic of all alcoholics but is more strongly associated with those who take their lives. The absence of communication on this topic is noninformative, but its presence may signal danger. As a predictor, it helps in identifying those more seriously at risk but is of little *immediate* help, owing to the repetitiveness and chronicity that have characterized the communicative behavior of many of our suicides.

Only 5 of these 50 alcoholic suicides were not known to have communicated suicidal thoughts in any way. In 2 other cases (Numbers 39 and 45) the only reported communication was within minutes to hours of the fatal event. As previously reported (Robins, Gassner, et al., 1959) such communication is characteristically of more than one kind, made to more than one person on more than one occasion. Considering only the 43 with potentially useful communication, 30 (70%) had voiced the specific intent to take their life; 18 (42%) referred to a specific method of suicide. Twenty-four (56%) had stated they would be better off dead; 40% expressed a desire to die. Thirty-seven percent stated that they were a burden or that the family would be better off without them. Six (14%) said they were worthless or not needed; eight (19%) expressed feelings of hopelessness or having nothing to live for. Two put their affairs in order. Eighteen (42%) were reported to have voiced "dire predictions"—oblique references to their intent, understandable only in hindsight. Examples were: "I just wonder what is over on the other side when we leave here" (Subject 27). Subject 9 talked about putting his affairs in order. Subject 37 told his wife, "I can't stand this world." Regarding repainting the interior of the house he said "This is my last big job." Then, to his wife he said, "This is my last night here." It was.

6. In the original material (Dahlgren, 1945), patients with a diagnosis of chronic alcoholism or "psychopathia and abuse of alcohol" comprise 18 of 29 patients (including one woman) in the group "Psychopathias" (Table 29, p. 84). This same group is termed "personality deviations" in the follow-up study (Dahlgren, 1977). There were 3 suicides in this group (no women), representing 16.7% of the alcoholics (Table 5, p. 78). That must mean that all 3 suicides were by alcoholics ($3 \div 18 = 0.167$) and were 12% of the dead ($3 \div 25$). Although 3 of 18 patients is a very small sample on which to rest much confidence, based on all available information, it is probably near to a lifetime risk of suicide in suicide attempters.

7. The substantial family history of suicide in the background of suicide cases has occasioned debate over the question of nature (genes) versus nurture (environment). A role for inheritance has been carved out by twin studies (Haberlandt, 1967) and adoption studies (Schulsinger et al., 1979). An extensive family study of Old Order Amish in Ohio (Egeland and Sussex, 1985) showed suicides almost entirely confined to a small number of families with high genetic loading for affective disorders. This result is consistent with the intuitively satisfactory view that the inherited risk of suicide comes by way of inheritance of the predisposition to affective disorders. Schulsinger's adoption data do not support that mechanism. More recently, Mitterauer (1990) has presented impressive evidence from family history studies of these two phenomena that shows their transmission to be independent of one another. Eight of 10 of my

alcoholic suicides with a known or probable family history of suicide had a diagnosis of major depressive disorder as well. That frequency of depression is not different than for the entire material. The family history data are altogether inadequate for any further study.

Chapter 9

1. In logistic regression analysis, a logistic transformation of the dependent variable is made, which yields the logit or log odds. The multiplicative factor by which the odds increase or decrease with changes in the predictor variables is then determined. The measure of association between the independent variables and the response variable in the analysis is the odds ratio, which is the multiplication factor relating the predictor to the outcome. The computer analysis was conducted using the Catmod Procedure with the maximum likelihood option of personal computer version update 6.04 of the Statistical Analysis System.

2. T is a statistical test of the equality of two means. F is a test of the equality of standard deviations. Both the mean ages and their standard deviations are very different from each other, confirming what is evident by inspection.

Chapter 10

1. The treatment of depression in the presence of alcoholism has not been well studied. The current negative view of the efficacy of tricyclic antidepressants in this application stems from trials of these drugs to influence drinking behavior, not depression as such. One recent study (Mason & Kocsis, 1991) addressed the critical question and found a significant *antidepressant* effect for imipramine in depressed alcoholics. Our present extensive pharmacologic armamentarium must be assumed to offer help. Study after study has shown that the depression leading to suicide has gone unrecognized and untreated (Barraclough, et al., 1971; Murphy, 1975; Mitterauer, 1981; E. Robins, unpublished data). Probably the most important single intervention that will reduce suicides overall is recognition and vigorous treatment of major depression. That this is truly possible has been demonstrated. The findings presented here offer hope that the outcome for alcoholics may be changed in the future.

Chapter 11

1. A larger minority of alcoholic suicides received inpatient treatment (Robins, Murphy, et al., 1959; Murphy & Robins, 1967; Murphy et al., 1979; Robins, 1981) than is found in these surveys of living persons. Of the 33 alcoholic and probable alcoholic suicides described by Robins (1981), 27% had had psychiatric treatment as either inpatients or outpatients. In the present series of 50 alcoholic suicides studied nearly 15 years later (Murphy et al., 1979), 32% had had inpatient psychiatric treatment. While access to treatment is undoubtedly greater today, it appears likely that alcoholics offered outpatient treatment may be less severely afflicted than those admitted to inpatient care.

2. The large follow-up study of Lindberg and Agren (1988) had not been published when the earlier version of this chapter was written for publication in the *Archives of General Psychiatry* (Murphy & Wetzel, 1990). The sample size is more than four-fifths that of the other studies in Table 11.7 combined. It contributes more than one-third of the person-years for the calculation. The risk for that sample alone is quite low (annual risk, 0.212%; lifetime, 4.04%). It brings the calculated annual suicide rate down from 0.326% to 0.284% and the lifetime risk down from 6.2% to 5.4%.

3. In the Epidemiologic Catchment Area (ECA) study (Regier et al., 1984, 1990), the mental health history and status of more than 19,000 persons aged 18 years and older were systematically assessed by interview in five cities across the United States. Between 10.7% and

15.9% of the population in five ECA sites (mean 13.5%) were judged to be suffering from alcohol abuse/dependency disorders according to DSM-III criteria (Robins et al., 1988, Table 1, p. 17). Given the very limited negative consequences of alcohol abuse required to meet DSM-III or DSM-III-R criteria for alcohol abuse disorder, a good case can be made that both the ECA study and the National Council on Alcoholism have substantially overestimated the prevalence of at least clinically relevant alcoholism. How large that overestimate may be is discussed on page 246.

A further datum on the question of overestimation is the fact that alcohol abuse/dependence was diagnosed most frequently of all psychiatric disorders in the age group 18–24 years in two of three ECA sites (St. Louis, Missouri, and New Haven, Connecticut) (Robins et al., 1984, Table 6, p. 955) and ranked behind only drug abuse/dependence and simple phobia (the latter overdiagnosed in all age groups) at the third site (Baltimore, Maryland). Alcohol abuse/dependence was again the leading diagnosis in the age group 25–44 in St. Louis and New Haven, ranking second only to simple phobia in Baltimore. The authors do not comment on this surprising finding.

Within the broader category of substance abuse disorders, the ECA study found 6.6–13.1% to have contacted a mental health specialist within a 6-month period (Shapiro et al., 1984, Table 7, p. 977). These were outpatient contacts only, and no estimate was given of inpatient treatment. It is likely that a large majority of persons meeting current (DSM-III or DSM-III-R) criteria for alcohol abuse disorder never receive formal treatment. In the present series of 50 alcoholics whose suicides occasioned their entry into the study, (Murphy et al., 1979), only 32% had had any psychiatric treatment, either in or out of a hospital. Similarly, of the 33 suicided alcoholics and probable alcoholics described by Robins, only 18% had had treatment (1981, Table 9.2, p. 426). In light of these facts, perhaps a more realistic risk figure can be derived from a more representative sample of alcoholics.

Chapter 12

1. Vehicular deaths are only very rarely investigated as possible suicides, and then only under special sponsorship. Two investigative teams (Pokorny, Smith, & Finch, 1972; Schmidt, Perlin, Townes, Fisher, & Shaffer, 1972) concluded that suicide was the likely mode of death in one out of seven fatal accidents investigated. All four of the adjudged suicides in Pokorny's study had communicated their intent in advance of the act. At least some of those suicides were impulsive, but alcohol was not always a factor. The method had been named in advance in some cases. A contemporaneous psychoanalytic interview study (Tabachnick, 1973) of *survivors* of single vehicle accidents failed to find evidence of significant psychopathology.

Despite the great likelihood that vehicular fatalities hide a proportion of suicides, such fatalities are so numerous that not even the most opulently funded medical examiner's office could afford to search for the suicides among them. The degree to which these suicides are impulsive and the contribution of alcohol to them are likely to remain uncertain.

2. Dahl (1985a, 1985b) carefully reviewed the literature on borderline personality disorder (BPD) and concluded that descriptive validity seems fairly well established. That means that a description has been given of features common to those patients who are given the diagnosis by clinicians. In that sense, it shares a common stance with the more firmly established diagnoses of psychiatry. BPD does not fare as well when it comes to construct validity, i.e., its status as an independent entity. Family studies tend to show no increase over the expected in family history of those with BPD. Moreover, there is a greater than expected family loading of affective disorders, substance use disorders, and, in some studies, antisocial personality disorders (ASPD). Descriptively, too, BPD is not well delineated from affective disorders or ASPD. Most importantly, BPD has not been shown to assort differentially in monozygotic versus dizygotic twins (Torgersen, 1984).

This is not to deny the concept of personality. Unquestionably, each person possesses a personality. Its characteristics are enduring. Common experience teaches us that fairly reliable predictions can be made regarding certain behavioral responses of a known individual, based on past experience. Past behavior may also predict future behavior in the short term in a patient diagnosed as having BPD. What has not been shown is that such behaviors are commonly enduring—except in those having another diagnosis, such as ASPD, substance abuse disorder, or major depressive disorder, to which those behaviors are attributable.

3. My most recent experience with BPD was with a 22-year-old man who, given that diagnosis, had spent 2 years at a high-profile eastern hospital specializing in intensive psychodynamic psychotherapy. Unimproved, the family out of money, he came to our psychiatric clinic where he met DSM-III-R diagnostic criteria for BPD as well as those of major depressive disorder. We cured him of his BPD symptoms in 2 weeks with a monoamine oxidase inhibitor (MAOI).

References

American Psychiatric Association. (1980). *Diagnostic and statistical manual of mental disorders*, (3rd ed.). Washington, DC: Author.

American Psychiatric Association. (1987). *Diagnostic and statistical manual of mental disorders. DSM-III-R* (3rd ed., rev.). Washington, DC: Author.

Arató, M., Demeter, E., Rihmer, Z., & Somogyi, E. (1988). Retrospective psychiatric assessment of 200 suicides in Budapest. *Acta Psychiatr. Scand. 77*, 454–456.

Armor, D. J., Polich, J. M., & Stambul, H. B. (1978). *Alcoholism and treatment*. New York: Wiley.

Åsgård, U. (1990). *Suicide among Swedish women. A psychiatric and epidemiologic study*. Stockholm: Kongl Carolinska Medico Chirurgiska Institutet.

Atkinson, M. W., Kessel, N., & Dalgaard, J. B. (1975). The comparability of suicide rates. *Br. J. Psychiatry, 127*, 247–256.

Barchha, R., Stewart, M. A., & Guze, S. B. (1968). The prevalence of alcoholism among general hospital ward patients. *Am. J. Psychiatry, 125*, 681–684.

Barr, H. L., Antes, D., Ottenburg, D. J., & Rosen, A. (1984). Mortality of treated alcoholics and drug addicts: The benefits of abstinence. *J. Stud. Alcohol, 45*, 440–452.

Barraclough, B. M. (1972). Are the Scottish and English suicide rates really different? *Br. J. Psychiatry, 120*, 267–273.

Barraclough, B., Bunch, J., Nelson, B., & Sainsbury, P. (1974). A hundred cases of suicide: Clinical aspects. *Br. J. Psychiatry, 125*, 355–373.

Barraclough, B. M., Jennings, C., & Moss, J. R. (1977, July). Suicide prevention by the Samaritans. A controlled study of effectiveness. *Lancet*, pp. 237–238.

Bazire, S. (1986). Interactions with monoamine oxidase inhibitors. *Pharm. J., 236*, 418–419.

Beaubrun, M. H. (1967). Treatment of alcoholism in Trinidad and Tobago 1956–65. *Br. J. Psychiatry, 113*, 643–658.

Beaumont, G. (1973). Drug interactions with clomipramine (anafranil). *J. Int. Med. Res., 1*, 480–484.

Beck, A. T. (1962). Reliability of psychiatric diagnoses: 1. A critique of systematic studies. *Am. J. Psychiatry, 119*, 210–216.

Beck, A., Brown, G., Berchich, R., Stewart, B., & Steer, R. (1990). Relationship between hopelessness and ultimate suicide: A replication with psychiatric outpatients. *Am. J. Psychiatry, 147*, 190–195.

Beck, A. T., Rush, A. J., Shaw, B. F., & Emery, G. (1979). *Cognitive therapy of depression*. New York: Guilford Press.

Beck, A., Steer, R., Kovacs, M., & Garison, B. (1985). Hopelessness and eventual suicide: A 10-year prospective study of patients hospitalized with suicidal ideation. *Am. J. Psychiatry, 142,* 559–563.

Beck, A. T., Ward, C., Mendelson, M., Mock, J., & Erbaugh, J. (1962). Reliability of psychiatric diagnoses: 2. A study of consistency of clinical judgments and ratings. *Am. J. Psychiatry, 119,* 351–357.

Berglund, M. (1984). Suicide in alcoholism. A prospective study of 88 suicides: I. The multidimensional diagnosis at first admission. *Arch. Gen. Psychiatry, 41,* 888–891.

Berner, P., & Kryspin-Exner, K. (1978). Wahnforschung und psychiatrische Hypothesenbildung. *Nervenartzt, 49,* 147.

Beskow, J. (1979). Suicide and mental disorder in Swedish men. *Acta Psychiatr. Scand., 277* (Suppl.), 1–138.

Bille-Brahe, U. (1987). Suicide and social integration. A pilot study of the integration levels in Norway and Denmark. In N. Juel-Nielsen, N. Retterstøl, & U. Bille-Brahe (eds.), Suicide in Scandinavia. A report on the internordic research project. *Acta Psychiatr. Scand. 76* (Suppl. 336), 45–62.

Blackburn, I. M., Bishop, S., Glen, A. I. M., Whalley, L. J., & Christie, J. E. (1981). The efficacy of cognitive therapy in depression: A treatment trial using cognitive therapy and pharmacotherapy, each alone and in combination. *Br. J. Psychiatry, 139,* 181–189.

Blackburn, I. M., Eunson, K. M., & Bishop, S. (1986). A two-year naturalistic follow-up of depressed patients with cognitive therapy, pharmacotherapy and a combination of both. *J. Affective Disord., 10,* 67–75.

Boman, M., Sigvardsson, S., & Cloninger, C. R. (1981). Maternal inheritance of alcohol abuse. Cross-fostering of adopted women. *Arch. Gen. Psychiatry, 38,* 965–969.

Böhme, K., Schonfeld, H., & von Weltzien, J. (1982). Life expectancy and causes of death after suicide attempts. *Psychiatr. Fennica,* pp. 127–141.

Bolander, A.M. (1972). Nordic suicide statistics. In J. Waldenström, T. Larsson, & N. Ljungstedt (eds.), *Suicide and attempted suicide. Skandia international symposia* (pp. 57–58). Stockholm: Nordiska Bokhandelns Forlag.

Bratfos, O. (1974). *Forlopet av alkoholisme. Drikkingen, den sosiale tilpasning og helsen.* Oslo/Bergen/Tromso: Universitetsforlaget. (English translation of the abstract kindly supplied by the author.)

Breed, W. (1967). Suicide and loss in social interaction. In E. S. Shneidman (ed.), *Essays in self-destruction* (pp. 188–202). New York: Science House.

Brent, D. A., Perper, J. A., & Allman, C. J. (1987). Alcohol, firearms, and suicide among youth. Temporal trends in Allegheny County, Pennsylvania 1960 to 1983. *JAMA, 257,* 3369–3372.

Brooke, E. M., & Atkinson, M. (1974). Ascertainment of deaths from suicide. In E. M. Brooke (ed.), *Suicide and attempted suicide,* Geneva: World Health Organization.

Brown, S. A., & Schuckit, M. A. (1988). Changes in depression among abstinent alcoholics. *J. Stud. Alcohol, 49,* 412–417.

Buydens-Branchey, L., Branchey, M. H., & Noumair, D. (1989). Age of alcoholism onset. I. Relationship to psychopathology. *Arch. Gen. Psychiatry, 46,* 225–230.

Buydens-Branchey, L., Branchey, M. H., Noumair, D., & Lieber, C. S. (1989). Age of alcoholism onset. II. Relationship to susceptibility to serotonin precursor availability. *Arch. Gen. Psychiatry, 46,* 231–236.

Cadoret, R., & Winokur, G. (1974). Depression in alcoholism. *Ann. N.Y. Acad. Sci., 233,* 34–39.

Cahalan, D. (1970). *Problem drinkers.* San Francisco: Jossey-Bass.

Chia, B. H., & Tsoi, W. F. (1972). Suicide in Singapore. *Singapore Med. J., 13,* 91–97.

REFERENCES

Choi, S. Y. (1975). Death in young alcoholics. *J. Stud. Alcohol, 36,* 1224–1229.
Chynoweth, R., Tonge, J. I., & Armstrong, J. (1980). Suicide in Brisbane. A retrospective psychosocial study. *Aust. N.Z. J. Psychiatry, 14,* 37–45.
Ciompi, L., & Eisert, M. (1969). Mortalite et causes de deces chez les alcooliques. *Soc. Psychiatry, 4,* 159–168.
Clark, W. B., & Midanik, L. (1982). Alcohol use and alcohol problems among U.S. adults: Results of the 1979 national survey. In National Institute on Alcohol Abuse and Alcoholism, *Alcohol consumption and related problems* (Alcohol and Health, Monograph No. 1, pp. 3–54). Washington, DC: U.S. Government Printing Office.
Cloninger, C. R. (1987). Neurogenetic adaptive mechanisms in alcoholism. *Science, 236,* 410–416.
Cloninger, C. R., Boman, M., & Sigvardsson, S. (1981). Inheritance of alcohol abuse. Cross-fostering analysis of adopted men. *Arch. Gen. Psychiatry, 38,* 861–868.
Combs-Orme, T., Taylor, J. R., Robins, L. N., & Holmes, S. J. (1983). Differential mortality among alcoholics by sample site. *Am. J. Public Health, 73,* 900–903.
Combs-Orme, R., Taylor, J. R., Scott, E. B., & Holmes, S. J. (1983). Violent deaths among alcoholics. A descriptive study. *J. Stud. Alcohol, 44,* 938–949.
Cooper, G. L. (1988). The safety of fluoxetine—an update. *Br. J. Psychiatry, 153,* 77–86.
Costello, R. M., & Schneider, S. L. (1974). Mortality in an alcoholic cohort. *Int. J. Addict., 9,* 355–363.
Covi, L., & Lipman, R. (1987). Cognitive behavioral group psychotherapy combined with imipramine in major depression. *Psychopharm. Bull., 23,* 173–176.
Dahl, A. A. (1985a). Borderline disorders—the validity of the diagnostic concept. *Psychiatr. Dev., 2,* 109–152.
Dahl, A. A. (1985b). A critical examination of empirical studies of the diagnosis of borderline disorders in adults. *Psychiatr. Dev., 3,* 1–29.
Dahlgren, K. G. (1945). *On suicide and attempted suicide: A psychiatrical and statistical investigation* (p. 142). Lund, Linstedts Univ. Bokhandel.
Dahlgren, K. G. (1951). On death-rates and causes of death in alcohol addicts. *Acta Psychiatr. Scand., 26,* 297–311.
Dahlgren, K. G. (1977). Attempted suicide—35 years afterward. *Suicide Life Threatening Behav., 7,* 75–79.
Dahlgren, L., & Myrhed, M. (1977). Alcoholic females. II. Causes of death with reference to sex difference. *Acta Psychiatr. Scand., 56,* 81–91.
Davies, A. M., & Kaplan-Dinur, A. (1962). Suicide in Israel: An epidemiological study. *Int. J. Soc. Psychiatry, 8,* 32–44.
Davies, D. L., Shepherd, M., & Myers, E. (1956). The two-years' prognosis of 50 alcohol addicts after treatment in hospital. *Q. J. Stud. Alcohol, 17,* 485–502.
deLint, J., & Levinson, T. (1975). Mortality among patients treated for alcoholism: A 5-year follow-up. *Can. Med. Assoc. J., 113,* 385–387.
Dorpat, T. L., & Ripley, H. S. (1960). A study of suicide in the Seattle area. *Compr. Psychiatry, 1,* 349–359.
Dorpat, T. L., & Ripley, H. S. (1962). A study of suicide in King County, Washington. *Northwest. Med., 61,* 655–661.
Dreyer, K. (1959). Comparative suicide statistics: 1. International comparisons. *Dan. Med. Bull., 6,* 65–82.
Dubourg, G. O. (1969). After-care for alcoholics. A follow-up study. *Br. J. Addict., 64,* 155–163.
Dudley, W. H. C., Jr., & Williams, J. G. (1972). Electroconvulsive therapy in delirium tremens. *Compr. Psychiatry, 13,* 357–360.

Egeland, J., & Sussex, J. (1985). Suicide and family loading for affective disorders. *JAMA, 254,* 915–918.

Elkin, I., Shea, T., Watkins, J. R., Imber, S. K., Sotsky, S. M., Collins, J. F., Glass, D. R., Pilkonis, P. A., Leber, W. R., Docherty, J. P., Fiester, S. J., & Parloff, M. D. (1989). National Institute of Mental Health treatment of depression collaborative research program. General effectiveness of treatments. *Arch. Gen. Psychiatry, 46,* 971–982.

Ellerman, M. (1948). Social and clinical features of chronic alcoholism. *J. Nerv. Ment. Dis., 107,* 556–568.

Englebrecht, G. K. (1983). Alcohol as a possible variable in suicide. *Humanitas, 9,* 61–68.

Ettlinger, R. W. (1964). Suicides in a group of patients who had previously attempted suicide. *Acta Psychiatr. Scand., 40,* 363–378.

Ettlinger, R. (1975). Evaluation of suicide prevention after attempted suicide. *Acta Psychiatr. Scand.* (Suppl. 260), 1–135.

Ettlinger, R. W., & Flordh, P. (1955). Attempted suicide: Experience of five hundred cases at a general hospital. *Acta Psychiatr. Neurol. Scand., 103* (Suppl.), 1–45.

Feighner, J. P., Boyer, W. F., Tyler, D. L., & Neborsky, R. J. (1990). Adverse consequences of fluoxetine-MAOI combination therapy. *J. Clin. Psychiatry, 51,* 222–225.

Feighner, J. P., Robins, E., Guze, S. B., Woodruff, R. A., Jr., Winokur, G., & Munoz, R. (1972). Diagnostic criteria for use in psychiatric research. *Arch. Gen. Psychiatry, 26,* 57–63.

Fillmore, K. M., Bacon, S. D., & Hyman, M. (1979). *The 27-year longitudinal panel study of drinking by students in college, 1949–1976* (Report No. PB 300–302). Springfield, VA: U.S. National Technical Information Service.

Fillmore, K. M., & Midanik, L. (1984). Chronicity of drinking problems among men: A longitudinal study. *J. Stud. Alcohol, 45,* 228–236.

Finney, J. W., Moos, R. H., & Chan, D. A. (1981). Length of stay and program component effects in the treatment of alcoholism: A comparison of two techniques for process analyses. *J. Consult. Clin. Psychol., 49,* 120–131.

Fowler, R. C., Liskow, B. I., & Tanna, V. L. (1980). Alcoholism, depression and life events. *J. Affective Disord., 2,* 127–135.

Fremming, K. H. (1951). The expectation of mental infirmity in a sample of the Danish population. In *Occasional papers on eugenics, number seven.* London: The Eugenics Society and Cassell and Company.

Gabriel, E. (1935). Uber die Todesursachen bei Alkoholikern. *Z. Neurol. Psychiatr., 153,* 385–406.

Galen R. S., & Gambino, S. R. (1975). *Beyond normality. The predictive value and efficiency of medical diagnoses.* New York: Wiley.

Gillies, M., Laverty, S. G., Smart, R. G., & Aharan, C. H. (1974). Outcomes in treated alcoholics. Patient and treatment characteristics in a one year follow-up study. *J. Alcohol., 9,* 125–134.

Gillis, L. S. (1969). The mortality rate and causes of death of treated chronic alcoholics. *S. Afr. Med. J., 43,* 230–232.

Gillis, L. S., & Keet, M. (1969). Prognostic factors and treatment results in hospitalized alcoholics. *Q. J. Stud. Alcohol., 30,* 426–437.

Goodwin, D. W. (1979). Alcoholism and heredity. *Arch. Gen. Psychiatry, 36,* 57–61.

Goodwin, D. W. (1985). Alcoholism and genetics. The sins of the fathers. *Arch. Gen. Psychiatry, 42,* 172–174.

Goodwin, D. W., & Guze, S. B. (1989). *Psychiatric diagnosis* (4th ed.). New York: Oxford University Press.

Gove, W. R., & Hughes, M. (1980). Reexamining the ecological fallacy: A study in which

aggregate data are critical in investigating the pathological effects of living alone. *Soc. Forces, 58,* 1157–1177.
Guze, S. B., Cloninger, C. R., Martin, R., & Clayton, P. J. (1988). Alcoholism as a medical disorder. In R. M. Rose & J. E. Barrett (eds.), *Alcoholism: Origins and outcome* (pp. 83–94). New York: Raven Press.
Guze, S. B., & Robins, E. (1970). Suicide and primary affective disorders. *Br. J. Psychiatry, 117,* 437–438.
Haberlandt, W. (1967). Aportacion a la genetica del suicido. *Folia Clin. Int., 17,* 318–322.
Hagnell, O., & Öjesjö, L. (1975). A prospective study concerning mental disorders of a total population investigated in 1947, 1957, 1972. *Acta Psychiatr. Scand.* (Suppl. 263), 1.
Hagnell, O., & Rorsman, B. (1979). Suicide in the Lundby study: A comparative investigation of clinical aspects. *Neuropsychobiology, 5,* 61–73.
Hagnell, O., & Wretmark, G. (1957). Peptic ulcer and alcoholism. A statistical study in frequency, behaviour, personality traits, and family occurrence. *J. Psychomatic Res., 2,* 35–44.
Hamilton, M. (1960). A rating scale for depression. *J. Neurol. Neurosurg. Psychiatry, 23,* 56–62.
Hasin, D.S., Grant, B., & Endicott, J. (1990). The natural history of alcohol abuse: Implications for definitions of alcohol use disorders. *Am. J. Psychiatry, 147,* 1537–1541.
Hastings, D. W. (1958). Follow-up results in psychiatric illness. *Am. J. Psychiatry, 114,* 1057–1066.
Haver, B. (1986). Female alcoholics: I. Psychosocial outcome six years after treatment. *Acta Psychiatr. Scand., 74,* 102–111.
Helgason, T. (1964). Epidemiology of mental disorders in Iceland. A psychiatric and demographic investigation of 5,395 Icelanders. *Acta Psychiatr. Scand.,* (Suppl. 173), 116–132.
Helzer, J. E., Burnam, A. & McEvoy, L. T. (1991). Alcohol abuse and dependence. In L. N. Robins & D. Regier (eds.), *Psychiatric disorders in America.* New York: Free Press.
Helzer, J. E., & Pryzbeck, T. R. (1988). The co-occurrence of alcoholism with other psychiatric disorders in the general population and its impact on treatment. *J. Stud. Alcohol, 49,* 219–224.
Helzer, J. E., Robins, L. N., Taylor, J. R., Carey, K., Miller, R. H., Combs-Orme, T., & Farmer, A. (1985). The extent of long-term moderate drinking among alcoholics discharged from medical and psychiatric treatment facilities. *New England J. Med., 312,* 1678–1682.
Hesselbrock, M. N., Meyer, R. E., & Keener, J. J. (1985). Psychopathology in hospitalized alcoholics. *Arch. Gen. Psychiatry, 42,* 1050–1055.
Hetmar, O., Povlsen, U., Ladefoged, J., & Bolwig, T. (1991). Lithium: Long-term effects on the kidney. A prospective follow-up study ten years after kidney biopsy. *Br. J. Psychiatry, 158,* 53–58.
Higuchi, S. (1987). Mortality of Japanese female alcoholics: A comparative study with male cases. *Jpn. J. Alcohol Dependence, 22,* 211–223.
Holding, T. A., & Barraclough, B. M. (1978). Undetermined deaths—Suicide or accident? *Br. J. Psychiatry, 133,* 542–549.
Humphrey, J. A. (1977). Social loss: A comparison of suicide victims, homicide offenders and non-violent individuals. *Dis. Nerv. Syst., 38,* 157–160.
Humphrey, J. A., French, L., Niswander, G. D., & Casey, T. M. (1974). The process of suicide: The sequence of disruptive events in the lives of suicide victims. *Dis. Nerv. Syst., 35,* 275–277.
Hyman, M. M. (1976). Alcoholics 15 years later. *Ann. N.Y. Acad. Sci., 273,* 613–623.

Imber, S., Schultz, E., Funderburck, F., Allen, R., & Flamer, R. (1976). The fate of the untreated alcoholic. Toward a natural history of the disorder. *J. Nerv. Ment. Dis., 162,* 238–247.
Irwin, M., Schuckit, M., & Smith, T. L. (1990). Clinical importance of age at onset in type 1 and type 2 primary alcoholics. *Arch. Gen. Psychiatry, 47,* 320–324.
Jobes, D. A., Berman, A. L., & Josselson, A. R. (1987). Improving the validity and reliability of medical-legal certifications of suicide. *Suicide Life Threatening Behav., 17,* 310–325.
Juel-Nielsen, N., Retterstøl, N., & Bille-Brahe, U. (1987). Suicide in Scandinavia. A report on the internordic research project. *Acta Psychiatr. Scand., 76* (Suppl. 336).
Kapamadžija, B., Biro, M., & Sovljanski, M. (1982). Sociopsihijatrijska I patomorfoloska analiza 100 izvrsenih samoubistave. *Soc. Psihijatr., 10,* 35–56. (Jugoslavia)
Kapamadžija, B., Biro, M., & Till, E. (1981). Alcoholism, depression and suicide. In J. P. Soubrier, & J. Vedrinne (eds.), *Depression et suicide*. (pp. 463–466). Paris: Pergamon Press.
Kelleher, M. J., & Daly, M. (1990). Suicide in Cork and Ireland. *Br. J. Psychiatry, 157,* 533–538.
Kendell, R. E. (1983). Alcohol and suicide. *Subst. Alcohol Actions/Misuse, 4,* 121–127.
Kendell, R. E., & Staton, M. C. (1966). The fate of untreated alcoholics. *Q. J. Stud. Alcohol, 27,* 30–41.
Kessel, N., & Grossman, G. (1961). Suicide in alcoholics. *Br. Med. J., 2,* 1671–1672.
Kleber, H. D. (1990). The nosology of abuse and dependence. *J. Psychiatr. Res., 24,* 57–64.
Klein, D., Najman, J., Kohrman, A. F., & Munro, C. (1982). Patient characteristics that elicit negative responses from family physicians. *J. Fam. Pract., 14,* 881–888.
Klein, D. F., Gittelman, R., Quitkin, F., & Rifkin, A. (1980). *Diagnosis and drug treatment of psychiatric disorders: Adults and children* (2nd ed.). Baltimore: Williams & Wilkins.
Klerman, G. L., Lavori, P., Rice, J., Reich, T., Endicott, J., Andreasen, N. C., Keller, M. B., & Hirschfeld, M. A. (1985). Birth-cohort trends in rates of major depressive disorder among relatives of patients with affective disorder. *Arch. Gen. Psychiatry, 42,* 689–693.
Kliewer, E. V., & Ward, R. H. (1988). Convergence of immigrant suicide rates to those in the destination country. *Am. J. Epidemiol., 127,* 640–653.
Knop, J., & Fischer, A. (1981). Duodenal ulcer, suicide, psychopathology and alcoholism. *Acta Psychiatr. Scand., 63,* 346–355.
Kolmos, L., & Bach, E. (1987). Sources of error in registering suicide. In N. Juel-Nielsen, N. Retterstøl, & U. Bille-Brahe (eds.), Suicide in Scandinavia. A report on the internordic research project. *Acta Psychiatr. Scand., 76* (Suppl. 336), 22–43.
Kranzler, H. R., & Babor, T. F. (1990). The identification and treatment of alcohol abuse and dependence. *Ann. Clin. Psychiatry, 2,* 229–238.
Krause, U. (1963). Long term results of medical and surgical treatment of peptic ulcer. A follow-up investigation of patients initially treated conservatively between 1925–34. *Acta Chir. Scand.* (Suppl. 310), 1–111.
Kreitman, N. (1961). The reliability of psychiatric diagnosis. *J. Ment. Sci., 107,* 876–886.
Lader, M. (1983). Combined use of tricyclic antidepressants and monoamine oxidase inhibitors. *J. Clin. Psychiatry, 44* (9, Sec. 2), 20–24.
Lambie, D. G., Whiteside, E. A., Bell, J., & Johnson, R. H. (1983). Mortality associated with alcoholism in New Zealand. *N.Z. Med. J., 96,* 199–202.
Lemere, F. (1953). What happens to alcoholics. *Am. J. Psychiatry, 109,* 674–676.
Lesch, O. M., Lesch, E., Dietzel, M., Mader, R., Musalek, M., Walter, H., & Zeiler, K. (1986). Chronischer Alkoholismus—Alkoholgekrankheiten—Todesursachen. *Wiener Med. Wochenschr., 136,* 505–515.
Lindberg, S., & Ågren, G. (1988). Mortality among male and female hospital ized alcoholics in Stockholm 1962–1983. *Br. J. Addict., 83,* 1193–1200.

REFERENCES

Lindelius, R., Salum, I., & Ågren, G. (1974). Mortality among male and female alcoholic patients treated in a psychiatric unit. *Acta Psychiatr. Scand., 50,* 612–618.
Lippmann, S. (1986). Monoamine oxidase inhibitors. *Am. Family Practitioner, July,* 113–119.
Litman, R. E., Curphey, T., Shneidman, E. S., Farberow, N. L., & Tabachnick, N. (1963). Investigations of equivocal suicides. *JAMA, 184,* 924–929.
Longabaugh, R. (1988). Longitudinal outcome studies. In R. M. Rose & J. E. Barrett (eds.), *American psychopathological association series. Alcoholism: Origins and outcome* (pp. 267–280). New York: Raven Press.
Lönnqvist, J., & Achté, K. A. (1971). Excessive drinking in psychiatric patients who later committed suicide. *Psychiatr. Fennica,* pp. 209–213.
Mackenzie, A., Allen, R. P., & Funderburk, F. R. (1986). Mortality and illness in male alcoholics: An 8-year follow-up. *Int. J. Addict., 21,* 865–882.
Marley, E., & Wozniak, K. M. (1983). Clinical and experimental aspects of interactions between amine oxidase inhibitors and amine re-uptake inhibitors. *Psychol. Med., 13,* 735–749.
Martin, R. L., Cloninger, C. R., Guze, S. B., & Clayton, P. J. (1985a). Mortality in a follow-up of 500 psychiatric outpatients: I. Total mortality. *Arch. Gen. Psychiatry, 42,* 47–54.
Martin, R. L., Cloninger, C. R., Guze, S. B., & Clayton, P. J. (1985b). Mortality in a follow-up of 500 psychiatric outpatients: II. Cause- specific mortality. *Arch. Gen. Psychiatry, 42,* 58–66.
Mason, B. J., & Kocsis, J. H. (1991). Desipramine treatment of alcoholism. *Psychopharm. Bull. 27,* 155–161.
McCarthy, P. D., & Walsh, D. (1966). Suicide in Dublin. *Br. Med. J., 1,* 1393–1396.
McCarthy, P. D., & Walsh, D. (1975). Suicide in Dublin: I. The under-reporting of suicide and the consequences for national statistics. *Br. J. Psychiatry, 126,* 301–308.
McGlashan, T. H. (1983). The borderline syndrome: II. Is it a variant of schizophrenia or affective disorder? *Arch. Gen. Psychiatry, 40,* 1319–1323.
Mečiř, J., & Brežinová, V. (1960). The causes of death in alcoholics. *Acta Univ. Carol., 6,* 593–607.
Medhus, A. (1975). Mortality among female alcoholics. *Scand. J. Soc. Med., 3,* 111–115.
Miles, C. P. (1977). Conditions predisposing to suicide: A review. *J. Nerv. Ment. Dis., 164,* 231–246.
Miller, W. R., & Hester, R. K. (1986). The effectiveness of alcoholism treatment: What research shows. In W. R. Miller & N. H. Heather (eds.), *Treating addictive behaviors.* New York: Plenum.
Mitterauer, B. (1981). Mehrdimensionale Diagnostik von 121 Suiziden im Bundesland Salzburg in Jahre 1978. *Wiener Med. Wochenschr., 9,* 229–234.
Mitterauer, B. (1990). A contribution to the discussion of the role of the genetic factor in suicide, based on five studies in an epidemiologically defined area (Province of Salzberg, Austria). *Compr. Psychiatry, 31,* 557–565.
Morrison, J. R. (1982). Suicide in a psychiatric practice population. *J. Clin. Psychiatry, 43,* 348–352.
Murphy, G. E. (1972). Clinical identification of suicidal risk. *Arch. Gen. Psychiatry, 27,* 356–359.
Murphy, G. E. (1975). The physician's responsibility for suicide. II. Errors of omission. *Ann. Intern. Med., 82,* 305–309.
Murphy, G. E. (1984). The prediction of suicide: Why is it so difficult? *Am. J. Psychother., 38,* 341–349.
Murphy, G. E., Armstrong, J. W., Hermele, S. L., Fischer, J. R., & Clendenin, W. W. (1979). Suicide and alcoholism. Interpersonal loss confirmed as a predictor. *Arch. Gen. Psychiatry, 36,* 65–69.

Murphy, G. E., & Robins, E. (1967). Social factors in suicide. *JAMA, 199*, 303–308.
Murphy, G. E., Simons, A. D., Wetzel, R. D., & Lustman, P. J. (1984). Cognitive therapy and pharmacotherapy. Singly and together in the treatment of depression. *Arch. Gen. Psychiatry, 41*, 33–41.
Murphy G., & Wetzel, R. (1980). Suicide risk by birth cohort in the United States, 1949 to 1974. *Arch. Gen. Psychiatry, 37*, 519–523.
Murphy, G. E., & Wetzel, R. D. (1990). The lifetime risk of suicide in alcoholism. *Arch. Gen. Psychiatry, 47*, 383–392.
Musher, J. (1990). Anorgasmia with the use of fluoxetine (letter). *Am. J. Psychiatry, 147*, 948.
Nakamura, M. M., Overall, J. E., Hollister, L. E., & Radcliffe, E. (1983). Factors affecting outcome of depressive symptoms in alcoholics. *Alcoholism: Clin. Exp. Res., 7*, 188–193.
National Council on Alcoholism, Inc. (1987). Facts on alcoholism and alcohol-related problems.
Nelson, F. L., Farberow, N. L., & MacKinnon, D. R. (1978). The certification of suicide in eleven western states: An inquiry into the validity of reported suicide rates. *Suicide Life Threatening Behav., 8*, 75–88.
Nicholls, P., Edwards, G., & Kyle, E. (1974). Alcoholics admitted to four hospitals in England: II. General and cause-specific mortality. *Q. J. Stud. Alcohol., 35*, 841–855.
Nielsen, B. G., Juul, S., & Munk-Jorgensen, P. (1987). Alkoholisme og mortalitet. Mortalitet blandt forstegangsklienter ved arhusianske alkoholambulatorier i 1972 og 1982. *Ugeskr. Laeg., 149*, 1559–1562.
Nørvig, J., & Nielsen, B. (1956). A follow-up study of 221 alcohol addicts in Denmark. *Q. J. Stud. Alcohol., 17*, 633–642.
Noyes, R., Perry, P. J., Crowe, R. R., Coryell, W. H., Clancy, J., Yamada, T., & Gabel, J. (1986). Seizures following the withdrawal of alprazolam. *J. Nerv. Ment. Dis., 174*, 50–52.
Nunomura, A., Shingae, R., Ikeda, A., Ohta, K., & Miyagishi, T. (1989). A study on death of alcoholics. *Jpn. J. Alcohol Drug Dependence, 24*, 89–99.
Nuttall, E. A., Evenson, R. C., & Cho, D. W. (1980). A comparison of suicide and undetermined deaths in psychiatric patients. *Suicide Life Threatening Behav., 10*, 167–174.
O'Carroll, P. W. (1989). A consideration of the validity and reliability of suicide mortality data. *Suicide Life Threatening Behav., 19*, 1–16.
Ohara, K., Suzuki, Y., Sugita, T., Kobayashi, K., Tamefusa, K., Hattori, S., & Ohara, K. (1989). Mortality among alcoholics discharged from a Japenese hospital. *Br. J. Addict., 84*, 287–291.
Öjesjö, L. (1981). Long-term outcome in alcohol abuse and alcoholism among males in the Lundby general population, Sweden. *Br. J. Addict., 76*, 391–400.
Öjesjö, L., & Hagnell, O. (1980). Prevalence of male alcoholism in a cohort observed. *Scand. J. Soc. Med., 8*, 55–61.
Ornstein, P., & Cherepon, J. A. (1985). Demographic variables as predictors of alcoholism treatment outcome. *J. Stud. Alcohol, 46*, 425–432.
O'Sullivan, K., Rynne, C., Miller, J., O'Sullivan, S., Fitzpatrick, V., Hux, M., Cooney, J., & Clare, A. (1988). A follow-up study on alcoholics with and without co-existing affective disorder. *Br. J. Psychiatry, 152*, 813–819.
Ovenstone, I. M. K. (1973). A psychiatric approach to the diagnosis of suicide and its effect upon the Edinburgh statistics. *Br. J. Psychiatry, 123*, 15–21.
Overall, J. E., Reilly, R. L., Kelley, J. T., & Hollister, L. E. (1985). Persistence of depression in detoxified alcoholics. *Alcoholism: Clin. Exp. Res., 9*, 331–333.
Palola, E. G., Dorpat, T. L., & Larson, W. R. (1962). Alcoholism and suicidal behavior. In D. Pittman & C. Snyder (eds.), *Society, culture, and drinking patterns* (pp. 511–534). New York: Wiley.

Pell, S., & D'Alonzo, C. A. (1973). A five-year mortality study of alcoholics. *J. Occup. Med.*, *15*, 120–125.
Penick, E. C., Powell, B. J., Liskow, B. I., Jackson, J. O., & Nickel, E. J. (1988). The stability of coexisting psychiatric syndromes in alcoholic men after one year. *J. Stud. Alcohol*, *49*, 395–405.
Persson, J., & Magnusson, P. H. (1989). Sickness absenteeism and mortality in patients with excessive drinking in somatic outpatient care. *Scand. J. Prim. Health Care*, *7*, 211–217.
Pickens, R. W., Svikis, D. S., McGue, M., Lykken, D. T., Heston, L. L., & Clayton, P. J. (1991). Heterogeneity in the inheritance of alcoholism. A study of male and female twins. *Arch. Gen. Psychiatry*, *48*, 19–28.
Pokorny, A. D. (1983). Prediction of suicide in psychiatric patients. *Arch. Gen. Psychiatry*, *40*, 249–257.
Pokorny, A. D., Miller, B. A., & Cleveland, S. E. (1968). Response to treatment of alcoholics. A follow-up study. *Q. J. Stud. Alcohol*, *29*, 364–381.
Pokorny, A. D., Smith, J. P., & Finch, J. R. (1972). Vehicular suicides. *Life-Threatening Behav.*, *2*, 105–119.
Polich, J. M., Armor, D. J., & Braiker, H. B. (1981). *The course of alcoholism. Four years after treatment*. New York: Wiley.
Pope, H. G., Jonas, J. M., Hudson, J. I., Cohen B. M., & Gunderson, J. G. (1983). The validity of DSM-III borderline personality disorder. A phenomenological, family history, treatment response, and long-term follow-up study. *Arch. Gen. Psychiatry*, *40*, 23–30.
Prout, C. T., Strongin, E. I., & White, M. A. (1950). A study of results in hospital treatment of alcoholism in males. *Am. J. Psychiatry*, *107*, 14–19.
Rathod, N. H., Gregory, E., Blows, D., & Thomas, G. H. (1966). A two-year follow-up study of alcoholic patients. *Br. J. Psychiatry*, *112*, 683–692.
Razani, J., White, K. L., White, J., Simpson, G., Sloane, R. B., Rebal, R., & Palmer, R. (1983). The safety and efficacy of combined amitriptyline and tranylcypromine antidepressant treatment. *Arch. Gen. Psychiatry*, *40*, 657–661.
Regier, D. A., Myers, J. K., Kramer, M., Robins, L. N., Blazer, D. G., Hough, R. L., Eaton, W. W., & Locke B. Z. (1984). The NIMH epidemiologic catchment area program. Historical context, major objectives, and study population characteristics. *Arch. Gen. Psychiatry*, *41*, 934–941.
Regier, D. A., Farmer, M. E., Rae, D. S., Locke, B. Z., Keith, S. J., Judd, L. L., & Goodwin, F. K. (1990). Comorbidity of mental disorders with alcohol and other drug abuse. Results from the epidemiologic catchment area (ECA) study. *JAMA*, *264*, 2511–2518.
Retterstøl, N. (1972). Discussion (the papers by Bolander and Retterstol). In J. Waldenström, T. Larsson, and N. Ljungstedt (eds.), *Suicide and attempted suicide. Skandia International Symposia* (p. 99). Stockholm: Nordiska Bokhandelns Forlag.
Rich, C. L., Fowler, R. C., Fogarty, L. A., & Young, D. (1988). San Diego suicide study: III. Relationships between diagnoses and stressors. *Arch. Gen. Psychiatry*, *45*, 589–592.
Rich, C. L., Fowler, R. C., & Young, D. (1989). Substance abuse and suicide. The San Diego study. *Ann. Clin. Psychiatry*, *1*, 79–85.
Rich, C. L., Young, D., & Fowler, R. C. (1986). San Diego suicide study: I. Young vs. old subjects. *Arch. Gen. Psychiatry*, *43*, 577–582.
Richelson, E. (1989). Antidepressants: Pharmacology and clinical use. In T. B. Karasu, et al. (eds.), *Treatments of psychiatric disorders*. Washington: American Psychiatric Association.
Ripley, H. S., & Dorpat, T. L. (1981). Life change and suicidal behavior. *Psychiatr. Ann.*, *11*, 219–226.

Roberts, A. H. (1963). The value of E.C.T. in delirium. *Br. J. Psychiatry, 109,* 653–655.
Robins, E. (1981). *The final months. A study of the lives of 134 persons who committed suicide.* New York: Oxford University Press.
Robins, E., Gassner, S., Kayes, J., Wilkinson, R. H., Jr., & Murphy, G. E. (1959). The communication of suicidal intent: A study of 134 consecutive cases of successful (completed) suicide. *Am. J. Psychiatry, 115,* 724–733.
Robins, E., Murphy, G. E., Wilkinson, R. H., Jr., Gassner, S., & Kayes, J. (1959). Some clinical considerations in the prevention of suicide based on a study of 134 successful suicides. *Am. J. Public Health, 49,* 888–899.
Robins, L. N., Helzer, J. E., Przybeck, T. R., & Regier, D. A. (1988). Alcohol disorders in the community: A report from the epidemiologic catchment area. In R. M. Rose & J. Barrett (eds.), *Alcoholism: Origins and outcome* (pp. 15–29). New York: Raven Press.
Robins, L. N., Helzer, J. E., Weissman, M. M., Orvaschel, H., Gruenberg, E., Burke, J. D., Jr., & Regier, D. A. (1984). Lifetime prevalence of specific psychiatric disorders in three sites. *Arch. Gen. Psychiatry, 41,* 949–958.
Rose, R. M. (1988). Blaming the patient. In R. M. Rose & J. E. Barrett (eds.), *Alcoholism: Origins and outcome* (pp. 127–141). New York: Raven Press.
Rosen, D. H. (1976). The serious suicide attempt: Five-year follow-up study of 886 patients. *JAMA, 235,* 2105–2109.
Rosenberg, M. L., Davidson, L. E., Smith, J. C., Berman, A. L., Buzbee, H., Gantner, G., Gay, G. A., Moore-Lewis, B., Mills, D. H., Murray, D., O'Carroll, P. W., & Jobes, D. (1988). Operational criteria for the determination of suicide. *J. Forensic Sci., 32,* 1445–1456.
Ross, H. E., Glaser, F. B., & Germanson, T. (1988). The prevalence of psychiatric disorders in patients with alcohol and other drug problems. *Arch. Gen. Psychiatry, 45,* 1023–1031.
Ross, H. E., Glaser, F. B., & Stiasny, S. (1988). Sex differences in the prevalence of psychiatric disorders in patients with alcohol and drug problems. *Br. J. Addict., 83,* 1179–1192.
Rounsaville, B. J., Dolinsky, Z. S., Babor, T. F., & Meyer, R. E. (1987). Psychopathology as a predictor of treatment outcome in alcoholics. *Arch. Gen. Psychiatry, 44,* 505–513.
Roy, A., DeJong, J., Lamparski, D., Adinoff, B., George, T., Moore, V., Garnett, D., Kerich, M., & Linnoila, M. (1991). Mental disorders among alcoholics. Relationship to age of onset and cerebrospinal fluid neuropeptides. *Arch. Gen. Psychiatry, 48,* 423–427.
Runeson, B. (1990). Psychoactive substance use disorder in youth suicide. *Alcohol and Alcoholism, 25,* 561–568.
Runeson, B., & Beskow, J. (1990). Borderline personality disorder in young Swedish suicides. *J. Nerv. Ment. Dis., 179,* 153–156.
Rush, A. J., Beck, A. T., Kovacs, M., & Hollon, S. (1977). Comparative efficacy of cognitive therapy and pharmacotherapy in the treatment of depressed outpatients. *Cognitive Therapy & Research, 1,* 17–37.
Rutz, W., von Knorring, L., & Walinder, J. (1989). Frequency of suicide on Gotland after systematic postgraduate education of general practitioners. *Acta Psychiatr. Scand., 80,* 151–154.
Sainsbury, P. (1973). Suicide: Opinions and facts. *Proc. R. Soc. Med., 66,* 579–587.
Sainsbury, P., & Barraclough, B. (1968). Differences between suicide rates. *Nature, 220,* 1252.
Salum, I. (1972). Delirium tremens and certain other acute sequels of alcohol abuse. *Acta Psychiatr. Scand.* (Suppl. 235), 15–19.
SAS Institute, Inc. (1988). *SAS procedures guide, release 6.03 edition.* Cary, NC: Author.
Saunders, W. M., Phil, M., & Kershaw, P. W. (1979). Spontaneous remission from alcoholism—A community study. *Br. J. Addict., 74,* 251–265.

Schmidt, C. W., Jr., Perlin, S., Townes, W., Fisher, R. S., & Shaffer, J. W. (1972). Characteristics of drivers involved in single-car accidents: A comparative study. *Arch. Gen. Psychiatry, 27,* 800–803.
Schmidt, W., & deLint, J. (1972). Causes of death of alcoholics. *Q. J. Stud. Alcohol., 33,* 171–185.
Schneider, P. B. (1954). *La tentative de suicide. Etude statistique, clinique psychologique et catamnestique.* Neuchatel, Paris: Delachauz et Niestle, S.A.
Schou, M. (1986). Lithium treatment: A refresher course. *Br. J. Psychiatry, 149,* 541–547.
Schuckit, M. A., & Gunderson, E. K. E. (1974). Deaths among young alcoholics in the U.S. naval service. *Q. J. Stud. Alcohol, 35,* 856–862.
Schuckit, M. A., Irwin, M., & Mahler, H. I. M. (1990). Tridimensional personality questionnaire scores of sons of alcoholic and nonalcoholic fathers. *Am. J. Psychiatry, 147,* 481–487.
Schuckit, M. A., Li, T.-K., Cloninger, C. R., & Deitrich, R. A. (1985). Genetics of alcoholism. *Alcoholism: Clin. Exp. Res., 9,* 475–492.
Schuckit, M. A., & Winokur, G. (1972). A short term follow up of women alcoholics. *Dis. Ner. Syst., 33,* 672–678.
Schuckit, M. A., Zisook, S., & Mortola, J. (1985). Clinical implications of DSM-III diagnoses of alcohol abuse and alcohol dependence. *Am. J. Psychiatry, 142,* 1403–1408.
Schulsinger, F., Kety, S., Rosenthal, D., & Wender, P. (1979). A family study of suicide. In M. Schou & E. Strömgren (eds.), *Origin, prevention and treatment of affective disorder* (pp. 278–287). New York: Academic Press.
Selzer, M. L., & Holloway, W. H. (1957). A follow-up of alcoholics committed to a state hospital. *Q. J. Stud. Alcohol, 18,* 98–120.
Shapiro, S., Skinner, E. A., Kessler, L. G., Von Korff, M., German, P. S., Tischler, G. L., Leaf, P. J., Benham, L., Cottler, L., & Regier, D. A. (1984). Utilization of health and mental health services. Three epidemiologic catchment area sites. *Arch. Gen. Psychiatry, 41,* 971–978.
Shaw, G., Waller, S., McDougall, S., MacGarvie, J., & Dunn, G. (1990). Alcoholism: A follow-up study of participants in an alcohol treatment programme. *Br. J. Psychiatry, 157,* 190–196.
Sheehan, J. J., Wieman, R. J., & Bechtel, J. E. (1981). Follow-up of a twelve-month treatment program for chronic alcoholics. *Int. J. Addict., 16,* 233–241.
Simons, A. D., Murphy, G. E., Levine, J. L., & Wetzel, R. D. (1986). Cognitive therapy and pharmacotherapy of depression: Sustained improvement over one year. *Arch. Gen. Psychiatry, 43,* 43–48.
Smith, E. M., Cloninger, C. R., & Bradford, S. (1983). Predictors of mortality in alcoholic women. A prospective follow-up study. *Alcoholism: Clin. Exp. Res., 7,* 237–243.
Spitzer, R. L., & Endicott, J. (1975). Schedule for affective disorders and schizophrenia—Lifetime version. In *Biometrics research.* New York: New York State Psychiatric Institute.
Spitzer, R. L., Endicott, J., & Robins, E. (1978). *Research diagnostic criteria (RDC) for a selected group of functional disorders* (3rd ed.). New York: Biometrics Research Division, New York State Psychiatric Institute.
Stengel, E. (1960). Some unexplored aspects of suicide and attempted suicide. *Compr. Psychiatry, 1,* 71–79.
Stengel, E. (1972). A survey of follow-up examinations of attempted suicides. In J. Waldenström, T. Larsson, & N. Ljungstedt (eds.), *Suicide and attempted suicide* (pp. 250–262). Stockholm: Nordiska Bokhandelns Forlag.
Stengel, E. (1973). A matter of communication. In E. Shneidman (ed.), *On the nature of suicide* (pp. 74–80). San Francisco: Jossey-Bass.

Sullivan, W. C. (1900). The relation of alcoholism to suicide in England with special reference to recent statistics. *J. Ment. Sci., 46,* 260–181.
Sundby, P. (1967). *Alcoholism and mortality.* Blindern, Oslo: Universitetsforlaget.
Tabachnick, N. (ed.) (1973). *Accident or suicide: Destruction by automobile.* Springfield: Thomas.
Tashiro, M., & Lipscomb, W. R. (1963). Mortality experience of alcoholics. *Q. J. Stud. Alcohol, 24,* 203–212.
Teicher, M. H., Glod, C., & Cole, J. O. (1990). Emergence of intense suicidal preoccupation during fluoxetine treatment. *Am. J. Psychiatry, 147,* 207–210.
Teoh, J.-I. (1974). An analysis of completed suicides by psychological post-mortem. *Ann. Acad. Med., 3,* 117–124.
Theret, L., Facy, F., & Pascalis, J. G. (1989). Le patient alcoolique suicidaire: Profil, facteurs de risque et revue de la litterature de 1955 a 1988. *Annales Medico-Psychologiques, 147,* 1092–1094.
Thorarinsson, A. A. (1979). Mortality among men alcoholics in Iceland, 1951–74. *J. Stud. Alcohol, 40,* 704–718.
Tollefson, G. D. (1983). Monoamine oxidase inhibitors: A review. *J. Clin. Psychiatry, 44,* 280–288.
Torgersen, S. (1984). Genetic and nosological aspects of schizotypal and borderline personality disorders. A twin study. *Arch. Gen. Psychiatry, 41,* 546–554.
United Nations, Department of Economic and Social Affairs. (1952). *Demographic yearbook, 1951.* New York: Author.
United States Department of Commerce, Bureau of the Census. (1985). *Marital status and living arrangements: March 1985.* (Current Population Reports. Population Characteristics. Series P-20, No. 410.)
United States Department of Health, Education and Welfare. (1973). *Vital statistics of the United States* (Vol. II, Section 5: Life tables). Washington, DC: Author.
United States Department of Health, Education and Welfare. (1979). *Vital Statistics of the United States, 1979.* (Vol. II, Pt. A, Section 1: General mortality, Table 1–22). Washington, D.C.: Author.
United States Department of Health and Human Services. (1990). *Vital Statistics of the United States, 1988* (Vol. II, Pt. A, Section 1: General mortality, Table 1–22). Washington, DC: Author.
Vaillant, G. E., & Milofsky, E. S. (1982). Natural history of male alcoholism: IV. Paths to recovery. *Arch. Gen. Psychiatry, 39,* 127–133.
Vallance, M. (1965). Alcoholism. A two-year follow-up study of patients admitted to the psychiatric department of a general hospital. *Br. J. Psychiatry, 111,* 348–356.
van Dijk, W. K., & van Dijk-Koffeman, A. (1973). A follow-up study of 211 treated male alcoholic addicts. *Br. J. Addict., 68,* 3–24.
Virkkunen, M. (1971). Alcoholism and suicides in Helsinki. *Psychiatr. Fennica,* pp. 201–207.
Viskum, K. (1975). Ulcer, attempted suicide and suicide. *Acta Psychiatr. Scand., 51,* 221–227.
Waller, D., & Edwards, J. (1989). Lithium and the kidney: An update. *Psychol. Med., 19,* 825–831.
Walker, D. G. (1989). Lithium and the kidney (Editorial). *Psychol. Med., 19,* 825–831.
Warshauer, M. E., & Monk, M. (1978). Problems in suicide statistics for whites and blacks. *Am. J. Public Health, 68,* 383–388.
Watts, C. A. H. (1961). The problem of suicide in general practice. *Proc. R. Soc. Med., 54,* 264–266.
Wells, J. E., & Walker, N. D. (1990). Mortality in a follow up study of 616 alcoholics admitted to an inpatient alcoholism clinic. *N.Z. Med. J., 103,* 1–3.

Welte, J., Abel, E., & Wieczorek, W. (1988). The role of alcohol in suicides in Erie County, NY, 1972–84. *Public Health Reports, 103,* 648–652.
Westlund, K. (1963). Mortality of peptic ulcer patients. *Acta Med. Scand., 174* (Suppl. 402), 1–99.
Wetzel, R., Reich, T., Murphy, G., Province, M., & Miller, J. (1987). The changing relationship between age and suicide rates: Cohort effect, period effect or both? *Psychiatr. Develop., 3,* 179–218.
Whitehead, P. (1972). Notes on the association between alcoholism and suicide. *Int. J. Addict., 7,* 525–532.
Whitlock, F. A. (1971). Migration and suicide. *Med. J. Aust., 2,* 840–848.
Wieser, S., & Kunad, E. (1965). Katamnestische Studien beim chronischen Alkoholismus und zur Frage von Sozialprozessen bei Alkhoholikern. *Nervenarzt, 36,* 477–483.
Williams, G. D., Stinson, F. S., Parker, D. A., Harford, T. C., & Noble, J. (1987). Epidemiologic Bulletin no. 15, Demographic trends, alcohol abuse and alcoholism 1985–1995. *Alcohol. Health Res. World, 2,* 80–83.
Woodruff, R. A., Jr., Guze, S. B., & Clayton, P. J. (1973). Alcoholics who see a psychiatrist compared with those who do not. *Q. J. Stud. Alcohol, 34,* 1152–1171.
Woodruff, R. A., Guze, S. B., Clayton, P. J., & Carr, D. (1973). Alcoholism and depression. *Arch. Gen. Psychiatry, 28,* 97–100.
Woody, G. E., Luborsky, L., McLellan, A. T., O'Brien, C. P., Beck, A. T., Blaine, J., Herman, I., & Hole, A. (1983). Psychotherapy for opiate addicts. Does it help? *Arch. Gen. Psychiatry, 40,* 639–645.
Woody, G. E., McLellan, A. T., Luborsky, L., & O'Brien, C. P. (1985). Sociopathy and psychotherapy outcome. *Arch. Gen. Psychiatry, 42,* 1081–1086.
World Health Organization. (1956). *Epidemiological and vital statistics report 9, 1956.* Geneva: Author.
World Health Organization. (1968). *World health statistics report 21, 1968.* Geneva: Author.
World Health Organization. (1971). *World health statistics annual.* Geneva: Author.
World Health Organization. (1977). *Manual of the international statistical classification of diseases, injuries, and causes of death* (ICD, 8th revision). Geneva: Author.
Zung, W. W. K. (1965). A self-rating depression scale. *Arch. Gen. Psychiatry, 12,* 63–70.

Index

Abstinence, 229
Abstinence,
   as goal of treatment, 234
   as means to social rehabilitation, 226–27
   as result of treatment, 228–29
   its relationship to suicide, 226, 234
   predicted by dependence, 247
Abuse of spouse. *See* Spouse abuse
Abuse vs. dependence. *See* Alcohol abuse vs. dependence
Addiction/dependence, psychopathophysiology of, 255
Addiction, narcotic, 34–36
   psychopathophysiology of, 255
Addictive drinking, 99
Affective disorder. *See* Depression; bipolar illness
Age at death, mean, 93
   tabulated, 96, 146, 160, 184
Alcohol abuse, age of onset. *See* Alcoholism, age of onset
   not always alcoholism, 247
   spontaneous remission of, 226
Alcohol abuse vs. dependence, 17, 33, 291–92 (note 1, ch. 4)
Alcohol blood levels. *See* Blood alcohol levels
Alcoholic cirrhosis. *See* Hepatic cirrhosis
Alcoholics, at risk of suicide, 246
   Type 1 vs. Type 2. *See* Alcoholism
Alcoholics Anonymous, 65, 78, 84, 89, 107, 111–12, 114, 119, 124, 172, 227
Alcoholism, age at death, mean, 94, 144, 161, 186
   death, ceiling effect on, 161
   age at greatest risk of suicide, 249
   age of onset, 26, 34, 100, 149, 161, 186, 291*n*4
      tabulated, 96, 146, 160, 184
   comorbidity with, 9, 162, **192–94,** 214, 218, 224, 230, 247–48, 250
   diagnosis of, 9, 16–17, 23–24
   diagnostic criteria, 17, 23–24, 258–59
      DSM-III, 17
      DSM-III-R, 17, 258–59
   diagnosis missed, 227–29
   disease concept, 15–17
   drug abuse in, 9
   duration to suicide, tabulated, 94, 144, 160, 184
   familial, 93, 98
   family history, 200–10
      tabulated, 237, 241, 242, 243, 244, 245
   followup studies, 239
      suicide risk calculated from, 237–46
   genetic theories of, 93, 98
   mean duration to suicide, 93, 100, 149, 161, 186
   medical care for, 227
   population prevalence, 246
   prevalence of, ECA estimate, 246, 295–96 (note 3, ch. 11)
      NCA estimate, 246, 296
   remission from, 226, 247, 291–92
   role in suicide, 8–10, 286–90
   specific treatment received for, 227
   spontaneous remission of, 226, 247
   suicide risk calculated from, 237–46
   suicide risk in women, 8, 34, **163–186,** 223, 290*n*12, table 7.1, 182–83
   treatment considerations, 229–33
   treatment results in, 228
   Type 1 vs. Type 2, 98–99, 148–49, 292
Alone. *See* Living alone
Antabuse, 65, 78, 84, 89, 107, 112, 114, 119, 124, 166, 230
Antidepressant therapy, 230–31

Antisocial personality disorder, contribution to suicide, 248, 253–54
    difficulty in retrospective diagnosis, 25–26, 98
    suspected, 62–64
    Type 1 vs. Type 2 alcoholics and, 292
Arrests, history of, tabulated, 96, 146, 160, 184
Ascertainment of suicide, coroners' practices in, 290–91
    general, 10–14, 290–91n13,15
    impact of method on, 12, 14
    impact of missed cases, 14–15
    U.K. vs. U.S., 10
    Scandinavia, 10
Attempted suicide. *See* Suicide attempt
Automobile fatality, 54, 86–87

Benzodiazepine therapy, 232
Bias, selection, in replication study, 27–30
Bipolar illness, 56–59, 118–20, 150–53, 162
Blood alcohol levels in suicides, 36, 42, 53, 55, 64, 66, 69, 77, 80, 85, 88, 90, 106, 108, 110, 113, 120, 122, 125, 130, 132, 138, 141, 147, 155, 157, 160, 165, 167, 168, 170, 173, 175, 178, 181
Borderline personality disorder, 253–54, 296–97n2

Cancer, 117–18, 123–25
    unsupported belief of, 43, 44, 49, 60–61, 126, 177
Case number
    1 (100–03); 2 (67–69); 3 (83–86); 4 (86–88); 5 (133–35); 6 (111–13); 7 (153–55); 8 (113–16); 9 (60–62); 10 (171–73); 11 (88–91); 12 (42–44); 13 (62–64); 14 (155–58); 15 (69–72); 16 (168–71); 17 (103–106); 18 (72–74); 19 (74–77); 20 (128–30); 21 (77–81); 22 (135–38); 23 (179–86); 24 (56–59); 25 (173–76); 26 (44–48); 27 (48–50); 28 (36–39); 29 (51–53); 30 (39–42); 31 (91–93); 32 (116–18); 33 (81–83); 34 (53–56); 35 (139–41); 36 (123–25); 37 (64–67); 38 (106–09); 39 (130–32); 40 (109–11); 41 (141–48); 42 (158–61); 43 (150–53); 44 (176–78); 45 (125–28); 46 (34–39); 47 (163–65); 48 (118–20); 49 (165–68); 50 (120–23)
Case selection, 21–24
Chronic obstructive pulmonary disease. *See* Emphysema, pulmonary
Cirrhosis, hepatic, 35, 45, 68, 70, 75, 82, 89, 98–99, 109, 114, 116, 156
Civil state, tabulated, 202–11
Cognitive behavioral therapy, 230–31

Communication, suicidal, **199–200,** 201, 294
    varieties of, 295n5
Comorbidity, as risk factor, 9, 162, 193, 194, 218, 224, **247–48**
    defined, 284
    psychiatric, 8–9, **192–94,** 218, 247–48
Coroners' ascertainment practices, 290–91n13, 15

Delirium, acute, 70–72, 167
Delusional disorder, 133–35
Dementia, 35, 82, 89–90, 91, 109–11, 112–13, 114, 128–30, 159–61, 162, **198**
Depression, as risk factor for suicide, 192–94
    cognitive behavioral therapy of, 230–31
    complicating alcoholism, 99, 149, 161, 185, 230, 293n2
    tabulated, 98, 148, 161, 185
    pharmacotherapy of, 231–33
    population prevalence of, 218
    preceding alcoholism, 153–55, 174–76, 193
    prevalence in living alcoholics, 194
    role in suicide, 193–94, 218
Depressive syndrome, tabulated, 97, 147, 161, 185, **201–11**
Diabetes mellitus, 97, 147, 161, 185
Diagnosis of alcoholism, missed, 227–28
Diagnostic criteria, alcoholism, 16–17, 23–24, **258–59**
Disulfiram (Antabuse), 65, 78, 84, 89, 107, 112, 114, 119, 124, 166, 230
Divorce, history of, 36–7, 39, 54, 77–8, 86, 91, 116, 123, 128, 133, 142, 158, 165, 171, 176
    threatened, 46–48, 49–50, 55–56, 59, 77, 85, 90, 103, 105–106, 113, 115, 117–18, 127, 129, 137–38, 140, 172–73
Drinking, as risk factor for suicide, 192, **214–23**
    loss of control of, 89, 99, 149
Duodenal ulcer, 40, 63
    history of, 114, 129, 153–55, 180

ECA. *See* Epidemiologic Catchment Area Study
ECT, 232
Education, tabulated, 94, 144, 160, 184
Electroconvulsive therapy (ECT), 232
Emphysema, pulmonary, 92, 117–18, 122, 130–31, 154, 156–57, 180
Employment status, tabulated, 97, 147, 161, 185
Enablement, 126, 195, 227
Epidemiologic Catchment Area (ECA) Study, 27, 194, 215–18, 227, 246, 295–96n3

Family history of alcoholism, 200–01
    tabulated, 94, 144, 160, 184

of depression, tabulated, 94, 144, 160, 184
of suicide, 201
  tabulated, 94, 144, 160, 184
of suicide, underreporting, 200
Fear of hospitalization. *See* Hospitalization, fear of
Fighting, tabulated, 96, 146, 160, 184

Genetics of alcoholism, 93, 98
of suicide, 294–95*n*7
Gastric ulcer, 153–55

Hamilton rating scale for depression, 293
Head injury, history of, 51, 101–02, 109–11, 112–13, 137, 156, 159–60
Health impairment, 197–98
  tabulated, 96, 146, 160, 184, 201–211
Hepatic cirrhosis. *See* Cirrhosis, hepatic
Hepatocellular disease. *See* Cirrhosis, hepatic
Heredity. *See* Alcoholism, genetic theories of, also suicide, genetic evidence for
Homicide, past history of, 50–53
Homicide, suicide, 150–53
  attempted, 61–62
Hospitalization, 227
  fear of, 37–39, 58, 72, 112–13, 115, 169–70
Hypomania, 151

Imprisonment, history of, 51, 116
Impulsive suicide, 111, 125, 251–52
Informants, differential reporting of events, 26
  limitation of availability, 26, 27–29
  limitation of knowledge, 26
  physicians as, 26
  self-exculpation, 29
Interpersonal loss. *See* Loss, interpersonal
Interview form (Appendix B), 260–82
Interview, securing, 23

Jail, in relation to suicide, 46–47, 79, 107–09

Lack of social support. *See* Social support, lack of
Legal troubles, current, 55–56, 63–64, 87–88, 108–09, **198–99**
Lifetime risk of suicide in alcoholism, 236–49
  meaning of, 248–49
  in suicide attempters, 200, 236–49, 256, 294*n*6
  in various geocultural areas, 246
Limitations of this investigation, 25–27
Lithium carbonate, 231
Liver disease. *See* Cirrhosis, hepatic

Living alone, 195, 202–10
Living circumstances, tabulated, 95, 145, 161, 185, 201–11
Living with spouse, **195–96,** 202–10
Loss, anticipated, 191–92
  interpersonal, **5,** 30, 43–4, 48–50, 74–77, 85–86, 89–91, 91–93, 112–13, 116–18, 126–28, 128–30, 142–48, 150–53
    as risk factor for suicide, 5
    nonreplication claimed, 190
    replication, 6, 21–30, 189–90: limitations of study, 25–27; sources of bias, 27–30
    associated with poor social support, 201
    greater than six weeks, 39–40, 52–53, 59, 69–72, 82–83, 156–58
    infrequent in depressive suicide, 5, 6
  other than interpersonal, 59, 62–64, 69–72, 86–88, 112–13, 116, 117–18, 120, 125, 192
  self-esteem, 36, 67, 70–72, 103, 108–9, 110–11, 122–23, 128, 132, 134–35, 192
  threatened, 38–39, 41–42, 46–48, 54–56, 59, 61–62, 63–64, 72, 79–80, 88, 108–9, 112, 115, 124–25, 126–28, 138, 140–41, 165, 169–71, 172, 191–92
Loss events, timing of, 24–25

Major depression, current, tabulated, 203–09
  suicide in, 9
Malignancy. *See* Cancer
MAOI. *See* Monoamine oxidase inhibitors
Marriages, tabulated, 85, 145, 161, 185
Marital separation. *See* Separation, marital
Manic-depressive disorder. *See* Bipolar illness
Missed cases, 27–29, 91
  diagnosis, alcoholism, 227–29
Monoamine oxidase inhibitors, treatment with, 231–32
Murder-suicide, 150–53
  attempted, 60–62

Narcotic addiction, 34–36
Numbering of cases, 33–34

Peptic ulcer disease and suicide, 293*n*3
Personality disorder and suicide, 253–55, 288
Personality disorder diagnosis, 64, 166, 296–97*n*2
Physician awareness of alcoholism, 227–29
  awareness of depression, 234–35, 255
  contact with suicidal alcoholics, 227
Physician education, impact on suicide rate, 255
Polysubstance abuse and suicide, 293–94*n*4

Prediction vs. description, 215–20
Progeny, tabulated, 95, 145, 161, 185
Psychiatric comorbidity. *See* Comorbidity
Psychoactive substance abuse, **199,** 254–55
Psychological autopsy, 7
Psychopathophysiology of addiction, 255
Pulmonary emphysema. *See* Emphysema, pulmonary

Reasons for suicide, tabulated, 203–11
Releasors of suicide, 256
Replication of interpersonal loss in alcoholics, description of, 6–7
Replication study, 21–30
Risk factors for suicide, 250
  cumulative, 219
  dementia, **198,** 203–11
  drinking, 192
  health problems, **197–98,** 203–11
  interpersonal loss, **189–91,** 203–11
  interpersonal loss, anticipated, **191–92,** 203–11
  interpersonal loss, threatened, 201–11
  living alone, **195,** 202–10
  psychiatric comorbidity, **192–94,** 201, 203–11, 247–48
  poor social support, **194–96,** 201–10
  suicidal communication, **199–200,** 201–22
  unemployment, 196–97, 201
  loss, other, 192, 203–11
Risk of suicide, annual, in alcoholism, 241–45
  lifetime, in alcoholism, 241–45, **246**
Risk prediction, 233

Schizoaffective disorder, diagnosis of, 175
Schizophrenia, diagnosis of, 59, 64, 164–65, 286
Seizure disorder, 68, 84–85, 89, 109
Selection bias, replication study, 27–30
Separation, marital, 41, 49–50, 57–59, 70, 74–77, 78, 85, 89, 115, 116–18, 126–28, 129–30, 136–38, 139, 150, 166
Social disruption. *See* Loss, interpersonal
Social support, in suicides with acute loss, 201
  lack of, **194–95,** 201
  tabulated, 95, 145, 161, 185, 201–11
Spontaneous remission of alcohol abuse, 226
Spouse abuse, tabulated, 96, 146, 160, 184
Statistical methods, vii, 5, 295
Substance abuse, psychoactive, **199,** 254–55
Substance abuse vs. dependence, 17, 33, 291–92 (note 1, ch. 4)
Suicidal communication. *See* Communication, suicidal

Suicide ascertainment. *See* Ascertainment of suicide
Suicide attempt, 40, 49, 51, 54, 63, 79, 84, 87, 122, 164, 168, 169, 172, 175, 177, 180
  as communication, 200
  lifetime risk of suicide, following, 256, 294n6
  history of, tabulated, 203–11
Suicide, a clinical problem, 227
  ambivalence in, 252–53
  contribution of alcoholic women, 34, 186
    limitations on studying, 25
  community studies of, 9
  defined, 10–11
  described, 286–90 (notes 1–12, ch. 2)
  family history of, 201, 256
    tabulated, 94, 144, 161, 184
    underreported, 201
  genetic evidence for, 294–95n7
  impulsive, 111, 125, 251–52
  in absence of psychiatric illness, 5, 9
  in alcoholism, **8–10,** 33–185
  lifetime risk, in alcoholics, 236–249: vs. general population, 248
    in population at large, 248
  missed cases, 14, 22, 27–29, 290–91n13–15
  mortality vs. overall mortality in alcoholics, 182–83
  peptic ulcer disease, and, 293n3
  personality disorder and, 253–55, 288
  physician education and, 255
  planning for, 253
  prediction of, 233–34
  polysubstance abuse and 293–94n4
  principal psychiatric diagnoses in, 8–10
  rates, reliability of, 11–14
  reasons for, tabulated, 203–11
  role of psychiatric illness in, 4, 9
  vehicular, 296 (note 1, ch. 12)
  viewed as accident by informant, 80, 130, 157
  viewed as homicide by informant, 56, 127
Suicide note, contents, 41–42, 50, 63, 88, 102–03, 106, 118, 127, 140, 143–46, 152, 167, 170, 173, 175, 181
Suicide prevention efforts, 233
Suicide rates, cross-cultural differences, 12–14, 244–45
  immigrants, 13–14
  reliability of, 11–15, 234
Suicide, releasors of, 256
Suicide risk. *See* Suicide, lifetime risk
Suicide risk, women, 182–83
Suicide studies, community, **9,** 286–90
Suicide interview form, 260–82

Transvestism, 87–88

Underestimation of suicide, 11
  of family history, 200
Unemployment, 196–97
  tabulated, 201–11
Uxoricide, 51–53
  attempted, 61, 250

Widowed, 43, 51, 156, 176
Women alcoholics and suicide, 8, 34, **163–86,** 223, 289, table 7.1 (182–83)

Zung depression scale, 293n2